FROM LEBANON TO CALIFORNIA

FROM LEBANON TO CALIFORNIA

A Marriage of Two Cultures

AN AUTOBIOGRAPHY

BY

HENRY J. ZEITER, M.D.

Copyright © 2006 by Henry J. Zeiter, M.D.

Library of Congress Control Number: 2005907017
ISBN :   Hardcover   1-59926-307-6
              Softcover   1-59926-306-8

This book was printed in the United States of America.

To order additional copies of this book, contact:
Xlibris Corporation
1-888-795-4274
www.Xlibris.com
Orders@Xlibris.com
29809

CONTENTS

III—CLEANSING OF BODY AND SOUL

PREFACE AND ACKNOWLEDGEMENTS

Writing this book over the past two years has been most enjoyable, though the memories may have caused me to shed a nostalgic tear or two. All the same, I am grateful for having learned from the tribulations of a lifetime, while being glad that both formal schooling and working for a living are over. The luxury of time now allows me to reflect on events gone by and what is still to come. The best part of all is being able to enjoy my good fortune in tranquility with my wife, my family and friends, and with God.

A human being is not merely defined by the work he does or by the place in which he lives. He is, above all, a being of thought, seen and known best in his higher mental and spiritual activities. It is impossible to understand and explain a life through material circumstances alone. One must rather take into account emotional, cultural, and religious influences that have shaped the life. An outside biographer, or worse yet a ghost writer, cannot give a full account of the inner essence of the subject. Only he himself can dig deep into his own mind and heart and give an adequate report of hidden thoughts and feelings. And that is particularly so when the story teller is not coloring the truth. A propos, Saint Augustine's *Confessions* has remained the classic example of an honest account of the turmoil of a life spent in authentic spiritual growth.

A list of proper names is to be found at the end of the book. I have tried to make it brief but complete: family names, material pertaining to Lebanon and events in the text, and a few historical figures of particular significance in the story. A genealogical family tree provides an additional visual resource. The list and the family tree give the reader an easy reference for following the cast of characters—a courtesy, I might mention, that Tolstoy never afforded his readers in *War and Peace*. (No comparison of merit intended, of course!) I have also included pertinent photos of family members and places described in the text.

I wish to thank my wife Carol for her help in the final editing and for enduring the frequent emotional and mental absences that I put her through while writing the story. I thank my son Philip for reviewing the text and making suggestions. I am grateful to my friend Joseph Pearce for his kindness in offering to write an introduction to my story. I thank my typist, Julie Flocchini, who, I am happy to say, consequently obtained a permanent job at Zeiter Eye Clinic. I thank my many technical computer helpers, especially Doug Honn, Sheryl Frieders, and young Michael Honn. Providentially, they are neighbors in our friendly Timberlake cul-de-sac in Lodi, California. I would particularly like to thank my editors, Bridget Neumayr and Dave Shaneyfelt, for bringing this book to fruition. They provided many revisions and patiently endured my frequent additions and changes. I myself take responsibility for any errors in the book.

Finally, I wish to thank my father and mother, and my brothers and sister for having inspired me throughout my life. I pray for them all.

I hope all my readers, and especially my family, find this story entertaining (perhaps even instructive!) as we all continue our search for happiness before reaching our final destiny.

Henry J. Zeiter
September 21, 2005

INTRODUCTION

by Joseph Pearce

I first met Henry Zeiter in 2004 at Thomas Aquinas College in Santa Paula, California. I had flown from my home in Florida to give a talk and he, as a long-serving member of the College's board of governors, was a guest of honour at the subsequent dinner. I had the great pleasure of sitting next to him and was struck immediately by the magnanimity of the man and by the magnitude of his knowledge. He waxed lyrical on art, literature, music, history, politics and philosophy. Had he not been constrained by my own woeful ineptitude he might have switched effortlessly in his lyrical loquaciousness to one or other of the several languages in which he is fluent, including French, Arabic, Italian and Spanish. Nonetheless we spoke, in English, of our many shared interests. Having confessed, almost apologetically, my great admiration for the music of Wagner, and particularly my enduring love for the masterful opera *Tannhauser* , I was heartened to discover that he was that rarest of oddities, a Catholic Wagnerian. Our conversational perambulations continued and I learned that his catholicity of taste extended to Bach, Beethoven, Brahms and a host of other giants of the western musical tradition.

As we worked our way through the courses on the menu we simultaneously worked our way through the corpus of western literature, discussing Dante and discoursing on Dostoyevsky. We lingered on the literature of the French Decadence and I was again heartened to discover a kindred spirit who shared my passion for the lurid lucidity of Baudelaire and Huysmans. Moving onto the dessert and into the desert of the twentieth century I was deeply impressed by the breadth and depth of his knowledge of the key figures of the Catholic literary revival. He reminded me, in fact, of Maurice Baring, another Catholic Wagnerian and one of the unsung giants of the very revival we were discussing, whose work is awash with high culture beyond the reach of our cultureless age. If Baring is largely forgotten today it is not because he is not worth reading but because the modern age cannot read on the level at which he wrote. Modernity is culturally illiterate; it is not worthy of him or the culture in which he was steeped. As I read through the manuscript of Dr. Zeiter's autobiography it reminded me very much, in spite of the many and obvious differences, of Baring's wonderful autobiography, *The Puppet Show of Memory*. Maurice Baring and Henry Zeiter have much in common, and we, who are common, have much that we can learn from them if we wish to ascend the heights of the civilization of which they and we are co-inheritors. Such were my first impressions of Henry Zeiter, and such was the deep impression he made upon me. As the meal ended a valuable friendship began.

Incidentally, and to allow myself the indulgence of a superfluous tangent, I cannot resist the comparison between my edifying cultural and culinary sojourn with Dr. Zeiter and the very different sort of culinary experience endured by the controversial poet, Roy Campbell, recounted graphically in his satirical poem, *The Georgiad*. May it suffice to say that my literary dinner with Henry Zeiter had nothing whatever in common with Roy Campbell's experience with the pretentious bores of Bloomsbury:

> Dinner, most ancient of the Georgian rites,
> The noisy prelude of loquacious nights,
> At the mere sound of whose unholy gong
> The wagging tongue feels resolute and strong,
> Senate of bores and parliament of fools,
> Where gossip in her native empire rules;
> What doleful memories the word suggests—
> When I have sat like Job among the guests,
> Sandwiched between two bores, a hapless prey,
> Chained to my chair, and cannot get away . . .
> O Dinners! take my curse upon you all,
> But literary dinners most of all . . .

Roy Campbell also wrote disparagingly about what he termed the "Peter Panic," the modern fear of growing old and the modern mania for staying young. There is in our myopic and meretricious age no interest in growing old with dignity, still less in treating the elderly with any dignity. Euthanasia is the logical product of youthanausea, the sickness of youth that sacrifices the dignity of the old on the altar of its own narcissistic self-worship. Youthful folly with its fallacious fancies has usurped the wisdom of the ages, and the wisdom of the aged. We no longer listen to our elders, believing that adolescents know best. "One's children want independence after being told what to do for the first eighteen years of their lives," writes Dr. Zeiter. "Their children are even further removed from our injunctions. Nowadays the young actually distance themselves from the old and the wise, as if only their peers (who know nothing!) can teach them about life." This, of course, is the height of inanity from which, as a culture, we fall into the depths of insanity. It is tragic. It is comic. This book, which is so much more than a mere autobiography, is an antidote to all such nonsense. As we turn the pages of this life we find ourselves in the presence of a learned elder from whom we can learn so much about our world, our culture, our heritage, our destiny, ourselves. We are also in the presence of a gifted storyteller who punctuates his narrative with sagacious anecdotes. The journey takes us from Lebanon to Latin America, and thence to Canada and, finally, to California; but it also takes us on a journey into the faith and philosophy of western civilization, and hence into an understanding of the meaning of life and consequently an understanding of ourselves. It is a journey beyond ourselves so that we can come to fully know ourselves.

I repeat and reiterate that this is so much more than a mere autobiography. In this edifying and efficacious life we meet not only Dr. Zeiter's family—his ancestors, his parents, his siblings, his wife, his children—we meet a host of his friends, many of whom he knows intimately, such as Aristotle and St Thomas Aquinas; St John of the Cross and Dante; Brahms, Beethoven and Bach; Eliot, Joyce and Hemingway. We discover also, perhaps to our surprise, that many of these people knew each other. Thus we discover that it was James Joyce who introduced Dr. Zeiter to St Thomas Aquinas: "Ironically, it may have been the unhappy arch-heretic—as he called himself—James Joyce who deepened my love of Thomas Aquinas."

Like my own father, from whom I learned more than from any other learned elder, Dr. Zeiter can recite Thomas Gray's Elegy by heart. He courted a girl named Penelope by reciting impassioned lines from Pope's translation of the *Odyssey*. (One can't help but wish that he had also met a girl named Beatrice!) He also courted, more successfully, his future wife by taking her, on their first date, to a performance of Verdi's *Requiem*, after which they discussed metaphysics in general and Thomistic metaphysics in particular. Perhaps Dr Zeiter's next book should be entitled *Aristotle and the Art of Seduction* or *Thomism for Lovers* or *Use the Muse to Improve your Love Life* or *Homer Sexual!* It is indeed typical of Dr Zeiter's culture-saturated soul that he begins a refreshingly candid discussion of his and his wife's "mid-life

crisis," which almost destroyed their marriage, by reciting the opening lines
of Dante's *Inferno*:

> Midway upon the journey of our life
> I found myself within a forest dark,
> For the straightforward pathway had been lost . . .

T.S. Eliot once wrote that he was so much in awe of Dante that all he
could do in his presence was to point in the inimitable Florentine's direction
and remain silent. At times I find myself so much in awe at Dr Zeiter's mode
of expressing profound thoughts that I can only imitate Eliot's silent reverence
by pointing at the inimitable doctor and remaining silent. Thus, for instance,
this is Dr Zeiter on civilisation and culture:

> The civilization that Greece bequeathed is testimony to the fact
> that the formative elements of history are basically cultural and
> intellectual rather than economic. History is guided over the
> centuries by the ideas and beliefs of select luminaries, by the cultural
> waves they produce with their notions of what is good, true and
> beautiful, and through the disciplines they employ to propagate
> these beliefs such as philosophy, religion, literature and art. A secular
> society, like the one ours is becoming, attempts to build a culture
> devoid of its origins. That has always pointed to the slow, but
> inevitable death of the civilization. It has been almost a century
> (1922), since T.S. Eliot foresaw the horrors of a godless, secular
> society just around the corner (Hitler, Stalin, Mao), and warned in
> *The Wasteland*, "I think we are in rat's alley / Where the dead men
> lost their bones . . . We who were living are now dying." And
> again, in *The Hollow Men*, "We are the hollow men / We are the
> stuffed men / Leaning together / Headpiece filled with straw." The
> traditions that have propped up our culture over the past two
> millenia have deteriorated considerably since Eliot's dire warnings.
> Have we become a slowly expiring civilization?

And here's Dr Zeiter extolling the praises of classical music:

> I have always proselytized on behalf of classical music, just as a
> religious missionary would preach the good news, because I
> firmly believe that great art and sublime music are joyful and

spiritually uplifting. For this reason, I find great satisfaction in sharing artistic and musical experiences. They lead to the love of Beauty and, as a consequence, to the love of God.

And how's this for putting Eliot, Joyce and Hemingway in a nutshell?

T.S. Eliot progressed from being an agnostic American author to belief in the traditional tenets of Anglo-Catholicism, and he became a prophetic poet, the most celebrated of the first half of the twentieth century. Joyce left his traditional country and faith for a life of restless wandering in continental Europe. He was a linguist of the first order and established a new style of writing, but he lost his bearings and his soul in the process. Hemingway never had a faith to start with, and after several adventures he turned morose and ended up committing a skeptic's suicide.

And here's what Dr Zeiter has to say about the crass reductionism of modern democracy, a reductionism that was condemned by Chesterton as "the Coming Peril" of "the standardization by a low standard":

The world has bit by bit lost the sense of the sacred. There is a tendency in democracies to bring down to a common level whatever is noble and elevated. Even God is now brought down to the level of friend and brother in exclusion of his awe-inspiring fatherhood as the mighty Creator of everything. Joseph Pieper has written a book on the new Church architecture in which he describes how shallow and sterile it has become compared to the Gothic and Renaissance temples of worship. He thought that modern church construction had lost the sense of the sacred. Just look at the tattered or immodest way people dress for Sunday Mass. There is an atrophied sense of respect left for the holy or the sacred.

It is clear that Dr Zeiter shares Chesterton's disdain for the vulgarizing tendencies of the secular fundamentalist version of democracy. It is equally clear, as the whole *raison d'etre* of this present volume testifies, that he would agree with Chesterton's counter-vision of tradition-oriented democracy as espoused in his seminal *Orthodoxy*, in which Chesterton describes tradition as the extension of democracy through time, the proxy of the dead and the enfranchisement of the unborn.

Dr Zeiter is steeped in Tradition and passes this tradition to us as he learned it from his own father, the "wise philosopher," who counseled him against arguing obvious points with obtuse people: "Son, remember the old Lebanese proverb, 'I argued with a wise philosopher and won, but when I argued with a donkey, I lost'."

Although we live in an age of donkeys who think that they know, the proverbial truths of tradition remain as perennial reminders of the permanent things. Again, we cannot do better than to quote Dr Zeiter quoting his own father, on this occasion his father's "favorite four verses":

> *He who doesn't know, and knows he doesn't know is ignorant: teach him.*
> *He who knows, but doesn't know that he knows is asleep: wake him.*
> *He who knows, and knows that he knows is wise: follow him.*
> *But he who doesn't know and thinks that he knows is a fool: shun him.*

I reiterate and repeat: this book is so much more than a mere autobiography. It can teach those who know they don't know; it can awaken those who don't know that they know; and it can lead those who know that they know. It will only be shunned by the fool who knows no better.

For those who may never have the opportunity of long and enlightening dinners with Henry Zeiter, this book is the next best thing. You will enjoy the inimitable company of the author and will grow in the wisdom he offers. What is more, you will be truly blessed.

JOSEPH PEARCE
Naples, Florida
December 24, 2005

Joseph Pearce is writer in residence at Ave Maria University. He is the author of *Literary Converts* and of *Literary Giants*, and has published biographies of Tolkien, C.S. Lewis, Oscar Wilde, Soltzenitzin, Chesterton, Belloc, and others.

SIT BY THE LAKE WITH ME

Many things will I remember
As I pour out my soul . . .
When will I come to the end of my pilgrimage?
And enter the presence of God?
Like the deer that yearns for running streams,
So my soul is yearning for you, my God.

P salm 42 fittingly begins the story of the "many things" I remember
journeying from my native Lebanon to Venezuela, Canada, and finally
the United States. Many are the memories of my "pilgrimage" in my adopted
country: the pilgrimage of a young man through professional life, through
emotional development, and through the sudden fear of death. Finally I have
reached the relative ease of retirement.

Retirement is an appropriate time to reminisce about childhood, indeed
about one's entire life. Some sunny afternoons, I sit in my chair surveying the
serene lake on which we live. I am reminded of the elderly man in the yellow
straw hat seated in a chair looking at the Mediterranean, with his brown walking
cane lying at his side, in Claude Monet's *Terrace at Sainte-Adresse*. Was he
daydreaming about the sand castles he once built with his playmates on the
beach below? Or is he recalling his adolescent years as he looks to his left at the
young lady with the parasol conversing with her gentleman friend? Or is he
reliving the adventures of his travels across the seas, as he looks at the boats on
the horizon? I've always loved that painting and longed to solve the enigma of
the elderly gentleman.

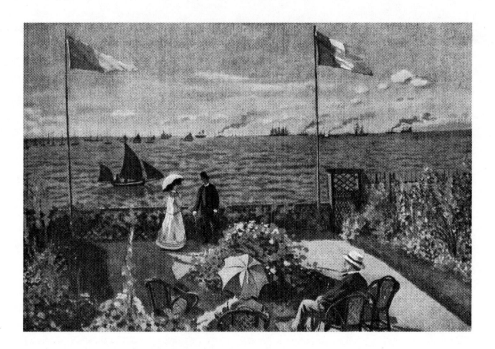

Claude Monet—Terrace at *Sainte-Adresse*, 1886

Sometimes, I look at the lake as in a haze and see episodes of the past flashing in front of me. The first reminiscence invariably leads to others, till the darkness of evening falls on the lake and I have to turn in for supper or other mundane matters.

Our memory of times past is said to become sharper as we get older, a time when short term memory becomes a problem. As a matter of fact, languages spoken in childhood and forgotten since then, begin to return with their entire lexicon. At an age when other young people had to work either to help with their family's finances or to put themselves through school, I spent my days with eyes wide open observing things around me. I became an expert at killing time, alone or in the company of friends. I literally let the hours disappear in front of my eyes, only to recreate them later to my own liking, or nostalgically to ruminate on them.

Now I am enjoying leisure once again. I would like to invite the reader to sit by the lake, as it were, and reminisce with me. We all have to undergo life changes with their share of turmoil and pain. When we reach the age of recollection we wonder whether all we did was worthwhile or a waste of a lifetime. Perhaps we are not too different, you and I, my "*hypocrite lecteur, mon semblable, mon frère*" (Baudelaire).

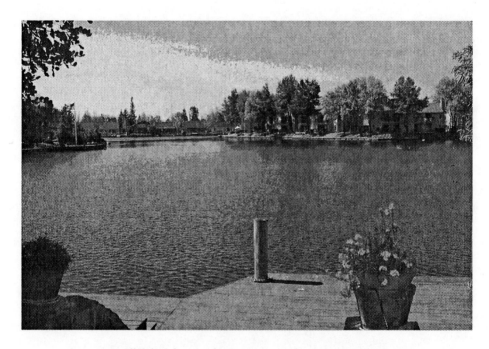

Mallard Lake, Lodi, Ca—A meditative moment
from our terrace by the lake

I

CHILHOOD IN LEBANON

ZEAITER-MUKA
(1800 – 20

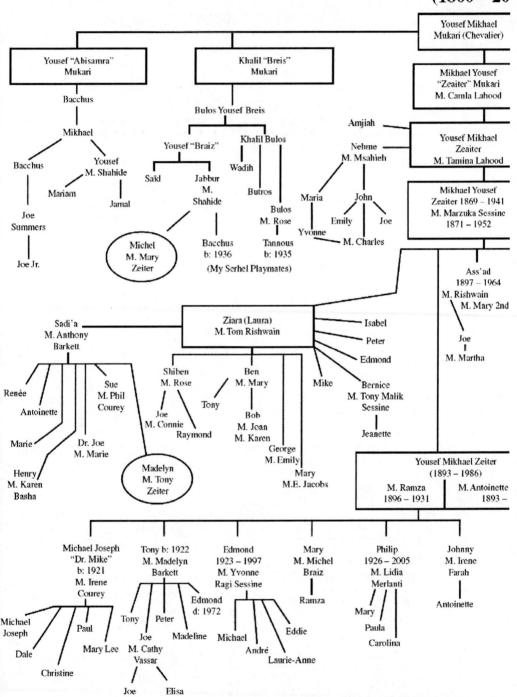

RI FAMILY

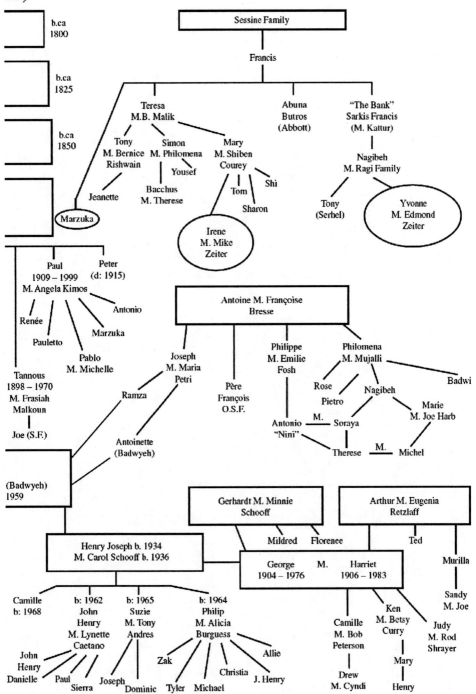

RI FAMILY family tree / genealogy chart

Sessine Family — Francis

b.ca 1800 · b.ca 1825 · b.ca 1850

Teresa M.B. Malik — Abuna Butros (Abbott) — "The Bank" Sarkis Francis (M. Kattur)

Tony M. Bernice Rishwain — Simon M. Philomena — Mary M. Shiben Courey

Yousef · Jeanette · Bacchus M. Therese · Marzuka

Tom · Shi · Sharon · Irene M. Mike Zeiter

Nagibeh M. Ragi Family — Tony (Serhel) — Yvonne M. Edmond Zeiter

Paul 1909–1999 M. Angela Kimos — Peter (d: 1915)

Renée · Pauletto · Antonio · Marzuka · Pablo M. Michelle

Tannous 1898–1970 M. Frasiah Malkoun — Joe (S.F.)

Ramza · Joseph M. Maria Petri · Antoinette (Badwyeh)

Antoine M. Françoise Bresse

Père François O.S.F. · Philippe M. Emilie Fosh · Philomena M. Mujalli

Rose · Pietro · Nagibeh · Marie M. Joe Harb · Badwi

Antonio "Nini" — M. — Soraya · Therese — M. — Michel

(Badwyeh) 1959

Gerhardt M. Minnie Schooff · Arthur M. Eugenia Retzlaff

Mildred · Florenee · Ted · Murilla

Henry Joseph b. 1934 M. Carol Schooff b. 1936 — George 1904–1976 — M. — Harriet 1906–1983

Sandy M. Joe

Camille b: 1968 · John Henry M. Lynette Caetano b: 1962 · Suzie M. Tony Andres b: 1965 · Philip M. Alicia Burguess b: 1964 · Camille M. Bob Peterson · Ken M. Betsy Curry · Judy M. Rod Shrayer

John Henry Danielle · Paul · Sierra · Joseph · Dominic · Zak · Tyler · Michael · Christia · Allie · J. Henry · Drew M. Cyndi · Mary · Henry

CHAPTER 1

ORIGINS

We might as well start the reminiscences at the beginning, the part of my life long past. In fact, I will start with what I remember being told as a child about the origins of our family.

My great-great-great-grandfather was the keeper of the cavalry for the Maronite "Patriarch of Antioch and all the Middle East" at the time of Napoleon Bonaparte in the early nineteenth century. The Patriarch's title has been the same since the time of the Apostles. The first bishop of Antioch was St. Peter, followed by Euodias, then Ignatius of Antioch. It is likely that my ancestors had the same occupation for decades. The family name was Mukari, meaning "horse keeper" in Arabic. Family members were all Maronite Catholics, i.e. Christians, probably as far back as St. Paul's voyages between Jerusalem and Antioch—possibly as far back as Christ himself, who is mentioned several times in the gospels as having gone to Tyre, Sidon, and Phoenicia to spread the "good news" and to cure the sick and heal the lame.

You see, for seven centuries after Christ and before the advent of Islam, the entire area was Christian. It was Ignatius, Bishop of Antioch, who first called the Church "Catholic" in his epistle to the converts in Smyrna (Ch. 8:2, AD 105), in view of its rapid spread throughout the then-known Mediterranean world. Then Islam came, conquering and converting by the sword the people of the low lands, that is, the plains and the coast. The crusades, four centuries later, were a belated attempt to recapture what Christendom had lost earlier. Some Catholics kept the faith by remaining buttressed in the high mountains and cliffs of Lebanon, particularly in the northern area near the famous "Cedars of God." And that is exactly where the Mukari family lived for the past two or three centuries. The family lived in Bdimane, the site of the Maronite Patriarch's residence to this day.

They were simple people who lived off the land in villages perched high on the cliffs of the *Kadisha* Canyon—"the Blessed Valley." It is an area full of the history and devotion of the early Church. The side canyons and cliffs below the villages were dotted with over twenty monasteries during the Middle Ages. Earlier, from the fourth to the seventh century after Christ, the same area was the abode of hermits and anchorites, the forerunners of Eastern monasticism. The original so-called "oriental monks," like St. Antony Abbot, or later St. John Maron, lived in the desert and became well known for their wisdom and asceticism. The rugged mountains of Lebanon were the refuge of many of these hermits and saints who sought to worship God in silence, away from the coastal cities of Tripolis (Tripoli of Lebanon), Byblos (Jbail), Berytus (Beirut), Sidon (Saida), and Tyre (Sur). They were seeking the Eternal far away from the noise and vanity of the world.

THE MUKARI FAMILY BECOMES THE ZEITER FAMILY

It is in these same mountains that the Mukari family lived, and it was there that I was born on July 31, 1934. Times were already "modern" in the coastal cities, but in the mountains, where we always spent our summer vacations, the quiet, simple life still remained. To this day, the monastery of Kos'haya and the convent of Qannubine remain as ancient landmarks of pilgrimage in the East. Kos'haya has had a revival of vocations and is still home to forty monks, while Qannubine has fifteen nuns in residence. During my childhood, my father's maternal uncle, Abuna (Father) Butros, was the abbot of Kos'haya. He was tall and handsome and sported a handlebar moustache with a well-groomed beard. He was a constant visitor at our summer home, which was a stone's throw from the monastery. I can never forget those childhood memories. The air I breathed in my early years was filled with devotion and mysticism.

Five generations ago, the family's name of Mukari underwent an unexpected change. My great-great-grandfather was nicknamed "Zeaiter." Before the name change, he was Mikhael Yousef (Ass'ad) Mukari, son of the original horse-keeper of the Patriarch, six generations before me. That Mikhael Yousef (Ass'ad) was father to Yousef Mikhael Zeaiter (Mukari), who begot Mikhael Yousef, my grandfather. Confusing? It was the custom to name the first born male by reversing the order of the first and middle names of the father. Since that was the case, the order of first and middle names of a grandfather corresponded with that of the oldest grandson. The generations in between simply reversed the order of first names every time, and this went on for generations making the accuracy of record keeping difficult.

One story was that the first Zeaiter always attended Sunday Mass wearing "*zahtar*" in his lapel. ("*Zahtar*" is the flowering tuft of the thyme plant.) The nickname stuck. After that, it became the family name, later modified to Zeiter, a German-sounding name (*Zeiter* is German for time-keeper). Apparently, before the name change that occurred five generations ago, great-great-great-grandfather Mukari had three boys who had distinctly different looks. One was blond, which in Arabic and Aramaic was called *abross* or *braiss*, and that branch of the family became Brais. Another child had a bronzed complexion, so he was called Abi-Samra, or "the one with the darker look," and that became the second branch of the family. The third child had curly hair, which in Arabic is *mzahtar*, and that could have been the name's beginning for our branch of the Mukari family. That is the other version of the origin of our name. Personally, I prefer to believe the story of the *zahtar* flower in the lapel; and that's the one I was told by Dad to be the more probable derivation.

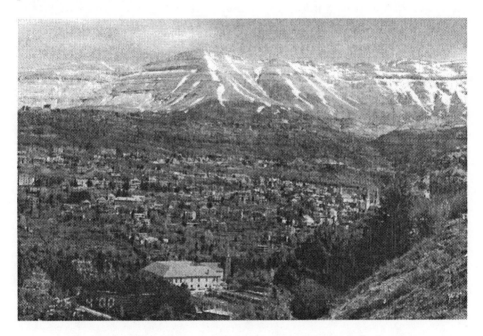

Snow still melting in August on Mount Lebanon with the town of Becharre in the center, birthplace of Lebanon's greatest poet, Khalil (or Kahlil—as he spelled it) Gibran. Below is the Kadisha Canyon (the blessed canyon), once home to over twenty monasteries. On this side of the gorge is the red-roofed residence of the Maronite Patriarch (of Antioch) in Bdimane, where my ancestors lived and worked as his horsemen (or *chevalliers*).

The curly haired son moved to another village, a few miles away, to work and marry. That village was Serhel (or Sereel), perched on the side of a forested mountain, overlooking the lower part of the impressive Kadisha (aka Qadisha) Valley or Canyon, verdant and lush, a few miles from the famous Cedars of Lebanon, higher up in the rugged mountains.

This first Zeiter-Mukari was married to a Camla Lahood, who bore him a son in 1850, whom they named Yousef Mikhael, most probably after his grandfather. Yousef Mikhael married a relative with the same family name as his mother, a Tamina Lahood. They were the parents of my paternal grandfather. They actually had three children, two sons, Grandpa Mikhael and his younger brother Nehme, and a daughter, Amjea, who immigrated to Australia and never married.

Mikhael, my paternal grandfather, was the oldest son, born in 1869. He married my grandmother Marzuka at the age of sixteen, when she was only fifteen. These were not unusual ages for marriage in those days. Yet for some unknown reason (my grandmother never told me), the two of them eloped by riding to the next village to be married by the priest there and returned home before anyone could find out. That marriage was blessed with six children, one of them being my father, Yousef.

One of the other sons, my uncle Pierre (Butros), fell from a tree into a ravine at the young age of seventeen, so I never got to know him. His death was fortunately the only one in the family over a span of many years. The other boys, Ass'ad, Tannous, and Paul, were all younger than Dad. The only daughter, my aunt Ziara (Laura), eventually married the young mayor of Serhel, Tommy Rishwain, and came to California. They raised ten children. Our extended family now numbers more than three hundred people who reside in the great San Joaquin Valley, in and around Stockton, California. My aunt's immigration to California was the family's second move to that state. Coming to California became a family trend that continued for an entire century. Grandma Marzuka first started the trend. Because of her strength of character and courage, she was the dominant figure in our family.

GRANDMA MARZUKA, CALIFORNIA PIONEER

At the beginning of the 20th century it was extremely unusual for a woman, let alone a married one with six children, to leave her family and immigrate to America in search of work and prosperity. As a matter of fact, several people from Serhel came to California about the same time: Yousef Nehme, Paul Abdallah, Sarkis Barket and Tom Barakett, to name but a few. But they were all men. Marzuka and her sister Teresa did the same thing around the year 1900. These two sisters of Abuna-Butros, the monastery abbot, left their children at home with their husbands, to pursue a risky adventure in America. I remember them as two very strong-willed women, emancipated and assertive—many decades before the feminist movement affected the United States, let alone the Middle East. Teresa lived 102 years; Marzuka died at the age of eighty; and Abuna-Butros, strong to the very end, was martyred in his monastery at the age of ninety-six, in 1978.

I think I was my grandmother Marzuka's favorite since I was the youngest grandchild who lived close to her during her final years. She used to sit and tell me at great length stories of the family and of California, "the land of milk and honey." She told me how she and her sister left the village on a hired donkey and traveled all the way to Beirut in 1898, the time of the Spanish-American War. From there they boarded a merchant vessel to Marseilles, France, continuing to New York on a passenger ship. Twenty years later my father Yousef and his brother Anthony were to take the same route, except that they also brought with them their new spouses. Marzuka's only daughter Ziara and her other two sons, Ass'ad and Paul, followed a few years later.

From New York, Marzuka and her sister Teresa took a train to Stockton, California. She worked hard and saved enough to accumulate a moderate sum. She was an entrepreneur at heart, a trait she bequeathed to her whole progeny. She went from farm to farm as a peddler selling the few small items that she could carry in her peddler's bag. Her sister Teresa normally accompanied her. The sisters did this for several years. It was the only thing they knew how to do; they would walk from farm to farm around San Joaquin County, knocking on doors and selling their wares—hair brushes, nylon stockings, combs, towels, and so forth.

Grandma Marzuka would often tell me how tired she would be at the end of each day, after walking over fifteen miles in the heat of California's Central Valley. When she figured that she had saved enough money to take care of her family back home, she decided to return to Lebanon. Meanwhile, Grandfather Mikhael did not remain idle back in the little village. While taking care of their young children, he was working the land of their small farm, as the family had done for centuries. Several years after Marzuka's return, her little fortune was spent on the family, so she decided to return to America, unaware that in just a few more years the world would be engulfed in the first of two devastating wars.

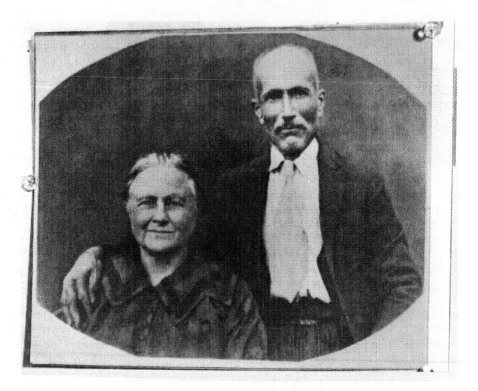

Grandparents Marzuka, d.1952, and Mikhael Zeaiter
(Zeiter), d.1941; circa 1939

Around 1913 Grandpa emigrated with his brother Nehme and Bacchus Malik, his brother-in-law (Teresa's husband), as soon as their wives returned to Lebanon from California the second time around. The men went to Mexico, saved some money by working as laborers in the New World, and returned to Lebanon just as World War I was ending. By that time, their children, were old enough to get married and start their own families.

MY DAD—ALMOST A MONK

My father was the only one of his family to sense a religious vocation. He wanted to follow in the footsteps of his uncle, Abbot Butros. So through the abbot's influence he entered the Monastery of Kos'haya in the Kadisha Valley, not far from his hometown in the Mount Lebanon range. During the war years between 1914 and 1918, he prepared for the priesthood by studying grammar, rhetoric, history, philosophy, and theology. The initiates had a few classes at the monastery during the summer, but in the winter all the seminarians were sent to study formally at the College of Saint Antony of the Desert, the monastic order's university in Beirut. This well-respected institution was also known as *Madrasat Al-Hikmeh* (the School of Wisdom), which in a way explains my father's lifelong dedication to that supreme virtue.

Dad received an outstanding education. It later inspired him to write many books. I have in mind, particularly, a series entitled *The School of Life*, which was inspired by his thorough knowledge of the biblical Books of Wisdom, (Job, Psalms, Proverbs, Ecclesiastes, the Song of Songs, Wisdom and Ecclesiasticus—the Book of Sirach), a love he instilled in me as a child, when I was barely able to understand such things.

But he never finished seminary training and, of course, never took final vows. He told me years later, "Son! When I saw many of the monks following the monastery rule only loosely and not living according to their vows of poverty, chastity, and obedience, I said to myself, if I am not going to live according to my religious vows, but according to the world, I might as well live *in* the world, get married, and have children." He went on to affirm, "I intended to educate my children with what I knew and send them to private schools for the other pertinent knowledge." Later he often told me, "I wanted to work only long enough to enable me to support my family in moderate style." And that was what he did. He eventually came to America, worked hard, and went back to Lebanon to live according to the Aristotelian dictum of *Eudemonia*—a life of moderate means, lived peacefully, virtuously and without being ostentatious.

In 1918 he left the seminary and returned to the village of Serhel, just a few kilometers down the Kadisha Gorge. By that time his mother was back from her adventure in America and his father had returned from Mexico. He took care of the family farm as well as he could, which was his responsibility as the eldest son. Like the Prodigal Son's older brother, he stayed home and helped his father, while his younger brother took off on his foolish adventure.

Soon, Dad could see no future in farming the poor mountainous land, and wanted to become a teacher or a doctor. Four years before, Grandma had come back from America for the second time, bringing back with her another small fortune. She converted the golden Liberty and St. Gaudens twenty-dollar coins into Ottoman gold coins, as Dad was to do fifteen years later in 1932, after his own return from America. She gave each son five hundred *Ismallieh* (the Turkish gold coins), and told them to make their future by multiplying the amount fivefold through education and hard work. She wanted my father to go to Beirut and enter medical school to become a physician of note. This is what he was "supposed to do" with the gold coins she gave him. But God had other plans for him.

Dad took the money and on his way to Beirut he fell in love and got married instead. In those days, if you had a vocation in medicine you didn't get married till the end of medical school, lest your career never come to fruition.

I have known many friends and relatives who got married during medical training; half of them finished their studies, but the other half were soon overtaxed, quit school, and continued to struggle for the rest of their lives with family and children, living a hand-to-mouth existence. Be that as it may, Dad descended to the big city, Tripoli, to buy supplies for home and acquire two new suits to wear in medical school. And that's when he exchanged a professional future for a business one. (Actually, he was interested in the advances of medicine all his life, just as he remained deeply religious in spite of becoming a successful, albeit respected businessman.)

THE SEAMSTRESSES

When he was visiting Tripoli, he bought some needed farm supplies, and even a horse he liked. But there was still the matter of the suits he wanted to buy to wear in medical school. He asked some friends to recommend a good tailor, and they naturally directed him to their cousins' place, which turned out to be the shop of his future wife. Ramza Bresse was a seamstress, in partnership with her older sister Antoinette (*Badwyeh* in Arabic). My father told me that when he entered the little shop he found two sisters of about his age, sewing and making clothes; the younger one was cute and attracted his attention. After several visits for the measurement and fittings of the two suits he had ordered, he worked up enough nerve to ask the younger one to marry him—out of the blue. "Just like that," he told me.

City girls were educated and proper in those days and would never dream of marrying an unsophisticated mountain man (a *montagnard*). But both girls soon found out that he was well educated, and had the means to support a family; after all his parents had just returned from America! In the Middle East that always meant a secure and comfortable lifestyle for the progeny.

The "young one," as he always called Ramza, accepted his proposal, but on one condition. "My sister and I are orphans," she told him. "Before our parents died we promised them that we would always stay together and look after each other. We further promised that if one of us decided to marry, the other one would remain single to help her sister's family, no matter what." Dad told me later how wonderfully that worked out since one sister would always help the other with the many children. As life would have it, he ended up marrying both—not at the same time, of course, but in succession. He married the "younger one," Ramza, in 1920. Since he had to support both sisters, and start a family, he immediately started thinking of immigrating to America, as his mother and father had done before him.

The sisters didn't tell him the details of their family history until after the wedding, though he knew some of that history from the cousins who had led him to their shop in the first place. My maternal grandparents, Mary and Joseph (Mariam and Yousef) Bresse were of Italian and French descent, respectively. The family name Bresse was derived from Bresse, a wine-making area in France (between Dijon and Lyon), famous for its Macon Villages brand. The parents lived as émigrés in Alexandria, Egypt, where the sisters were born in the 1890s.

Yousef and Mary both spoke Arabic with a French-Italian accent, which gave them away as not being fully Arabs. They spoke several languages, which they also taught their daughters. They had moved to Lebanon very early in the twentieth century and settled in El Mina, the ancient port city of Tripoli, Lebanon. My enduring and tender memories of childhood include traveling on Sunday afternoons with our whole family, in a horse-drawn carriage, the several kilometers from Tripoli to El-Mina to visit my mother's family. Oh what beautiful memories! It seems to me as if these trips were always on days that were sunny, bright, and cheerful. The angels of adventure and excitement were always in the air.

PÈRE FRANÇOIS AND MY MOTHER'S OTHER RELATIONS

My maternal grandparents' family consisted of four children: Joseph (my maternal grandfather), Philippe, the philatelist, Philomena, the only daughter, (whose children and grandchildren were very close to my family as we grew up,) and a Franciscan abbot, "Père" (Father) François. I often went with Mom to visit great-aunt Philomena after school. Mom was very loving and a lot of fun to be with. On the way, Mom would always stop at the delicatessen to buy me a vanilla and chocolate sundae. I would relish it so much that I would clean the ice-cream cup with my spoon down to the last drop and then tell the deli owner that I had saved him from having to wash the cup.

Père François, or Father Francis, was the youngest of my mother's uncles. He was the Franciscan order's provincial (ruling head) for the whole Middle East. His office and monastery were far to the south, in Tyre, the old maritime capital of the Phoenician empire, where the ancient world discovered our alphabet, the purple dye and the art of navigation. He would often come to visit us wearing his thick, woolen, ankle-long Franciscan brown robe, tied at the waist with a white cord, looking like St. Francis of Assisi in so many paintings. He was an impressive Renaissance man. Père François wrote many books, including a dictionary for six languages: French, Latin, Italian, English, German and Arabic, with French as the leading language. We used to have a copy of the dictionary at the house and I would marvel over its order and precision. But at some point in our travels we lost track of it. I have always regretted its loss.

Père François was tall, with white hair and a gray, well-groomed mustache and goatee. If his brother Philippe, the philatelist, was impressive, say an eight on a scale of ten, Père François was a ten. Uncle François always had stories to tell. Most of them were historical tales of "elevated" themes. By elevated I mean the sort of thing Baron Von Sweeten told Mozart in the movie *Amadeus*. Mozart was saying that he was sick and tired of people writing and composing operas about themes like honor, valor, and the Greek gods, when the Baron reminded him that these are the ideals that "elevate" life from the mediocrity it tends to fall into. The story epitomizes Père François' respect for the *noble* things in life. He would weave together stories of heroism to make the ideals that were noble in life exciting for the young children in the family.

Père François had a great sense of humor. He had an optimism tempered with the wisdom that comes from life's experiences. He declared that life was neither a tragedy nor a comedy, but contained elements of both at the same time. It was the sort of thing that Bach, Beethoven, Shakespeare, Goethe, Cervantes, Swift and Mozart, particularly the latter in *Don Giovanni*, had all portrayed in their late works—works known for treating of happiness and sunshine amidst adversity and suffering. So these were the beliefs that Père François imparted to us children, always tinged with *comic seriousness*. He was always the person that my parents would go to for advice and direction.

Philomena, his older sister and my mother's only aunt, I remember as a bedridden person, with her spinster daughter, Rose, always taking care of her. In my childhood I saw the same relationship between great-aunt Teresa, Marzuka's sister, and her daughter Hafiza. I have no idea whether these relationships were happy or sad, but I am reminded of them every time I read this parable of Gibran Khalil Gibran.

Apparently, there was a spinster daughter living with her elderly sickly mother. They were both somnambulant; so one night they got out of their beds at the same time, and with their arms outstretched in front of them, went walking in their garden. At one moment during their sleep-walk, the mother touched a pair of outstretched hands. Figuring out they must have been her daughter's, she exclaimed: "Ah! You miserable daughter of mine, I almost died when delivering you, and ever since you have begrudged anything I have asked of you; I can't stand you any longer." And the daughter upon hearing these words, (while still asleep,) said to the mother: "You demanding tyrant, you've robbed me of the best years of my life, while I wait on you night and day. You have been my jailer all these years."

As Gibran tells it, the cock crowed and both awakened from sleep and recognized each other. Then the mother said to the daughter "Oh! My darling sweetheart, come into the house, I don't want you to get a cold; I'll fill a bag with warm water and place it on your cold feet." And the daughter replied: "I am fine Mother! It's you I am worried about, you love of my life. Take my shawl and put it on your shoulders to protect you from the cold."

Aunt Philomena and her dutiful daughter, short and emaciated Rose, lived together in a tiny second-story apartment not far from our large flat in Zehrie, an upscale neighborhood in Tripoli. Auntie had a son, Badwi, who was a prankster. He was in his forties when I was a child. He always teased me, but one day he finally got my goat. I was walking on the sidewalk, not far from Philomena's apartment, when he sneaked up behind me, messed up my well-combed hair, and smacked me playfully, but hard, on my rear. Without a moment's hesitation, I turned around and kicked him with all my might on the shin of his left leg. The lower third of the tibia has one of the poorest circulations in the body, so the gash my boot caused on his leg took three months to heal.

These sudden outbursts of anger, brought on by taunting or other people's illogical comments, were to plague me often throughout my life. Anger commonly leads to loss of self-control, and that can be devastating to the people who count most in one's life. Poor Badwi! He never bothered me after that incident, and we subsequently became good friends. He was named after St. Anthony of *Padua* or simply *Badwi*.

Incidentally, in Arabic every *P* is pronounced as a *B*, because there is no *P* in the alphabet. I realized this only later in life, when my mother, who was called Antoinette when addressed in French, was called Badwyeh (the Paduan) when spoken to in Arabic. I figured that she couldn't have been named "Bedouin" which in the Arabic feminine gender is Bad-a-wyeh. That would have been a surname in a Moslem family, not in a Catholic, Franco-Italian one. It is still difficult for the old Lebanese in America to pronounce the letter *p*. Years later, I was at my paternal uncle Tannous' house visiting when I heard him tell his children: "Kids, tomorrow is Blum Sunday (meaning to say Palm Sunday), I think I'll take you to the San Francisco Zoo." From the other room, his wife Frasiah corrected him: "You've been in this country for over forty years and you still murder the language. It's not Blum Sunday, dummy! It's Balm Sunday!" Their children roared with laughter.

The other children of Philomena Mujalli (that was her dead husband's family name) were Pietro and Nagibeh, her second daughter next to Rose. It was primarily to visit the progeny of that family that we took the Sunday horse-carriage trips to the port city of El-Mina. Nagibeh's daughter Soraya was married to Nini (nickname for Antonio), son of her great-uncle Philippe, the philatelist.

GREAT UNCLE PHILIPPE

I remember visiting great-uncle Philippe, a debonair Franco-Italian gentleman. He was a commercial philatelist dealing in rare stamps, and he was always telling jokes. Upon entering his shop, my eyes would dance across myriads of exciting displays on the walls and windows. There were sheets of multicolored stamps inside glass cases, on the walls, and in all the drawers. He had a multitude of envelopes, each filled with colorful stamps from every country. There were big stamps and little stamps, square and rectangular stamps, even triangular stamps that I had never imagined. My older brothers tell me that he had rare stamps too, each valued at several thousand dollars. He was a widower by the time I knew him, and he had several children and grandchildren who were my playmates when we visited.

As I neared the age of thirteen I had a crush on Therese, one of Philomena's granddaughters, who was one year younger than me. One summer she was sent up to Serhel to spend her vacation with us, the last summer we spent in Lebanon before emigrating. In our mountain summer home there was a wooden ladder going up to the flat, white-painted Eastern Mediterranean roof. (Dad always painted the cement-roof white, as it kept the house cooler in the summer.) One day as Therese was ascending the ladder to the roof, a few steps ahead of me, I couldn't help but notice her cute lavender silk panties underneath her swirling, chiffon white skirt. It was an exciting novel sight for me. So every day, that whole summer of adolescent bliss, we went up to the roof to see the sunrise and the sunset, with her ahead, and me behind her on that blessed ladder. I was in adolescent heaven daily. Therese eventually married her cousin Michel Harb, son of Marie Harb, her mother Soraya's sister. One still has to get a special dispensation from the bishop to marry one's first cousin, but many of these people were second and third cousins of ours through Mom's family. My brother Philip and I were the only ones in the extended family not to marry a relative or a Lebanese. I was to marry a Polish-American and Philip an Italian.

Michel Harb, eventually to be Therese's husband, was first in love with my sister Mary. That was in 1948, when we were all recent immigrants in Caracas. But she wouldn't marry him. While I lived in Caracas, Michel Harb went overboard in being nice to me—since he wanted to marry my sister! We would tour the city in his little green Nash Metropolitan automobile. We loved American movies and would list the movie stars in order of apparent greatness.

The best actress, we decided, was Bette Davis. "She's not pretty," he told me, "but she can really act." Following her on our imaginary list were Ingrid Bergman, Greer Garson, Sophia Loren, Deborah Kerr, and Jeanette McDonald, in that order. The greatest film actors we thought were the Shakespearean-first actors, Laurence Olivier, John Gielgud, Ralph Richardson, and Alec Guinness; and may be Gary Cooper and James Mason.

Back in 1995, on one of my last occasional visits to the relatives in Venezuela, I saw Michel for the last time. He was already emaciated because of advanced cancer. It was nostalgic to recall old memories with him. He said, "Henry! Do you know that all of our favorite British actors have converted from Anglicanism to the Roman Catholic faith?" I don't believe that's true of all four, although many renowned British poets, actors (including Alec Guinness), and philosophers in the past two centuries have come back to Roman Catholicism, England's original church (before the Reformation of Henry VIII).

At the time of the Oxford movement in the nineteenth century, the great scholar John Henry Newman, the poet Gerard Manley Hopkins, and countless others crossed over to the Catholic Church; the conversions became a deluge in the early twentieth century and still continue to this day. Michel would have been happy to read a recent book by Joseph Pearce, *Literary Converts*, in which the author intertwines the lives of many of these English literary figures. It is a marvelous history of the interactions between Chesterton, Belloc, Baring, Benson, Knox, Sheed, Waugh, C.S. Lewis, Muggeridge, and countless others, many of whom became High Anglicans first, and then took the next logical step toward Roman Catholicism.

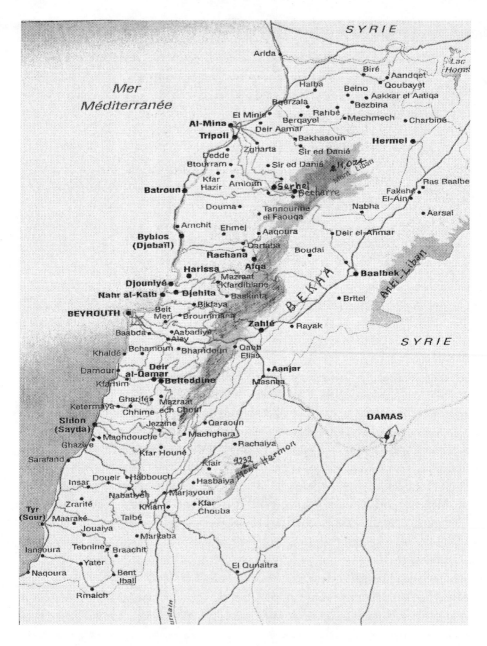

Map of Lebanon, showing from left to right the Mediterranean Sea, the coastal cities (Tripoli north, Beirut center, Sidon and Tyre south), then the Mount Lebanon range running longitudinally (10,174 ft. elev. at Qurnut-as-Sauda. Serhel is just 10 miles due west from the peak), next the fertile Bekaa

Valley, separated from arid Syria by the so-called Anti-Lebanon Range (9,232 ft elev. at Mount Hermon to the south). The layout is a miniature of California's region (the comparison is more obvious on the next map), moving from the Pacific Ocean cities of Eureka, San Francisco, Los Angeles or San Diego (located north, central, and south), then east to the coastal range, then the fertile central valley, next the Sierra Nevada range (14,495 ft. elev. at Mount Whitney) and finally to arid Nevada. In both places the sun rises over the mountains and sets in the sea. Both Lebanon and Northern California have a temperate Mediterranean climate with four distinct seasons, and grow in their central valleys, vineyards, fruit trees, and enough vegetables to supply their respective countries.

CHAPTER 2

LIFE FROM DEATH

D ad and his first wife Ramza (my aunt, or "the younger one," as he called her) were deeply in love. Shortly after their wedding, Dad obtained passports for himself, Ramza, and Antoinette to travel to the United States. He presented his plan to go to America to Grandmother Marzuka as a fait accompli. She did not like what she heard, he told me many years later. He was the oldest and the most educated one in the family, and she wanted his know-how on the farm and around the house. However, she did not stand in his way, realizing she had undertaken the same adventure (twice!) before him. Because he was leaving home, his brother Tannous and his wife Frasiah decided to emigrate with him.

The group embarked, in Beirut, on a ship to Marseilles, France, in 1920. In Marseilles, while sightseeing, Dad lost his way back and had forgotten the name of their hotel. However, he remembered that in the park next to the hotel there was a statue of a man on a horse, with a javelin in his raised right hand. So he hailed a taxi and described the statue to the driver; in ten minutes he was back at his hotel.

He did the same thing to me fifty-odd years later (in 1968). When he was seventy-five I took him with me to Paris. He didn't wait on the second landing of the Eiffel Tower as we had agreed. I went up to the third floor of the tower to see the sights from there, after having told him I would come down and get him if the view from up there was any better. When I came down I couldn't find him anywhere. He was gone! I became petrified because I knew he wouldn't remember the name of the hotel. But again when he found himself lost, he recalled a statue next to the hotel and described it to the taxicab driver—surely the grandson of the first driver in Marseilles, fifty years earlier!—who then took him to the hotel. I waited in the security office of the Eiffel Tower for a whole hour after it had been closed to the public, when suddenly the captain on guard called me over and said to me in French, *"Monsieur, il y a un vieux au téléphone; c'est peut être votre père!"* I picked up the telephone to discover my father was back at the hotel. What a relief it was!

Returning to my parents' trip to America brings us back to Marseilles, where they boarded a ship headed for Quebec City in Upper Canada. They disembarked twelve days later and stayed there several months. They all hated the cold weather in that city. I recall my mother telling me how on one of their peddling routes she reached a very high bank of snow and could not descend to the road below. She used to chuckle at the memory of putting one of her peddling bags beneath her to use it as a sled. Whoosh, she went down, landing below on the road she wanted to take. Dad followed suit, she told me. Ramza stayed home almost the entire winter, as "she was delicate and always cold," I was told. They stayed only six months in Quebec, and when summer came, they moved down to Windsor, Ontario, next to the Great Lakes, a considerably warmer area.

Ramza was pregnant when they left Lebanon, so she delivered her first child, a son, whom they baptized Michael Joseph—his grandfather's name. He was born Canadian, but they soon moved to Detroit where there was plenty of work at the Ford Motor Plant. Dad worked there for three years before he saved enough money to open a grocery store on Larned and Townsend Streets, not too far from the bridge to Belle Isle Park. In the meantime, Ramza continued having children. After Michael, came Tony, then Edmund, then Mary, their first and only daughter, followed by Philip, and finally Johnny—all born in Detroit.

Around 1923, Dad was joined in the grocery business by his brother Tannous. This was after they had both worked at the Henry Ford assembly plant for a few years and saved the money they needed to go into business for themselves. Dad recounted memories of those days quite often. On Fridays after work, he would stop at the Fisher Theater on Woodward Avenue (Detroit's main drag) to see *the* show, before heading home: "The Fisher Roquettes," a locally famous dance troupe featuring girls who would "kick their legs high up to the sky!"

One day two mafia-looking types came to the grocery store. Uncle Tannous was temporarily tending it alone because Dad had gone out to shop for supplies. These characters told Uncle Tannous that he needed "protection," and they would gladly provide it—for an outrageous monthly sum, of course. When Uncle told them to get lost, they grabbed him and carried him to the large freezer where he and Dad normally hung half sides of beef and pork. They shoved him in and locked the door from the outside. He was there for over an hour before Dad returned. When Dad entered the store he heard pounding from inside the freezer. He opened the door and there was his brother with icicles on his moustache, scared half to death on one side and half frozen on the other. Fortunately, they never saw the hoodlums again.

Dad was the older of the two and Tannous respected him. Just as Dad used to stop by the Roquettes' show on the way home from work, Tannous spent his time after hours in the pool hall. Late one evening, Tannous' wife, Frasiah, came to my Dad to complain that her husband stays in the pool hall until midnight every night. "Look what hour it is Joe," she said. "Please, do something about your brother." Dad grew furious as he drove toward the pool hall. Upon entering the hall he grabbed the cue stick from his brother's hand and whacked him with it, breaking it against his butt. Tannous didn't say a word. He knew that he was at fault, so he put his tail between his legs and went home to his wife, and never again played pool after nightfall.

Ramza, the younger sister, was having children so fast that it was hard to keep up with food, clothing, and life's essentials; so Antoinette took on a job as a seamstress for a tailor named *Amato*, who was Italian-American. He was old and his wife, like Sarah and Elizabeth in the Bible, had been barren for many years.

One New Year's Eve, my parents were invited to the Amatos'. Everybody was dressed in their finest for the occasion. Mrs. Amato was wearing a beautiful long white silk dress. It was embroidered with bright stones and sequins. She did not have any children, so she begged Ramza to let her hold her year-old child. He started crying and, while fussing, copiously urinated on her dress. Ramza was quite embarrassed and didn't know what to say. Her sister, Antoinette, always on her toes, reacted immediately to save the day. She told Mrs. Amato that what just happened was a good omen. "In the old country," she told her, "they say that when a baby 'passes water' on a lady she is bound to get pregnant within the year." The woman had been barren throughout her twenty years of marriage; but sure enough, four months later she was pregnant with her first child, a baby boy. From that day on Amato the tailor couldn't do enough for Antoinette to keep her happy. "For starters, I got an immediate raise," she told me.

PRE-DEPRESSION PROFITS

As a child, I was told many more stories of life in those days, but I forgot most of them. Somehow though, visiting my brothers always conjures up a sweet nostalgia for the years gone by, and one memory or another return to our recall. My brother Mike tells me that he went to a parochial school in Detroit for three years. He remembers that Dad was writing articles for Lebanese-Arabic newspapers in Boston and New York. At that time, Gibran Khalil (sic) Gibran was also writing articles for the same papers. (Incidentally, the correct spelling is *Khalil*, not the customary *Kahlil*. The mix-up probably originated when an immigration official misspelled the poet's name on the original entrance papers. That is commonly the reason many family names differ between cousins, or even siblings, living in the U.S. Our case is a perfect example of that, as we have spellings as diverse as Zeaiter, Zeiter, Zaiter, Zetter, and Ziter within the extended family). Dad said he and Gibran knew of each other through the papers to which they both contributed articles. Twice they met at a Lebanese reunion (a *Haflah*) in Detroit, where Gibran was the invited speaker.

In time, Dad built a four-unit apartment building on a lot he had bought next to the grocery store. Shortly after, he bought a full-fledged gas station nearby. He told me many years later that he sold the complex just before the crash of 1929. He received forty-five thousand dollars, which in those days was a considerable sum. At the time he told me this I myself was quite involved with real estate, and I remember being on a flight with him from San Francisco to Detroit—to visit my brother Mike in Windsor. I asked Dad, "What would you say was the annual income from the property that you sold?" He said that it totaled about five thousand, five hundred dollars annually. Interestingly, fifty years later when I was buying and selling apartment complexes, the sale price for real estate was always about eight times the gross annual income. This was a formula that had been in use for many years, at least during my time. It was called the "multiplier of eight," and when I mentioned that to Dad, he wanted to know what it meant. I explained to him that for property with an annual income of fifty-five hundred dollars, the sale price should be eight times that much, which comes to forty-four thousand dollars, a sum quite near the price he sold his property for. Of course, both the income and the corresponding value of the property would be much higher now, I explained to him, but the multiple of eight worked the same for him then as it does for us now.

Dad was mystified. He was pensive for a few minutes; then he turned and said to me, "Son, I am essentially a monk, a poet, and a writer. I opened these stores because I had to make a living, and I've never known much about multiples or prices. That was simply the amount offered to me at the time and I took it because your aunt Ramza was very sick. The doctors had told me to sell everything and take her back to Lebanon."

As it turned out, the depression started three months later in October 1929. It first hit the stock market and then real estate. If my father had sold the complex a year later, he would not have gotten even half the price. Every time I commented on his ability to make serendipitous gains, he would tell me, "Son, it was the work of the Holy Spirit. I never knew much about business, and I always hated it. That is why I retired at the age of thirty-seven to raise my family in the fear of God, using my leisure time to write poetry." And that pleasant avocation occupied him until his death, when he was just entering the ninety fourth year of his life.

Anyway, back in Detroit, Ramza was debilitated and sick and getting worse as time went on. So they visited two different doctors for consultation. Both were Lebanese-Americans, and both told my father to take his wife back to Lebanon "where the air was cleaner." So he took all of the children out of school, sold his store and real estate, and bought tickets for Ramza, Antoinette, and the children. The family sailed to Lebanon in 1930.

RETURN TO LEBANON

Upon reaching Beirut, they took a Ford Model-T taxi up to Serhel, via Tripoli. Dad told me years later that "there was no sense tarrying in the capital city," where he would have had to stay in costly hotels and eat in expensive restaurants. "I had made just enough money to live on in moderate comfort," he said to me, "and I wanted nothing to do with working day and night all over again, which I knew would happen to me if I spent my savings unwisely."

All of his acquaintances who stayed behind in the U.S. eventually lost most of what they owned in the depression of the thirties, and had to start working even harder than before to recover their losses. He related that fact to me as a lesson that I ought to learn about human covetousness. He rarely advised me directly; instead he would give me examples from his life or would embellish old proverbs in his inimitable way. He was thirty-seven years old when he retired from working for a living and started living for what he considered essential in life: God, family, poetry, and peace of mind.

For the first year after the family returned to Lebanon they stayed in my grandparents' home. It was a simple house, as I remember from my childhood days in the village. I was often at my grandmother's and can picture now the place with its surroundings as if it were in front of me. The abode consisted of two huge rooms, bounded by adobe walls and roof. There was a simple kitchen, but it was outside on the patio. The toilet was in an adjoining stone building that was in fact the chicken corral. For a bath, they used a tub and changed water between the children's baths. The house was dark during the day, with one tiny window in each room, letting in just enough light for one to get around without stumbling. It was really not very different from a house one sees in "Western" movies; and it wasn't large enough for nine people.

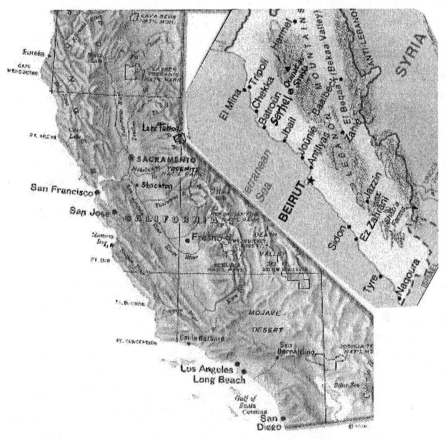

Both in Lebanon and California, the sun rises over mountains to the east, traverses an agricultural valley in the center, and sets into the sea/ocean, having passed over a second range of mountains near the coast. See also the previous map and caption

So eventually, the family had to move to more spacious quarters and leave the grandparents in the old house. They had brought plenty of money with them for that purpose, so they began to plan a palatial home that became the pride of the small village. After a few months in the ancestral home, autumn came and Dad had to take the children down to Tripoli where the good schools were located. For eighteen years thereafter, winter term was passed on the lovely coast of the Mediterranean in Tripoli; summer vacations were enjoyed in the mountains at three thousand feet above sea level. Summer was normally cool in the village, as it was tucked away in the shadows of the huge mountains of the Lebanon range.

In Tripoli, Dad built an eight-unit apartment house in the Zehrie District close to the big river, Abu Ali. It took him only four months to complete the project. He was the architect, developer, and construction supervisor all in one. The apartments were built in the old style with high ceilings, and they were quite large having four bedrooms each.

We all grew up in one of the apartments on the third floor. From the balconies, but especially from the roof, we could see the Mediterranean Sea to the West (along with the many orange groves on the coast) and the snowcapped mountain crests to the east. The memory of this view from the roof has remained with me throughout my life. At that moment I started appreciating the natural beauty of the mountains and the sea. Years later, when living in the Midwest, I couldn't wait to move to California (after I had seen how similar to Lebanon it was). What better combination could there be than the majestic mountains descending to the sea? That's how it is in both Lebanon and California.

Before summer came, Dad started building the summer villa in Serhel. He chose the highest hill above the village and built a house that he had designed himself. It was embellished by eight Greco-Roman Doric columns in front, and marble floors on the inside. But most of all I liked the inside walls which were decorated by an artist whom Dad had brought in from Italy for the project. As a child I would explore from my bed the rows of cats and birds and curlicues that were painted on the walls of my bedroom. Each room carried its own motif—it was ingenious!

LE CHATEAU DE MON PÈRE (MY FATHER'S CASTLE)

When I go back to visit I always stay at the villa, still in great shape; and I sleep in my old room, perhaps on exactly the same bed I was born in. Memories of times past float in front of me as I look up at the painted figurines of my childhood years. The colors have not faded over the years. I have an association connected with every little figure on the wall; whether it is Mom bringing me milk in the morning, or Dad tossing me up in the air and making me giggle with happiness, or my sister Mary reading me a story from an illustrated book of Aesop's *Fables*. It is still my favorite place in the whole world. As construction progressed, Mom made sure that the front door and windows were wide enough to look out on the impressive valleys and mountains beyond. She loved light—lots of sunshine—and had the front door and windows open to the view throughout the day. She would look out from the front rooms, the living room, or the veranda and exclaim, *shi bi farfeh al'aleb*, literally meaning, "Oh, my heart! Lighten up your mood!"

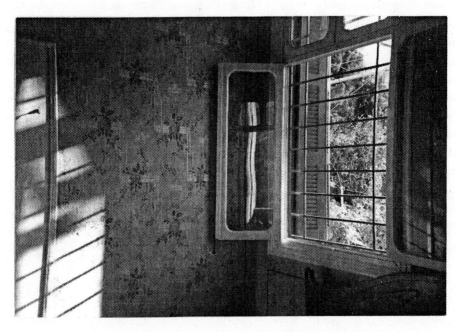

The bedroom I was born in, with yellow roses painted on all four walls. Every morning the sunbeam would enter the room from the window on the right. As the sun continued to rise, the reflection on the wall would descend towards the floor. In the evening I would watch on the opposite wall the golden-orange rays of the setting sun rise higher and higher until they disappeared. I always thought of this, even as a child, as a sign of the evanescence of our own life.

The view was magnificent. Later, I would swoon over Lorrain, Constable, Watteau, Fragonard, and particularly, Turner, all great landscape painters, and I would search for their canvases in every museum I would visit. J.M.W. Turner was an impressionist long before anyone had ever heard of the term impressionism. The Tate Gallery (Turner's Museum) in London has always been a destination of pilgrimage for me. Among the four Transcendentals— Truth, Goodness, Beauty and Being—Beauty (the platonic ideal of Beauty) has remained my favorite.

I recall reading James Joyce's "A Portrait of the Artist as a Young Man." I latched on to every word of his on what constitutes beauty. He quotes Saint Thomas Aquinas throughout (Joyce attended an Irish Jesuit school in Dublin). St Thomas defines beauty as: "*Pulchra sunt quae visa placent*" (Beautiful are those things, the sight of which pleases). And then he goes on to name the necessary constituent elements of beauty: *integritas, consonantia et claritas*, that is, "wholeness, harmony, and radiance (clarity)." Ironically, it may have been the unhappy arch-heretic—as he called himself—James Joyce who deepened my love of Thomas Aquinas.

Later, in 1957, I visited Yosemite National Park for the first time. I had been away from my Lebanon Mountains and the scene from my mother's front door for nearly ten years. I shed tears of happiness when I beheld the magnificent views at Yosemite. The surging flood of emotions I experienced that day formed a peak experience. I did not realize why I was so overtaken with joy until I returned to Lebanon eleven years later. On the old road to Serhel there is still a place where, all of a sudden, a breathtaking view of canyons and mountains opens up before the eye. On that first trip back to Lebanon (1968), I took one look at the scenery and was transported back to the magnificent views of Yosemite. All of the captivating Yosemite scenes from eleven years earlier (1957) flooded my mind in an instant of supreme bliss.

I realized then why I had cried when I first saw Yosemite Valley. As children we habitually spend our time looking down at frogs and butterflies and ants. We rarely look up to take in the wider picture. Nonetheless, the larger impressions, seen only peripherally, become deeply embedded in our subconscious. When I saw Yosemite for the first time, I failed to recognize its similarity to the surroundings of Serhel. But eleven years later, when I returned to Lebanon and looked at the Serhel landscape with adult eyes, the "déjà vu" experience was immediate. There was no way to ignore it. I am still emotionally captivated with Serhel, Yosemite, Yellowstone, the Grand Canyon, the Alps, and places of extraordinary natural beauty. All this comes to mind now—what was faithfully stored in memory and imagination during fourteen years of a happy childhood in Lebanon is now liberated and brought into consciousness.

RAMZA'S END

When the villa in Serhel was in the last stages of construction, tragedy hit the family. Ramza, the mother of six children, was ill. Her coughing increased and was now tinged with blood, a symptom known as hemoptysis. The doctors were now certain that she had advanced tuberculosis. Since no anti-tuberculosis drugs were available then, she was taken to the Bhannes Sanatorium in the mountains overlooking Beirut, about seventy miles south of Serhel and Tripoli. Dad went down every weekend to see her. Her sister, Badwyeh (Antoinette) took care of the children as she had been doing for years. People often commented on how well she took care of her sister's children: "Better than she would have taken care of her own." Until the end of her life, she remained devoted to her sister's children and their children. Not to mention me, her own child.

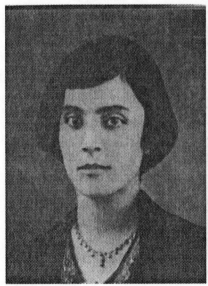 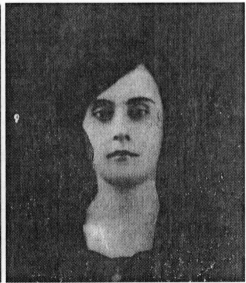

The younger sister, Ramza Bresse, age 25, in 1920

My mother, Badwyeh (Antoinette) Bresse, aged 27

Six months later, early in 1932, Ramza died. She was buried in the Tripoli Cemetery, just beneath the great crusader castle of St. Giles. That imposing structure dominates the hills behind Tripoli and was built by Count Raymond de St. Giles in 1140. Ramza lies beneath the ground that witnessed the fight between the cross-like sword of the crusaders and the rising crescent of Islam, an antagonism still raging nine centuries later.

During this time Dad had been very fortunate to have Badwyeh care for the children. It allowed him to visit Ramza in the sanatorium at least once a week before her death. It also enabled him to complete the apartments in Tripoli and the Villa in Serhel.

He soon began to replant the terraced tracts of land belonging to the family with vines, and olive and almond trees. In time he bought more land in Serhel's outskirts and planted it with vineyards. Meanwhile, in front of the villa he planted every kind of fruit-producing tree imaginable. I remember eating the various fruits each summer at the very time they ripened. Each fruit had its own time and season. There was no refrigeration. For instance, it was said that white grapes began to ripen on July 20th, the feast of Saint Elias; and that one could begin to taste red grapes starting on Transfiguration Day (August 6) about two weeks later. Everything was connected to a saint's feast day. The experience kept us close to the land and to the Church calendar. The family estate was a veritable Garden of Eden before the fall!

A GOLDEN OPPORTUNITY

When all the construction was over there was still plenty of money left from the original sale in Detroit. The question was what to do with it. The Depression had made banks shaky all over the world. Dad decided to buy gold coins just as people had done for centuries. I remember seeing these Turkish gold coins years later. My father hid them in various secret spots in the apartment in Tripoli. He used to pay our tuition for a trimester at the private school with one gold coin. The gold coins showed the signature of the Turkish sultan in Istanbul (Constantinople). I have one of the same coins in my hand right now. The likeness of the sultan on the obverse side is a simple impression of a head wearing a "tarbush," but the signature on the reverse side is the most flamboyant I have ever seen.

I bought a few of these coins in the early 1980s. Dad's gold coins had protected the family from inflation when I was growing up, and I must have wanted to do the same in 1980 when worldwide inflation became a threat. Thank God for American fiscal know-how. President Reagan appointed Paul Volker to the Federal Reserve Board, who turned out to be an economic genius. It is through his efforts that inflation was calmed, and the roaring eighties and nineties ensued—an era which saw the birth of many new millionaires (among them the dot-com entrepreneurs). Yet, as we all know by now, their prosperity was wiped out in a flash when the stock market bubble burst in the year 2000. One of my father's poems (a limerick) describes the rise and fall of such fortunes,

> *Life is an art composed of thought and deed;*
> *So Live on friend, and see how your wheel turns.*
> *One day is for you, the next against you;*
> *One day you're quite rich, and the next you're poor.*
> *So read on, friend, and if still not in awe,*
> *Know, and note full well, that you're still a fool.*
> —Joseph Zeiter, *The School of Life*, 1965, vol. I.

Sixteen years passed before Dad spent the last gold coin. He had not bought them for hoarding, however, for they were the one sure currency that people accepted as legal tender in times of inflation. The coins were used to pay for living expenses, and they were spent frugally. They each weighed a quarter of an ounce; and when gold was still pegged at twenty dollars the ounce, they were worth five American dollars each. Dad bought four thousand of them with the twenty thousand dollars he had left, after having built the villa and the apartment house.

Six months after Dad had converted his cash into gold coins, President Roosevelt devalued the dollar by raising the price of gold by two thirds. This meant that the worldwide price of an ounce of gold went up from twenty dollars to thirty-three dollars an ounce. So Dad made a sixty-six percent profit in a few months. The practical result from this event was that for sixteen years, from 1932 to 1948, with inflation raging in Lebanon, and during all the years of World War II, gold maintained its full value compared to the diminishing buying power of the local currency. Eight years later, when Dad had used half of the coins, the remaining half was worth just as much in local currency as all the coins together were worth when he had first bought them. It has been said that a one-ounce gold coin has always bought a well-tailored suit. It amuses me to note that when gold was twenty dollars per ounce, a well-tailored suit cost twenty dollars, and now that gold is worth over four hundred dollars per ounce, that is the price one pays for a well-tailored suit. Gold keeps up with inflation! Yousef Zeiter's gold adventure became even more interesting as time went on.

At first, my father put all the gold coins at the bottom of a huge urn. Urns were used to store various kinds of grains and staples for winter use, same as on

American farms at that time. In those days packaged staples did not exist. Dad used the bottom of the urn that contained beans for a hiding place. As the beans were used up for cooking, their level in the urn kept going down until it approached the bottom, where the coins were placed. One day, the maid, Watfah, ran to mother very excited. "*Ya sit* (Mrs) Badwyeh! *Ya sit* Badwyeh!" She screamed, *"Shoo hal 'agibe! Shoo hal 'agibe!"* ("What a miracle! What a miracle!")

"What is it my daughter?" my mother asked her.

"Oh, you should see this, I just put my hand in the jar to get some beans and behold! It came out full of gold coins. Blessed be the Lord! What holy household this is, where God turns beans into gold."

My mother tried hard to suppress a laugh and being quick witted said to Watfah, "Truly, God has blessed us my daughter. We will use the newly found gold as charity for the poor and the rest to pay for the children's private schooling!"

This was not far from the truth! But immediately and with the same breath, Mom turned to Dad and told him, "Yousef! Yousef! Quick, hide the coins somewhere else!" So Dad not wanting the miracle to be repeated again in the maid's hands, took the coins out of the jar, wrapped them in several small bags and hid them away again. It wasn't until a few years later that I discovered where they were hidden.

When I was a little child I was allowed to sleep on a little bed in my parents' room whenever I became afraid of the dark. There was a mirror-studded armoire in that room. (There were no built-in closets like the ones we have today.) The armoire was decorated with hundreds of small mirror facets on its front doors. The little mirror facets acted as multiple prisms refracting and reflecting the sunlight that entered the room through the big bright windows. The rays would be split up into their various spectral colors in the morning, filling the whole room with hundreds of little rainbows glistening on the walls and furniture of the bedroom. It created the effect that stained glass windows produce on the pews and columns of Gothic cathedrals. When I slept in that room the effect enchanted me. It was like waking up to see hundreds of butterflies flying all around me.

Late one morning as I was barely waking up, I noticed Dad from the corner of my eye, pushing the armoire away from the wall and doing something behind it. Then he pushed it back against the wall before leaving the room. I soon discovered Dad's secret. That day was the beginning of the trimester at school and he had to pay the Carmelite priests for my brothers' and sister's education. So I figured that this morning he had come to retrieve a gold coin from this new secret hiding place. Obviously, it must have been where he had hidden the gold after its discovery by the maid. Well, after a little investigating of my own, I discovered that he had made a trap door in the back of the armoire and had built a small, well-camouflaged wooden cubbyhole there to store the gold coins. It was quite ingenious! Years later, I was to secretly store gold coins in safety deposit boxes in the banks where I kept accounts in order to protect my family against the 20% inflation of the early 1980s. What children see, children do!

In 1948, when we emigrated from Lebanon, the gold stash was depleted, but Dad acquired new money by selling the apartments in Tripoli. From the proceeds of the sale, he took eighty thousand American dollars with him to Venezuela, which he shared with my brothers who wanted to enlarge their business there. Amazingly, that was about double the sum he had brought with him to Lebanon from America in the first place, even though he supported the whole family for over eighteen years with education in private schools and beautiful homes to boot. He had unwittingly stored his fortune in gold and real estate during inflationary times. What a lesson to learn!

GIBRAN KHALIL GIBRAN

On April 10, 1931, Gibran Khalil (Kahlil) Gibran died in America. He was the most famous and revered Lebanese author of the twentieth century. His body was taken back to Becharre, Lebanon, his hometown, for burial in a cave overlooking his beloved Kadisha Canyon—that was his personal request in his will. He bequeathed all his personal fortune and future royalties for the benefit of his beloved Becharre. The coffin was brought from America by ship and disembarked in Beirut. On its way to the mountains, the cortège stopped in Tripoli. Some two hundred thousand people crowded into the Central Plaza (*Tal*) and the streets beyond.

My older brothers love to tell the story of how Dad was asked to be the first speaker to eulogize Gibran. He did it with Arabic poetry. There is nothing that moves an Arab like poetry. They tell me that the applause lasted several minutes and after the other speakers had finished their speeches, Dad was hailed again to speak to a private group of poets and writers about his connections with Gibran in America.

That episode was one of the highlights of my father's life. As a poet himself, he idealized his fellow-poet's style. Gibran's fame increased after his death, particularly in the United States where his work both as poet and artist is now compared to that of William Blake. Still to this day, in the United States, Gibran's *The Prophet* and other works are showcased in the front windows of national bookstores as recommended gifts at Christmas. Gibran published works originally written either in Arabic or in English. He was well versed in both idioms. He was a master of a distinctly individual mystical style, drawn from biblical lore, as well as Arabic and Persian poetry. In all his published books one sees illustrations of his paintings in black and white, but in the Gibran Museum in Becharre, Lebanon, his original paintings are exhibited in all their brilliant colors.

MARRYING THE SISTER-IN-LAW

Two years after Ramza's death, and the completion of the construction in Tripoli and Serhel, Dad was still a widower. The family spent winter in Tripoli during the school season and the summers in Serhel, which always meant vacation time. Badwyeh lived with Dad and the children. It was a blessing to all members of the family since they were motherless and she loved them as if they were her own. As time passed they considered her to be more and more their own mother, even though they always called her "Auntie," using the English term they had first used back in Detroit.

The Franciscan uncle of Badwyeh (and Ramza) approached Dad, one late spring day in 1933. It was that time of year when the birds were flying in pairs, singing and cooing. "Yousef," Uncle said, "People are talking!" My dad looked back at him surprised:

"What are they talking about?" he asked.

"You are living in the same house with your sister-in-law," said Uncle François, "and people are talking about it!"

"If you believe that anything is going on between me and my sister-in-law, you are insane," replied Dad.

"No, Yousef," said the priest. "I know you are both honorable. But I also know that it would be best if she remained with you to take care of her nephews and niece. An aunt is much preferable to a strange stepmother."

Uncle François continued: "If that is so, then why not marry her."

Well, that fell on Dad like a ton of bricks. To my father, Badwyeh was like a sister. How could he marry so familiar a sister? If marriage were on his mind, he might have thought of a playful young woman who would revive his spirits. But the priest's suggestion was a practical solution. People told me later that

Père François was, in fact, afraid that Dad would marry a younger woman and then keep his niece Badwyeh as a taken-for-granted helper with the children. Père François knew that those circumstances would most probably lead to great problems for the children. A week later he approached Dad again. Dad told him that he had enough children and did not want to marry anybody, young or old.

"But Yousef," the Franciscan told him, "the woman is forty years old. The most change that could happen is that she may bear you one child, and no more. She may even be beyond child bearing. Also, if you don't marry her, she may leave you. Can you handle all six children by yourself?"

François knew that Badwyeh would never leave her sister's children. He knew that she would die for them, but that was a cunning ploy. The priest knew that introducing doubt into Dad's mind about his own security would probably induce him to marry the aunt of his children. Well, it worked. Shortly thereafter, the two got married and François' prophecy about the one child (me!) was fulfilled.

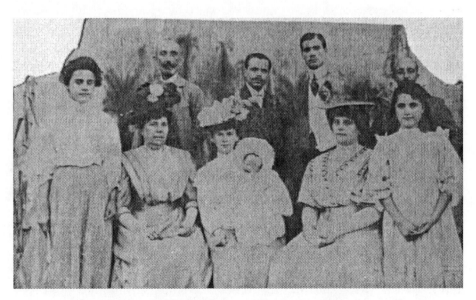

Early photograph of the Bresse Sisters' family circa 1912: Great Uncle Philippe Bresse (center back row), Badwyeh Zeiter (extreme left, front row) and Ramza Zeiter (extreme right). Uncle Philippe's wife is Countess Evelyn Foch (niece of Marshal Foch, supreme commander of the Allied Forces in World War I). She is seen holding her baby son Nini.

I was born ten months later on July 31, 1934, in the front bedroom of the villa in Serhel. I grew up loved by mother and father, and especially by my five brothers and one sister. I was the youngest by almost seven years after Brother Johnny, but I never felt like I was a stepbrother. The family was ready to have a new little brother in the house to play with. For me it was wonderful and providential that I grew up as the baby loved so much by my parents and siblings.

During my birth, all of the relatives were gathered around the house. My mother had been in labor for almost twenty-four hours, so by the time delivery occurred she was exhausted, but kept screaming at the top of her lungs. She was a primipara and had a particularly long and painful labor. Doctor Akrini had been called. He was the regional doctor. He lived in a town closer to the coast, but practiced medicine in that particular region of Mount Lebanon. He traveled on horseback with his doctor's bag, and that day he was late in coming.

By then half of the village was gathered about the house, probably alerted by my mother's screams. I don't know if it was only because of that or because we were the "first" family in the village. In Lebanon, a returned émigré from America was usually given respect, as nobility used to be in Europe. I was told about the great gathering of people by my older brothers. My cousin, Dr. Joseph Barkett, years later (as we became good friends in California), told me that his entire immediate family was on the terraced patio in front of the house that day, waiting for Mom to deliver. He was then a six-year-old boy. There were many other cousins there, and also many friends and neighbors. Most of them eventually emigrated from Serhel and went overseas to Venezuela, Michigan, California, or Australia. I am still in contact with a few of them, and they have all repeated the same story to me.

Finally, Dr. Akrini arrived wearing a white suit and riding a white horse. In a Wagnerian opera, that would symbolize my mother's rescue and/or the birth of a prince, such as Tristan, King Mark, or Lohengrin! Dr. Akrini always wore one of those white, wide-brimmed hats that English colonials wore in Egypt and India. He arrived just in time to help me emerge from nine months of darkness into a lifetime of light. I would often tell my parents that I came out that day screaming, meaning to say: "This place is dark and suffocating! Get me out of here!" It always gave them a good chuckle. Nonetheless, it was a long and difficult labor, but since the doctor arrived late and Mom was well along into the delivery, no forceps were used. By the time he arrived I was almost totally out of the birth canal. I thank God that my brains weren't tampered with!

I was baptized at St. Michael's church on September 3, 1934. My godmother was Sadi'a Barkett, my much older first cousin (and mother of Dr. Barkett), and my godfather was Constantine (*Ksantin*) who lived down in the valley by the river. They gave my name to the priest as *Henri Joseph*, the French spelling for Henry. My family always used the English version, Henry, but for all the years I attended the French School in Tripoli, the teachers and students always used the French version, Henri, pronounced *On-ree*.

CHAPTER 3

THE TIGER PILLOW

How is it that when we are young our thoughts and plans are for the present or the future? But when we turn old we begin to reflect back on memories from our childhood and youth. And as if to allow us to savor our memories, God increases our ability to remember events long past; yet He curtails our short-term memory, even to complete forgetfulness of what we were saying or doing just ten seconds before. This paradox is described in psychology as long-term memory retention versus short-term amnesia, or forgetfulness. It is a well-known phenomenon of aging. Is it a fluke or is it providential? Is it reward or is it punishment? Those who have lived healthy, happy lives by following the laws of God and man, now savor their past memories; whereas those who scoffed at goodness and virtue are stuck with the guilt associated with their past memories, even though they would prefer not to remember anything at all. I suppose it is a form of poetic justice.

As I write about my life, memories of past events flood my consciousness like the tumbling waters of Niagara Falls. One memory stimulates the recall of ten other related events. Things that I have not thought of for years now appear vivid in detail. So where do I draw the line? As I am preparing an outline for the story, every detail of life seems to lead to other events. Some events are trivial, while others are of great consequence in my life.

Time is a web of moments, all interlaced, forming the tapestry of an entire life. Both the details and the events together make up a lifelong experience. Yet their simple sum cannot explain the total gestalt of a lifetime's experience and thought. It has been proposed—first by the composer himself, and later by Hanslick, a music critic—that Brahms' long and elaborate Second Piano Concerto was made up of a myriad of short melodies, all beautiful and concrete. Yet the brilliant conception of this immense and complex one-hour work cannot be explained by the little melodic measures that make it up. In an article I published in 1954, I compared this concerto, and most of Brahms' works, to Gothic cathedrals in which the sculptured portals, the gigantic columns, and the stained glass rosettes considered separately cannot explain the whole. Only the totality and sacredness of the entire structure can portray the awesome grandeur of these hallowed medieval masterpieces. And so, I explained, is the case with all of Brahms' symphonic works, masterpieces of profound meaning and grandeur. And so it is with our life.

When I was in medical school, I wondered whether the infinite number of neural tracts and cells could explain abstract ideas or the freedom of the will. I concluded in the negative. I thought that the complexity of the human nervous system might possibly explain perception, instinct, memory, imagination, and even the emotions, but I could not believe that abstract ideas, subtle concepts, and free decisions could be fully explained scientifically. There is much more than meets the eye here. I had read and studied enough philosophy and psychology so not to swallow the pseudo-scientific reductionism of my classmates, who were sold on scientism as a religious faith that would one day explain everything on earth and in heaven. I did not buy into that.

One of my favorite authors, Hilaire Belloc, the early 20th century English writer and statesman, echoes my own sentiments on why we love what we love:

> *It has been proved in the life of every man that though his loves are human, and therefore changeable, yet in proportion as he attaches them to things unchangeable, so they mature and broaden. And on this account . . . does a man love an old house which was his father's, and on this account does a man come to love with all his heart, that part of earth which nourished his boyhood. For it does not change, or if it changes, it changes very little, and he finds in it the character of enduring things.*
> —Hilaire Belloc, *The Four Men* (1910)

I cherish the things and events of my childhood. In them I find the character of enduring things.

EARLIEST MEMORIES

My earliest memories up to the age of three are a little hazy and seem to flutter away like a mirage. I remember, as through a veil, a big man with hair uncombed and a beard of amorphous shape, Signor Leoni. He is seated on the floor in the living room of the villa in Serhel on a typically hot summer afternoon.

Around him, two brothers and I are enjoying the cool marble floor. My older brothers are listening to him talk, while I am engrossed in nothing intellectual. He is teaching them from a globe of the world, and I am lying down, leaning on a pillow with the image of a tiger woven on its cover. That image is much clearer to me now than is the rest of the scene. The teacher and my brothers may have been discussing deep subjects, but they are seen only as a mirage; while the tiger (*my* tiger) is vivid with brown stripes and bright yellow fur.

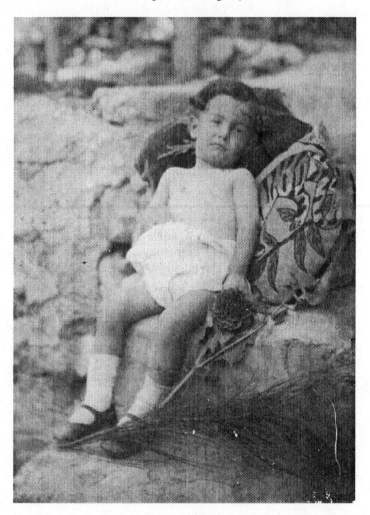

Henry, relaxing next to his tiger pillow, at age two, 1936

Dad had hired a teacher, Mr. Ferrer, from the Carmelite School in Tripoli to spend the summer with us in Serhel. He tutored my older brothers in math, French, and Italian. His compensation was my mother's Lebanese cooking and the fresh air of the mountains. I don't recall the teacher's name as being a French Ferrer. I always remembered it as Leoni, an Italian! Did my pillow tiger make me think for years and years that his name was Leoni? Two feline animals! My oldest brother says that yet another tutor was Rafael Khoury, a relative. I met him years later in Venezuela where he had immigrated. In contrast to the teacher in my imagination, he was rather small in stature, just slightly over five feet tall. However, he did have a distinctly leonine face, like Bert Lahr in "The Wizard of Oz."

These tutors left us after two or three summers, but the tiger pillow remained in the house until I was fourteen, when we left Serhel for America. From the age of four to the age of fourteen, whenever I looked at the woven tiger I recalled the setting of our group on the marble floor next to the tutor with the leonine face.

Not all of my earliest memories are as clear as this one. Later events in one's life may be more historically detailed and more factual than the earlier ones. Is one less significant or less true than the other? I doubt it. I remember that early scene, lying on the cool marble floor with my tiger pillow, with more tenderness and nostalgia than any other image that came after it.

Sometimes my brothers help me to remember. Recently, I begged my brother Mike, "Please, recall the story about Père François influencing Dad into marrying for the second time." Well, Mike told me that Dad was even more influenced by Afifeh, my mother's friend. Apparently, she worked hard on Mom to marry Dad. It seems my mother was no keener on getting married than was my father.

Now Afifeh was the wife of a certain French officer in Lebanon during the mandate that followed World War I. I vaguely recall the man as tall and imposing. I know that his name was General Prévot; at least, that's how we addressed him. In my mind, he was always a "General" of the occupying French Army, a slight misconception it seems, since I learned from my brother Mike that he was never higher than a major.

I remember their progeny well. They had four children: Francois, Robert, Maurice and Violette, the only daughter. François is now a successful businessman in Detroit and a close friend of mine. Robert became the general commissioner of the United Nations in the Middle East with headquarters in Beirut; he is now retired, and I rarely see him. The last time I met Maurice was in 1968 when he took me around northern France in his Peugeot and was very kind and hospitable to me. That was also the first time I visited Chartres Cathedral. I remember going up to the top of the left spire with him and his girlfriend, a certain Comtesse de Saussy (a town near Dijon, France). He now lives in Paris, practices sports medicine and was sports physician on-call to the Le Mans auto race for several years. As to his sister Violette, I have not seen her for years.

My dominant memory of Afifeh is a strange one. During my visit to her house in Tripoli, she once gave me a cookie out of an old box. I had just taken a bite out of the cookie when I noticed a small, half-bitten worm wiggling in it. It was a disgusting experience, especially to a boy aged eight. That day, Dad had just picked me up from my piano lesson at the Carmelite Sisters' Convent in Tripoli, next door to her house. The connection between the disgusting worm and my piano lesson has remained vivid in my imagination. Thank God it didn't ruin my love of music. I still see the worm coming out of the cookie, after I had just bitten into it. I can also still hear Dad telling me later that Afifeh, who was then a widow, was a "big miser" who probably has had that box of cookies unopened since her wedding reception, twenty years earlier. I remember exactly every word he said.

SUMMERS IN THE MOUNTAINS, WINTERS BY THE SEA

During those memorable summer days in Serhel, Dad had hired Rafael Khoury specifically to teach my brothers Arabic. Every now and then, Mr. Khoury would sneak in a few lessons in Aramaic (also known as Syriac, the language of the Maronite Mass and of Jesus himself). Dad never complained to him about that, since he himself had studied Aramaic when he was preparing to become a monk.

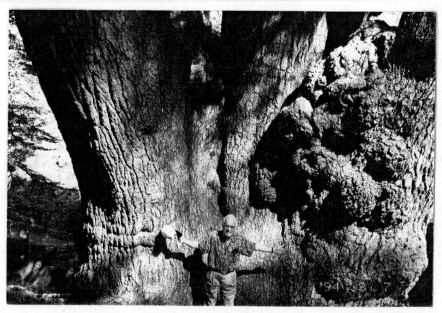

I am in front of the trunk of an ancient cedar, still living; it probably dates from the time of Christ. The famous cedars grow at an altitude of 6,600 feet. Serhel, our village, is ten miles southwest of the old cedars as the crow flies, at an elevation of 3,000 feet.

One early morning in 1939, when I was five years old, I recall that Anthony and Sadi'a Barkett's family had breakfast at our home just before their voyage to America. Some members of that family had not been back to see Serhel until a few years ago. I recall watching them come up the steep path from the village to stop at our house for breakfast. Mom fried about two dozen eggs for them, and Dad cut up "mountain oysters" (lamb testicles) and tossed them on top of the simmering eggs. That was supposed to be invigorating for the long trip to Tripoli, then Beirut, and finally America. Eating mountain oysters was supposed to improve one's libidinal life, just as pulverized deer horns are thought to do by the Japanese. Old wives' tales can be bizarre indeed!

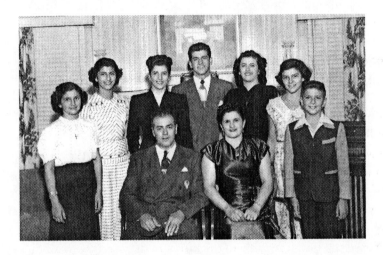

Anthony and Sadi'a Barkett seated, and their family, left to right, Su'ad, Antoinette, Madelyn, Dr. Joe, Renee, Marie, and Dr. Henry (circa 1947).

I can still picture the black Ford model-T on the hillside road above our villa, waiting to take the Barkett family away. I recall the kisses, hugs, and good-byes. Everybody was crying. I can still see them going up the path to the waiting vehicle—Anthony and Sadi'a, the parents, followed by Madelyn, Renee, Joe, Antoinette, Marie, and little Suad. Their son Henry had not been born yet. Madelyn eventually married my brother Tony and went to live with him first in Venezuela, and later in California. Joe grew up to become Dr. Joe Barkett, my cousin and friend in Stockton for the past forty years.

I used to be scared of the dark when we were up in Serhel. Both the kitchen and the bathroom were separated from the house by a breezeway. So, I would dash like lightning between the house and the annex, afraid of encountering a wolf or hyena. Wolves actually lived in the forest nearby and wolf stories abounded in Serhel. Hyenas, we were told, were particularly dangerous since, for them, "children are a delicacy." (And that was long before I had read Jonathan Swift's *A Modest Proposal*—the satirical essay about pickling Irish infants as a delicacy for the palate of the "insatiably voracious English.")

During the otherwise silent nights, one would hear on occasion the howl of the wolves and foxes, and the croaking of the frogs and toads. Particularly annoying during daylight hours was the chirp of the cicadas, which went on relentlessly all day. At night, however, the cicadas went to sleep and stopped their chirping. Several naturalists have connected the frequency of their chirps to the atmospheric temperature, and I think it was Henri Fabre, the French naturalist, who years ago developed a mathematical formula for this phenomenon.

In Serhel, the maids would be cooking or washing in the annex while telling me stories of my infancy. "Your mother fed you her milk for fourteen months," they would say. "Her milk was plentiful!" Indeed, I recall my mother as having been well endowed for that function. No anorexic was she! Not fat either! The maids would also tell me, "Your brothers and sister played with you constantly. You were their doll. When you were two, they would pick you up and toss you on your bed, and you would giggle and they would laugh. You often slept in your sister Mary's bed during the afternoon siesta. She would cuddle you and shower you with kisses. At night, you slept in a crib in your parents' bedroom at first; but later we made a makeshift bed for you to sleep on. We used the low, side table in the kitchen, dressed it with a small mattress and sheets, and placed it between your Mom's and Dad's beds." Mom and Dad usually slept in adjoining beds and only rarely in the same bed. Freud would have had a lot to say about all these arrangements, I am quite sure!

I remember how comfy my childhood years were. I recall the few times that I dozed in my sister's bed for the afternoon nap. She was ten years older than me and would read me stories in a French children's book called *Le Renard et les Autres Animaux*. I would listen for a short while and then drop off to sleep. I can still smell the perfume my sister used to wear. I was enthralled by how pretty she was. All this took place in Serhel during the summer. Oh, how I loved those enchanting summers! Was it the sweet smell of the almond blossoms in the garden outside, or was it my sister's perfume that enchanted me?

In the winter, all of my brothers were busy with schoolwork. I recall feeling very happy that I didn't have to do any schoolwork at that age. Yet by age six,

I already knew a great deal about geography, music, and history. My sister would read me children's historical novels. We always went to Sunday Mass at 9:00 a.m.; and when I attended the Christian Brothers' school in Tripoli, the whole class went to daily Mass. We were taught devotion, modesty, and piety at the Catholic school. I was always fascinated by the statues of St. Joseph and the Blessed Virgin Mary on either side of the altar.

RAGI DANIEL, THE PAINTER

In those years, Dad dabbled in several business enterprises, even though he was officially retired, but most of these ventures didn't turn out to be profitable. First, there was the coal mine. A friend of the family, Mr. Ragi Daniel, enticed Dad to prospect with him on an old, closed coal mine, not far from Serhel. After two years of mining, they could barely meet expenses.

Ragi Daniel was the village's Renaissance man. As a youth he went to Italy to study art and painting; when he returned several years later he was an accomplished oil and fresco painter. He was a man of taste, always interested in literature, philosophy, and rhetoric, having acquired a classical education in Italy. It was most beneficial to the village that he also learned how to prepare and paint frescoes, because after the failure of the coal mine and other business ventures, he decided to paint the inside of St. Michael's church, now the pride and joy of the village.

He asked the municipality to provide the art supplies and promised that he would paint the Church for free. After several years of work, he succeeded in decorating the village church with some of the most beautiful frescoes in the entire Middle East. Now, fifty years later, my wife and I have donated funds to have the frescoes retouched after they suffered water damage.

When I was a child the huge mural that Ragi had painted on the wall behind the high altar fascinated me. It showed a strong, youthful St. Michael the Archangel, dressed in blue with a vivid red cape, sword in hand, and a foot on top of Lucifer's head. Satan was being hurled into hell amid flames and smoke. Lucifer was depicted as bald-headed with elongated ears. Later on I discovered that the mural was similar to one of Guido Reni's paintings on the same theme. With all the walls and ceilings decorated by Ragi, the inside of the church looks like a miniature Sistine Chapel.

Every time I return to Lebanon I visit St. Michael's. It is the church where I was baptized September 3, 1934. I attend early morning Mass daily when I am visiting. Usually, two or three of the local widows show up. It is unfortunate that neither the peasants nor the well-to-do show up for Mass during the week. They all routinely come on Sunday; but they don't realize what they're missing when they don't receive Christ daily, when He is so available in the Blessed Sacrament.

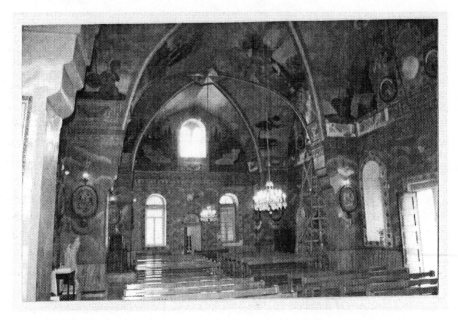

A section of the interior of St. Michael's Church in Serhel, painted by Ragi Daniel in 1950.

Ragi Daniel had another side. He loved to scandalize the simple folk of the village. They all thought he was an agnostic or an atheist. Dad knew, however, that Ragi was a faithful Christian, and all his antics were a show. Ragi would tell the village priests, Father Michael and Father Joseph, that attendance at Mass would increase dramatically if they distributed for Communion a big patty of fried *kibbe* (the Lebanese national dish). I remember Dad scolding him for saying such sacrilegious things in front of the poor, but deeply devoted and pious villagers.

Mr. Daniel went down to Tripoli in the winter, just like the rest of us. At the Maronite cathedral in Tripoli there would always be a guest preacher during Lent. These priests were great orators just like the Redemptorists, or the Passionists. They would go from church to church preaching the word of

God. There were always extra services in the evening during Lent. The visiting priest, usually a doctor of theology or of philosophy, would ascend the ornately engraved mahogany pulpit with all eyes fixed on him. The sermon would be in fluent, and elaborately brilliant, classical Arabic. That language lends itself perfectly to ornamentation and aggrandizement. Spanish poetry inherited that trait from the seven centuries Moorish occupation of Spain. The Greek language, too, must have had the same effect on literate ears, since St. John Chrysostom ("the golden-mouthed") used it in his fabled sermons. The effect of the great preaching of those days made a strong impression on me. I miss it terribly.

Well, Ragi Daniel was often present at these sermons and, while listening attentively, he would always cross his legs for comfort. In our country, to cross one's legs during a service was, and still is, frowned upon. One day while everybody had their eyes fixed on the preacher, the local priest happened to walk down the aisle and see Ragi sitting with his legs crossed. He tapped him on the leg on top and gave him a disapproving look. Ragi looked at him and asked, "What is the problem, Father?" "Your legs," said the priest. Ragi understood that the priest wanted him to uncross his legs. He looked up at him and said in a very low tone, "Father why should that bother you? The leg that is under the other supporting its fellow member generously and ungrudgingly for the past hour, has not complained, has it? It is carrying all the weight, yet it says nothing. Then why should *you* be bothered by it? Besides, you are interrupting our mutual enjoyment of this great preacher. We ought to listen to him instead of worrying about petty things; God only knows the good it would do our speech and our sermons!"

I recall Ragi and his wife, Elmoz, visiting us often. Ragi got along with my father very well because both were educated and had philosophical minds. Visiting the neighbors was a common practice in the evenings and at any time after Mass on a Sunday. I remember Ragi visiting us often, if only to hear the news on the short-wave radio that Dad had bought soon after its invention by Marconi. Just before my birth my father acquired the first short-wave radio in town, and people would visit us to listen to the latest world news. I recall with amusement that when villagers used to come down from Serhel to Tripoli for supplies and to visit us in the city, they would invariably look behind the huge radio—at first radios were manufactured to look like elegant pieces of furniture—in an effort to find the little announcer, or the little musician, who was talking or playing an instrument within the box that the Zeiters called "radio."

On New Year's Eve there was always a grand gathering and a glorious party at Ragi Daniel's home in Tripoli. It was the social highlight of the winter season. I have a well-preserved image of men dressed in black-tie evening clothes in one room, playing poker on a huge table lined with green felt, with young ladies watching them from the side. In another room, I see my brother Edmond, the "life of the party," singing "O Sole Mio" and "Santa Lucia" in his mellow tenor voice, and later people waltzing. Most of all I remember the dishes of bonbons, baklava, tiramisu, marie-eclairs, chocolate figurines, napoleons, and *mahmul*: a child's dream of sweets, satiation, and satisfaction. It was New Year's Eve and I could eat all I wanted!

There were glowing chandeliers hanging from the ceiling, and the elegant dancing and swirling reminds me of the spectacular scene in Tchaikovsky's opera *Eugene Onegin* when the nobility enter the hall and dance the brilliant polonaise. I can still hear the music. All the women at the party were in the room next to the plates of food and desserts, feeding me bonbons and éclairs, because I was "skinny little Henri," and they all wanted to fatten me into a red-faced Frans Hals Dutch urchin. Oh, how glorious was the aroma of a hundred perfumes emanating from all these well-coiffed ladies, dressed in their resplendent gowns! My mother would be sitting like a queen, content to see her child happy, the beloved toy of all her friends. The party would end after the New Year chimes rang. Then home to bed, where we all slept like logs until noon the next day.

UNCLE PAUL

The youngest of my Dad's brothers, Uncle Paul, was an entrepreneur in the similar vein of Ragi Daniel. He was a tall, good-looking man. He combed his abundant smooth black hair backwards, parted in the middle, just like in the *Great Gatsby* era of the early twenties. As a young man in Lebanon in the 1920s, he used to travel across Mount Lebanon's crests, from Serhel to Baalbeck, where he would go to exchange fresh fruits from our grandmother's garden in exchange for grains and produce from the fertile plains of the Bekaa Valley on the other side of the mountain range. The Bekaa has always been the bread basket of Lebanon. On the way back from the Bekaa area, his mule would be loaded with burlap sacks, full of grain and sundries, hanging on either side of the animal.

On one of his trips back from Baalbeck, he was crossing the mountain pass high up next to Qurnut-as-Sauda (Lebanon's highest peak, 10,174 feet above sea level) when he came across residual pockets of snow and ice still not melted in July. It so happened that it was one of the few times that he had come back from the Bekaa with a light load on his mule, and he started thinking that the ice would be "heaven-sent" if he could get it to the sweltering village in time. He always carried with him an ax for cutting wood and an old army knife for self-protection, so he used them to cut off chunks of ice from the glaciers and loaded these on the mule in the half empty burlap sacks. He used his whip on the mule only once, and from there on it was downhill all the way to Serhel. Upon arriving, he went straight to the main square and started selling the blocks of ice, unloading them off his mule.

A week later, back from a similar trip, he was better prepared to sell iced tea and cold lemonade (with plenty of ice) to the sweltering farmers returning from their fields. Once he realized the overwhelming need for ice-cold refreshments during the hot days of summer, he began to take extra burlap bags with him and a second mule, thus planning to brink back with him all the blocks of ice the animals could carry. He eventually established a small outdoor coffee house on the main square, which did quite well. The following summer, it occurred to him to send the boys from the village up to the mountains to get the ice, while he stayed in his coffee shop serving customers and catering to the backgammon players in the village square. He made enough money, to buy several suits, plenty of needed supplies and eventually a travel ticket, after he had decided to emigrate from Serhel and go into business with some of Serhel's emigrants who had preceded him to Caracas, Venezuela. Uncle Paul passed away in the year 2000 at the age of ninety. I always include him in my prayers.

VACATIONS IN SERHEL

When school was over in late June, we would pack and be driven up to our beloved mountains. In the summer months in Serhel, our parents would have a daily routine for us. After breakfast, we had to study until ten or eleven o'clock. Since none of us had watches, Dad would take a piece of white chalk and draw a line across the patio beneath the balcony. When the sun rays reached that line, we were free to stop studying. Nature was our time-keeper (aka *zeiter*, in German)! On Saturday, around ten in the morning, we would wait for the mailman who came to the village only once a week at exactly that hour. "Are there any letters from the relatives in America?" we would ask. Some days following morning study my brothers would go hunting. It was their favorite sport. After preparing the bullets and packing them with powder, my older brothers would take off into the nearby forest to hunt for wild rabbits, squirrels, and quail. I was reminded of that familiar morning scene in Serhel when I saw the French movie *La Gloire de Mon Père* in which the young boy watches his uncle pack the powder in the bullets before going hunting. The movie takes place in Provence, with scenery very similar to that of the Lebanese coastal mountains where I grew up. It is a delightful movie, along with its sequel, *Le Château de Ma Mère*.

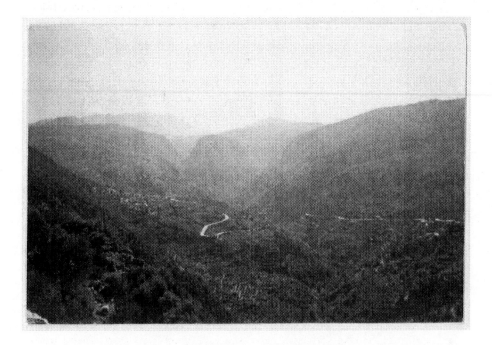

The lower part of the Kadisha Valley in North Lebanon, viewed from the old road coming from Tripoli on the Mediterranean. The village of Serhel is perched on a ridge at the far left. The Zeiter house is the one above the village to the very far left. Beyond are the rugged, verdant mountains of North Lebanon and the Kadisha Canyon.

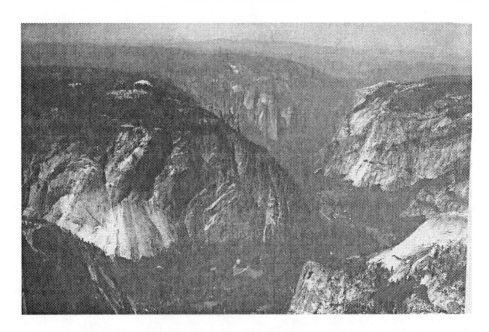

View of Yosemite Valley in California, which compares well with the lower Kadisha Valley and Serhel. Even the contours of the mountains can be superimposed one on the other. Except for the scenic village (Serhel) in the first valley, the similarity of scenary is astounding.

While my older brothers went hunting, the rest of us played in the fields around the house. I recall being fascinated by chameleons. I would watch them move on a vine branch ever so slowly with their tongues sticking out to catch insects. Passing from a shaded area to a sunny one, they would change color. They used this same kind of camouflage in order to match the color or hue of their surroundings. I would be chasing butterflies, lizards, and grasshoppers at one time or another during the day, but running away from bees and wasps.

The climate was exactly like that of the northern California foothills—cool in the morning, then hotter and hotter as the day progressed, then cool again in the evening. I can still feel the dryness in the air during the day, and the caressing western breeze that blew from the Mediterranean in the evening. As autumn approached, the air coming from the Mediterranean became much colder. It would rustle the pine and fir trees around our house in whiffs and spurts. The air would crackle with dryness as the day wore on. Or was it the monotonous chirping of the cicadas? The first few days of summer vacation their chirping irritated us, but after a week or so we would barely hear them. The noise they made would melt into the background of the day.

We always ate our main meal at noon. It was well prepared by mom and the cook (we always had one). Actually Mom would hire young girls from the village and teach them cleaning, washing, and cooking. They were from poor families who lived in adobe (mud) houses. As they got older they would leave us to get married and their younger sisters would take their places. Mom would complain about them leaving since she had to teach the new ones all over again. However, many stayed a long time with us. To this day, my sister Mary often complains about the maids quitting on her in Caracas. "Oh, I lost my maid yesterday! What am I going to do without her?" And for Mary it's crisis time!

As I grew up we had Watfah, Latifah, and Sa'dah, then Marie, and finally Mariam. I liked Mariam the best. I was eleven years old and she was about seventeen. I would always ask her about the birds and the bees. She educated me with all kinds of novel information that I promptly relayed to my friends, whose curiosity was just as great as mine. I would run out to tell the boys of the neighborhood what Mariam told me, especially Antoine, Bacchus, and Tannous. She was our source of learning about the puzzling enigma of life and birth.

Curiosity about our bodies and those of the opposite gender was not our only concern. Many things were new experiences at that age, including lighting up a dried branch of grapevine and smoking it. We experimented that way a few times when I was about ten. I remember playing with Antoine and Joseph, (sons of Tamar Mujalli,) a neighbor, and with their nieces Marie Therese and Irene Farah. Irene ended up marrying my brother Johnny. Marie Therese married Joe Lahoud, who owned a Mercedes agency in Quebec City. My little playmate, Joe Mujalli, is now dying of cancer at the age of sixty-five. The Farah girls were beautiful and still are, even now that they are in their sixties. We used to tease poor Antoine because he was a little effeminate. He ended up leading a rock band in Germany, and eventually getting a sex change. I was told later that he changed his name to Sonya. He died of AIDS in Germany.

Marie Therese was the oldest of the group. She taught Irene and me how to cut a dried, but porous, branch of vine and how to use it as a cigarette by lighting one end and puffing through the other. One inhaled nothing but smoke. It is no wonder that I've never tried to smoke cigarettes. After the newness wore off, we realized that it was making us sick and dizzy.

IN GRANDMOTHER'S GARDEN OF EDEN

In the village, after the main meal at noon, all the adults and siblings (including the maids) had a siesta, except for me. I couldn't sleep in the afternoon; I had an innate feeling that leisure time was a gift from God not to be wasted on sleep. I would observe the antics of grasshoppers, butterflies or lizards outside, or read fairy tales to myself, or simply daydream while lying on the cool marble floor inside the house, gazing at the drawings on the ceiling. I think it was due to times like these that I developed the habit (perhaps talent?) of enjoying solitude, observing little nothings, while meditating on life and feeling free from any anxiety or guilt in passing my time lazily. Oh, the difference between growing up in the country versus the busy city! It took the rigors, the frenzy, and the competition I discovered in medical school to derail me from the easy-going oriental lifestyle.

I had no idea that I was providentially preparing for the supreme joy of my days of leisure, both before and after my retirement in sunny California. My heart bleeds for the many people I encounter who are bored to death, following retirement, and want to go back to gainful work or to be busy doing something, anything. I sometimes say to myself what vacuous minds. Yet, I chase the judgmental thought out of my mind saying to myself, *chacun à son gout* (Fr.); *cada loco con su tema* (Sp.); to each his own. But working on one's own moral growth and spending time helping others less fortunate is a worthy goal to seek during retirement. As I learned later, "The life of money-making is one undertaken under compulsion, and wealth is evidently not the good we are seeking; for it is merely useful and for the sake of something else," wrote Aristotle in his *Ethics*.

The rest of the family, unwittingly practicing the talent that I just mentioned, would go on dozing for an hour or more every afternoon we were in Serhel. With no hassle in sight anywhere, I had all that time to be alone, free and happy. I distinctly remember, and can still feel, exactly as I felt then: lying there, with the refreshing coolness of the marble floor on my back, lazily daydreaming, one hot summer afternoon after another. The aura of those afternoons comes back to me every time I listen to a certain type of music, particularly Claude Debussy's *The Afternoon of a Faun*. This composer marvelously portrays, actually embodies in his impressionist composition, the languor of the hot summer days I am attempting to describe. His musical strains lead one into daydreams. One can slide into a faraway Eden, where God gave man everything to enjoy and no reason to work by the sweat of his brow. Debussy's composition amply demonstrates the ability of music (especially music without words) to embody the essence of a feeling at a moment in time. Claude Debussy's "impressionist" music and the delightful experience in my imaginative memory are one and the same.

At three o'clock in the afternoon, when everybody woke up, I was allowed to go down to the village to Grandma's house. That was the best time of all. Grandma Marzuka was the confident, capable woman who came to America, worked hard for several years, and returned to Lebanon with a small fortune. I would go down the mountain using a serpentine path between houses, fields, and terraces. I remember one spot on the route where there would be a hornets' nest every summer. I had to pass by it cautiously. It was in the terrace stonewall at the bend, not far from great-aunt Teresa's house. The moment I would get to that spot, I would take off like lightning. The wasps would come out buzzing after me, but always too late to get me. Yet feeling my own exhilarating propulsion, I never stopped until I reached Grandma's house.

Grandpa Michael had died several years before. Apparently, around 1941, in his seventy second year of life, he was up in a tree picking fruit when he fell from it and died. It was believed to have been a heart attack. I remember him as quiet and soft spoken, still wearing the old folkloric clothes, the *tarbush* (Turkish fez) and the *sherwal*, large billowy trousers with ample material at the crotch that made movement much freer while farming. He always felt that Grandma nagged, so he would often hold his hand up and make a scissor-like motion using his index and middle fingers, symbolizing the cutting off in the next world of tongues that talked too much. I remember him going up to the roof of their modest home in the evening and walking back and forth while reciting his rosary. He told me once that it was the only place where he found peace in silence.

Thinking back over my whole life, I believe I was happiest playing near my grandmother's garden. It seemed like the Garden of Eden. She had apple and pear trees, loquats and persimmons, almonds and walnuts, cherries and apricots, and all kinds of grapes, all interspaced between furrows of peas, peppers, cucumbers and melons. I would play with Bacchus and Tannous Brais in the vicinity of my grandparents' house. It was difficult to keep my white outfit clean, even though my mother would have warned me not to get dirty. I don't know why she always dressed a seven-year-old boy in white expecting him to keep immaculately clean. She was from the city, prim and proper, and would generally not let me play with the poor, dirty kids down in the village. When she said go and play, she said it with a certain hesitation. Two days each week, Grandma would ask me and my friends to walk up the hill and open the village water reservoir from five to six in the evening. That was her allotted time for irrigation; each farmer had a scheduled time to use the water.

One of our favorite tasks was to run up about a thousand paces from the village to open the reservoir, which was fed by a fresh water spring. We would go up to the spring first and drink from its pristine water; it had a mineral tang that I can still taste. It was also cold and refreshing, its water seeping all the way down from the snowy mountain tops of the Lebanon range. Then, before we opened the reservoir, Tannous would leap from the spring area above, right into the reservoir itself, splashing enough water to soak a small garden. I used to tell him, "Stop doing that, you're wasting a quarter of my grandma's water."

There was an opening at the bottom of the reservoir. It would be plugged with rags and mud, held down by a wooden post. We would remove the post and watch the water gush into the conduit at the bottom. Then we would run along the side of the ensuing water stream through bends and terraces in the field all the way down to Grandma's garden. She would be there with shovel in hand directing the water this way and that by opening certain furrows and closing others. At the end of the hour allotted to her, the water stream would slow to a trickle, and then it would stop. This meant that the reservoir was empty. One of us would go back up to the reservoir and plug it again, so it would be full the next day for the farmer whose turn it was to use it.

JIDDO'S EGGS

It would be six to seven o'clock in the evening by then. Since it was summertime, there would still be several hours of sunlight remaining. My reward for helping in the irrigation was always a couple of Grandma's eggs. She would give the other boys a penny each and send them home to their mothers.

I will never forget Grandma's eggs. They were fried in olive oil in a *taijan* (a clay skillet) over an open fire and she would squeeze tomatoes over them. One day as I was savoring my grandmother's delicious eggs with pita bread, I told her: "Your eggs are delicious Grandma! Even if you gave me a million dollars I wouldn't stop eating." Her reply was, "Try me for a nickel." That was the first time I realized that the foolish enthusiasm of youth compares poorly with the practical wisdom of old age.

I have been frying eggs for breakfast her way for the past fifty years. I make them for my sons and daughters, grandsons and granddaughters, nephews and nieces, grandnephews and grandnieces in Canada, Detroit, Venezuela, and California. They all call them "*Jiddo's* eggs," that is, Grandpa's eggs, (even though they should be calling them "Grandma's eggs"). I caught my son John Henry, about a year ago, having the audacity to tell the same story, but calling them "Daddy's eggs!" *His* eggs! Pure plagiarism, I say.

In my childhood, when I told my Grandma, "I love your eggs," she always had a loud chuckle. In the Arabic language eggs (*baidat*) also means, of all things, testicles. As a matter of fact, mountain oysters (sheep testicles) fried with eggs and vegetables make a treasured breakfast omelet in the Middle East—it's believed to increase one's libido, an old wives tale.

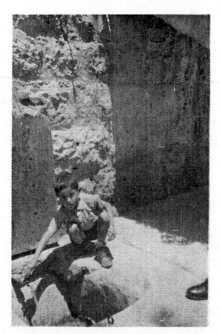

Here I was in 1940 opening a faucet below the summer villa. Dad had built a reservoir under the house, which in the winter gathered the rain water from the flat roof and saved it for the dry summer to water the garden and for laundry use. Drinking water was brought up from the fresh spring in the village and stored in pottery urns, which kept the water cold by evaporation through the semi-porous clay.

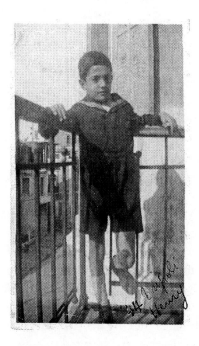

The back of this photo is marked, *A mon petit frère Henri, de sa soeur qui l'aime beaucoup, Marie, 1941* ("To my little brother Henri, from his sister who loves him very much, Marie"). Here I am standing on our third floor veranda in Tripoli. Such photos bring back precious memories of summer vacation time in Serhel and winter school and study time in Tripoli, Lebanon.

Grandma was not a big woman, but she was portly, and when she laughed her belly would shake up and down with every chuckle. She wore dark dresses and always had an apron on, as if prepared to cook at any moment. I remember her covering her hair with a scarf, wrapping it around her round face and tying it in a knot below the chin. Teresa, her sister, and Msahieh (Nehme's widow), her sister-in-law, always wore the same dark head-cover. Grandma was a generous almsgiver to any beggar who came by. Some of these transients trusted her enough to leave with her whatever little money they had collected on their rounds, for safekeeping. There was a fellow in town who gave everyone in the village an appropriate nickname. His appellations were uncannily accurate. Grandma was "the mother of beggars"; Uncle Paul, who had a bronzed complexion, was "the Egyptian"; and my godmother Sadi'a, one of Marzouka's granddaughters, was nicknamed "the nest of vipers" because she had a vile temper.

ACCIDENTS WILL HAPPEN

I remember one evening when, after eating Grandma's fried eggs, I went to the flat roof of Bacchus' house to play marbles with him. I shot a marble that went past him. When he lunged back to get it at the edge of the roof, he leaned too far and plunged over head down. If it weren't for the wall of the house next door that broke his fall, he would have been paralyzed for life. He bled like a stuck pig from a deep cut in his forehead. We took him to Mr. Butros al-Khoury, the village's old self-appointed doctor. At best he must have been a hospital orderly at one time. He sutured the wound with a sewing needle and wrapped up the head with a huge bandage.

I recall another serious injury around our house. Mom cut her hand accidentally while preparing dinner for us and a week later her hand got infected. The same self-appointed physician decided to treat the cut with leeches. Medical care in the village was still primitive in those days. I can still picture her hand in a pan full of crawling leeches sucking her supposedly poisoned blood. By the time my brother Mike (who was a medical intern then) got home, the infection had spread to her whole arm. Mike became upset with her for being so naïve, and he immediately drove her to his hospital in Tripoli for treatment; they got there in the nick of time to save her from dying of generalized septicemia.

One day there was a funeral for Tannous Brais' little brother who died of tetanus. The next day, Tannous, Bacchus, and I crept near the mausoleum, and finding the door ajar, went inside and opened the casket. The little body had worms crawling on it and the stench was unbearable. We were so startled we ran away leaving the casket open. For nights on end I would see him coming towards me through the open window of my bedroom.

SUMMER EVENINGS IN SERHEL

These grim memories are offset by my thoughts about the physical beauty of Serhel. At the sunset hour, I would go up to the roof of our house to watch the alpenglow on the mountain tops. The roof was the best vantage point. The reflected pinkish light from the setting sun on the opposite horizon would bathe the mountains in a heavenly glow. The bright reddish hue from the setting sun would rise up higher and higher on the mountain range until it disappeared from view altogether. I always understood (even at that age) how symbolic this event was of the winter of life when sight will be extinguished.

I still watch this phenomenon in the mountain crests of the California Sierra Nevada. When the show from the roof at Serhel was over, I would come down to the house and supper would be ready. The best time of the day was yet to come.

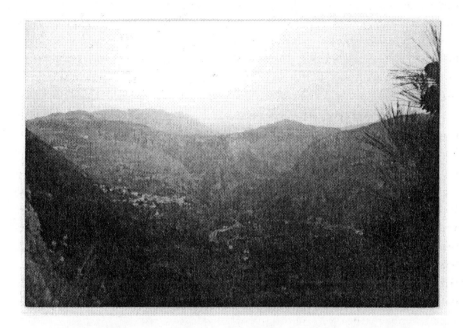

The final fifteen minutes of *alpenglow,* shining on Serhel and the mountain range beyond. I enjoyed this scene every summer evening. As the sun was setting on the horizon behind me, dark shadows would fill the valley, and the pink rays of alpenglow would cover the mountain crests in front of me. My eyes would delight in this phenomenon of nature.

Dad or Mom would light a Coleman kerosene lamp and set it on the patio in front of the house. When neighbors and friends saw it lit, they would come up from the village to pass the evening. There were no televisions, movies, or theaters, so we relied on each other for entertainment. The men would sit in one group and discuss politics, and the women would form another group, exchanging recipes or telling each other the latest gossip. As the place filled up with visitors, Dad would light another kerosene lamp and take it up to the flat Mediterranean roof. It would light up the trees in the forest nearby, just like a full moon. That's when the outlying villages would know about yet another party at the Zeiters'. The light would be seen from Tourza across the river and as far away as Beit Minzer, a village on top of another mountain across the deep valley.

The children would be in their glory, playing outside or being told stories by one of the elders. After one of these long days I would finally get tired enough to enter the *khaimeh* or "evergreen" tent that's on the roof, jump on a mattress, and go to sleep. My brothers would come later to join me. We would all wake up with the rising sun shining in our eyes, since the open entrance to the tent was always built facing east. We would still be half asleep coming out of the tent, greeted by the glorious view of huge mountains and waterfalls.

The evergreen tent (*khaimeh*) was a tradition in itself. A day or two after our arrival in Serhel for summer vacation, my brothers (with help from some of the older neighbors) would start building the tent on the flat roof. Their best helper was Michel (my brother-in-law now, married to my sister Mary) because he was familiar with the pine forest. One of the largest evergreen forests in Lebanon belonged to the municipality of Serhel. Michel and my brothers would go into the forest and cut some tree branches (pine, fir, and spruce) and drag them to the roof of the house. For a whole week they would build the structure that was to become our tent. They would use the denuded larger branches to construct the frame or skeleton of the tent. The smaller branches, full of green needles, would then be tied on the sides and roof of the tent, leaving a large opening for an entrance facing east.

The result was a sturdy structure that a strong wind could not shake. The tent was usually large enough to house about eight to ten mattresses, which we brought up from our bedrooms below and laid on the flat roof. The floor of the tent was actually the flat roof of the house. We slept tight in our tent every night from July until late September when the fog set in. It was cool, breezy, and fun—heaven on earth for us kids.

On the nights when my father went to Tripoli shopping, we would all sit on the rear patio of the house waiting for him to come home. We would stare at the road skirting the cliffs above, looking for the lights of the taxi that would be bringing him home. At first, the car lights would appear to be pinpoints, then would look like faraway flashlights; they would get bigger and brighter as the car got closer. The visual effect was akin to the sound effect Ottorino Respighi was to produce in the *Pines of Rome,* using the orchestra to depict the Roman legions marching closer and closer to Rome, at first appearing far away on the Appian way, with the music getting louder and louder as they got closer and closer, until the trumpets blare and the drums and cymbals crash loudly announcing their triumphant arrival beneath the raised canopy of the surveying emperor. The lights of the taxi and the roar of the motor seemed like this as they announced how far away Dad still was; when the lights of the car came into full view and were blinding us, we knew that Dad was home.

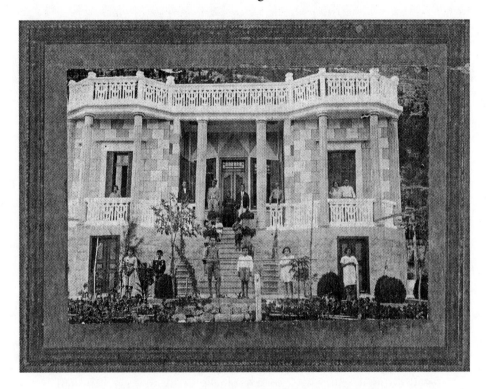

Our summer villa as it looked in 1933, shortly before my birth. Mom and Dad are on the right balcony. To the left of them, standing, are Grandpa Mikhael, M. Mansur (who ended up as a banker in Aruba), Grandma Marzuka (barely seen, dressed in black in front of the main door); Bacchus Farah (father of Irene, Brother Johnny's wife), and Tamar Mujalli (our next door neighbor). On the left balcony is Watfah, the maid who discovered the hidden gold coins in the jar of beans! On the steps are my brothers Johnny and Edmond. In front of the house (r. to l.): Madelyn Barkett in white (now my Brother Tony's wife; Tony was sick inside the house), my sister Mary, brothers Philip and Mike, six-year-old Joe Barkett (now Dr. Barkett), and Renee his sister. All of these people play a part in this book.

CHAPTER 4

INNOCENCE AND HAPPINESS

We always went down to Tripoli about mid-October because that was when the school year started in Lebanon. By the end of summer, we were still sleeping in our tent every night. Then autumn would arrive. The air would be crisp, requiring many covers, and we would cuddle up to each other for warmth. In Serhel, about six in the evening of a fall day, a low fog starts rolling in from the Mediterranean, just the way the fog rolls into San Francisco through the Golden Gate. That fog always meant that it was time to go back to Tripoli and start the new school year.

We all dreaded going back to school, especially me, even though I was good at schoolwork. After the age of ten, I was always seen with a book in my hand. All the people who knew me back then, still remind me, "Henry, you were always reading a book." It didn't mean I loved going to school, however. It only meant that I had to study harder to remain in first place; that can produce an aversion to going to school. However, when I got to college and medical school I began to enjoy school for the knowledge I was acquiring. Then school became fun.

Later in college I became familiar with Aristotle's famous first line from his *Metaphysics*: "All men by nature desire to know." How true this was for me! I've always quoted this line to my children. My sons John Henry and Philip now use it to start their talks and presentations. John Henry, an ophthalmic surgeon, loves to start conferences with this quotation, because it specifically refers to the importance of vision in acquiring knowledge. The entire passage from Aristotle seemed to summarize my childhood zeal to learn through the senses,

All men by nature desire to know. An indication of this is the delight we take in our senses; for even apart from their usefulness they are loved for themselves; and above all the sense of sight. For not only with a view to action, but even when we are not going to do anything, we prefer seeing (one might say) to everything else. The reason is that this, of all our senses, makes us know and brings to light many differences between things.

—Aristotle, Metaphysics, Book A (I), 980a

Those days in Tripoli I remember as carefree. I recall standing on the balcony of our third floor apartment in Tripoli on a gloriously sunny Mediterranean day, wearing the typical dark blue sailor outfit that kids used to wear. Those sunny winter school days in Tripoli during the Second World War, when Lebanon was at peace, unaffected by the rage going on in nearby Europe— those sunny days when little Henri was loved, happy, and carefree; those days of brightness and joy, days blessed by the absence of past or future concerns when only the present moment counted for anything—those days are etched in my memory and imagination forever. Such are the days to be desired and wished for throughout life. It is unfortunate that such days become difficult to come by as one gets older and over-concerned with working for a living, getting married, and raising a family, making ends meet, and worst of all over-philosophizing and asking irrelevant questions about the psychological reasons for everything one sees or does.

FATHER ANTHONY SHEINA

I remember returning to Lebanon several times in the 1990s when I was in my sixties. One morning, I went up—with Antoine Ragi (a cousin and caretaker of our house in Serhel) and Dr. Bill Latham from Stockton, who was visiting with me—to visit a hermit, Fr. Anthony Sheina, who lived near the Monastery of Kos'haya. We hiked our way up the cliffs of the Kadisha Canyon to get to his hermitage. I had always wanted to visit a modern-day hermit, having read a lot about these anchorites in Middle Eastern history. I had read Blessed John Cassian's fifth-century treatise on Eastern monasticism. That book influenced Saint Benedict in the founding of Western monasticism, long before the Moslem invasion of the Middle Eastern and North African Christian population.

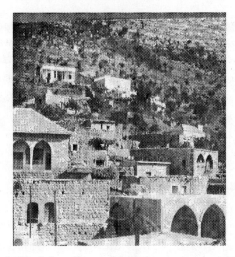

The eastern half of the village of Serhel as it was in 1932. Dad had just built our summer villa, the highest house above left. His parents' home was below the house that is seen farthest right.

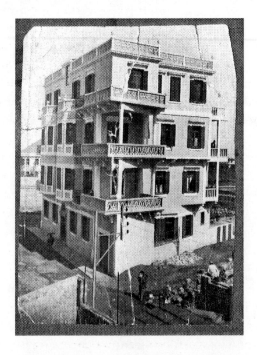

The almost completed apartment building Dad constructed in Tripoli in 1932 next to the Christian Brothers school. We lived on the third floor. From the roof, we could see the snow-capped mountains to the east, the blue Mediterranean to the west, and the orange groves surrounding the city.

In the 1990s William Darlymple of the British press followed St. John Cassian's early fifth-century route through Middle Eastern monasteries and hermitages and then wrote a travelogue about it entitled *From the Holy Mountain*. He started in Venice and traveled through Yugoslavia, Bulgaria, Mount Athos (in Greece), Anatolia, (present-day Turkey,) and finally Syria, Lebanon, Palestine, and the Coptic areas of Egypt. He found that (except for Mount Athos, Lebanon, and Egypt) many ancient monasteries, which had survived for over fifteen hundred years, even into the twentieth century, finally had to be closed, either because of antagonistic government pressures (Turkey) or simply because of the absence of vocations. The realization that so old a way of life should have finally fallen to the axe of twentieth-century secularism and disinterest brought tears to my eyes. The author felt the same way I did. In his travelogue he tells about visiting the same hermit we were visiting in Lebanon, not far from Serhel. Unfortunately after interviewing him, the British newsman wrote that he forgot to ask the hermit his name.

What a shame, because Father Anthony Sheina is well known all over the Middle East. There are not many hermits left anywhere, but this holy man was not even your usual hermit. I was told that he studied at the Sorbonne in Paris during World War II; that he lived in Paris for many years; and that he returned to Lebanon to become the Superior General of the Antonine Order of Maronite monks. Years later, he gave it all up and left the world to become a hermit in the Blessed Valley (Kadisha) of Mount Lebanon.

We arrived at six in the morning as we were told that Father Sheina sees visitors only before his 8:00 o'clock mass. Someone else was in his cell, so I waited, hoping he would see me next. About 6:30, the door opened and the man who was there before me came out and told me I was next. I entered the small cell and saw an old man, about eighty years of age. He was quite willing to converse. He welcomed me and said "If you're not going to Communion this morning, would you like to have some coffee?" I assured him that I intended to go to Communion at his Mass (which he celebrates next to his small room for a few villagers and guests at 8:00 a.m.). I told him that I was the great-nephew of Abuna Butros who was the abbot of Kos'haya three decades before. "Oh, I knew him well," he said. "He and I used to play *shash-bash* (Turkish for the numbers six (shash) and five (bash), a toss of the dice in backgammon). He used to beat me all the time. Your great-uncle was a champion backgammon player." Then he told me that my great-uncle was a modern Christian martyr—apparently at the age of ninety-six, my uncle had refused to deny Christ, and he was martyred by several Somali mercenaries who had been sent to Lebanon, bankrolled by Gadhafi during the civil war.

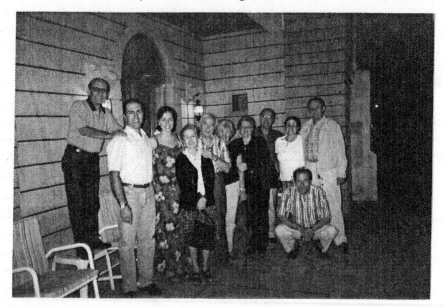

Family and friends in front of the Monastery of Kos'haya (Father Sheina's hermitage is one mile from it) following Mass during a 1998 visit (l. to r.): Brother Philip, Camille and Chantal (daughter of Bacchus Sessine), Mary, Mike and Irene, Lydia (Philip's wife) Michel Braiz (Mary's husband) and Therese and Bacchus Sessine, and his brother Yousef Sessine (crouching).

Then I asked Father Sheina if he had ever met Jacques Maritain (the prominent French Thomist and Aristotelian philosopher) during his stay in Paris, after the Second World War. He wanted to know why I was asking this. I told him that that's what I had heard. He then explained that he, Jacques Maritain and his wife Raissa, Etienne Gilson, Father Garrigou-Lagrange, and a few others formed an intimate group in Paris in the 1940s. They used to meet monthly, and even acted like a nonofficial advisory committee to Pope Pius XII during the war years and for a few years thereafter. (Besides Maritain, Etienne Gilson was another great Catholic historian-philosopher of the twentieth century; Reginald Garrigou-Lagrange, a Dominican and author of *The Three Ages of the Interior Life*, a classic in mystical theology, was perhaps the greatest theologian-philosopher of the past century.)

When Father Sheina revealed that he knew these deep thinkers intimately, I was in awe, having read many of their works. He spoke of them with the greatest humility. I then begged him to hear my general confession. Afterwards, he asked me if I was the son of Yousef Zeiter. When I assented, he told me, "He was a very good Christian writer." Then he got up and said, "I am going to vest for Mass. Use my missal during Mass if you wish."

I was thrilled he would lend me his well-used missal. There were now about twenty people gathered in the small chapel, waiting to hear the Mass celebrated by this holy man. When I started looking at his old missal, it had Aramaic on one side and Arabic on the other. I knew Arabic well, but I had never before tried to decipher Aramaic writing. I soon realized that I could (with effort) read some words in the text. Aramaic appears to be a cross between Arabic and Hebrew. The letters are all slanted backwards from upper right to lower left. Since the Arabic translation in the missal was on the opposite page, I began to figure out some of the meanings of the words. Some were different in pronunciation from Arabic, but since I had actually heard a lot of them when I was a youth going to the Maronite Mass, I found the task of "on the spot" translation easier than I would have thought. (Eight years later, when I first saw Mel Gibson's *The Passion of the Christ*, I was amazed to discover that I understood quite a bit of the Aramaic spoken in the movie.) After Mass, I reluctantly said goodbye to Father Anthony Sheina, the British newsman's hermit, and Antonio, Bill Latham, and I went down to visit the monastery itself.

SUNDAY CUSTOMS IN SERHEL

While in Serhel, Sunday was always our favorite day. We always went down to Mass at St. Michael's Church using a path that wound between the houses in the village. I remember that the women sat on one side of the aisle and the men sat on the other. This custom was still in place twenty years later when I went back with my wife and in-laws to visit. The priest would intone half of the Mass in Arabic and half in old Aramaic. The entrance hymn still rings in my ears, "*Lbaytokh aloho 'elet waq dom bemdilokh sogdet malkoch mayno hasoli khuldah tit loch*" (Aramaic), or "I have entered your house, O Lord, the Lord of my youth, and have worshipped before your throne." (The Latin equivalent is, *Introibo ad altare Dei . . .*) And just before the first scriptural reading the people would intone, "*Qadishat Aloho, Qadishat Hayetono, Qadishat lo moyouto,*" or "Holy are you, O God, Holy are you, O Strong One, Holy are you, O Immortal One"—hence *Kadisha* (aka *Qadisha*) Valley, the holy or blessed valley. Aramaic in the Eastern Church is similar to the use until recent times of the Latin language in the Latin-Rite Roman Catholic Church. I miss both Latin and Aramaic. I feel that by forcibly taking Latin out of the Mass, the Catholic hierarchy has taken away from the average American the opportunity of getting acquainted with a foreign tongue; actually, the mother language of Italian, French and Spanish.

Following Sunday morning Mass, everybody would return home for breakfast at about 9:00 a.m., but only after they had gathered first in front of the Church to exchange pleasantries. I would meet a few of the boys I knew, and we would play games. I recall one particular Sunday when I met with Yousef Sessine (a third cousin) and we went hunting for birds with a slingshot (*mughaita*). He was very good at it. He eventually became a successful businessman, first in Venezuela and later in Lebanon where he lives now.

At times, I would go with him or one of his brothers, Michael or Bacchus, to their house. Their father Simon was a poor farmer, who worked the land of Aunt Teresa, his mother. I saw both Simon and his wife Philomena on my last trip to Lebanon one year before they died. The picture I had of them when I was a child had vanished. They were emaciated and weak, looking as if they were ready to meet the old man with the sickle. I recalled the psalm: "In the morning we are a flowering bush, in the evening we are cut down with a sickle and tossed into the fire."

Teresa was the sister of Marzuka, my grandmother. The two sisters were strong and assertive. They went to America to make their fortunes, leaving their husbands at home. Upon returning to Lebanon, they brought enough money to acquire property, and they ruled the family with a strong hand. Marzuka softened her demeanor later in life, but Teresa never did. They were the titular heads of their families. Teresa ruled her husband, children and grandchildren with an iron fist. She was a tall and wiry woman and I remember her sitting with a long stick in her hand that she used to shoo off the chickens whenever they got too close. She would swing the eight-foot long stick here and there like a whip, chasing away anything in sight. This image is somewhat symbolic of her role in the family ruling the chickens in the roost.

I remember when her husband Bacchus died. He had an obstruction of the small intestine. By the time they called my brother Mike who was an intern at the hospital in Tripoli, it was too late; gangrene had set in.

ABUNA BUTROS

Teresa's brother, Abuna Butros, would often come from the monastery to visit her, and his other sister, Marzuka, about once a month. His routine never varied. He would have supper at Teresa's first. Immediately afterwards he would walk over to Marzuka's house to pass the evening and then fall asleep on the wooden bed on the porch. That wooden bed was always covered with a black canvas when Uncle Butros was not there. In the morning he would have breakfast at Mazurka's house, then hike up to our villa, have lunch with us and play backgammon with Dad, followed by a half-hour siesta. He would then end the day by going back to Teresa's for supper, and to bed at Marzuka's. He carried this routine for three days—never longer. On the fourth morning he would get up at 4:00 a.m. (as monks usually do to recite Matins), and disappear before anyone else woke up.

Uncle Abuna Boutros was a great backgammon player—the best. Once, when I was ten years old I asked him if he would play with me. He told me, "No!" When I asked him why, he said, "Because you are still a child. If I lose to you you'll laugh at me, and if I win you'll go to your mother crying, and she might think I did something to hurt you. You see, either way I lose; so I cannot possibly win playing with you. Go along and play with your friends now, and when you're old enough come back and then I'll be glad to play backgammon with you."

I distinctly remember walking away disappointed. From there I went to pick up the little table on which Grandma used to serve me her fried eggs. I barely moved the table from the wall when all hell broke loose. I hadn't noticed that grandma's big cat was behind the table nursing her five newborns. That cat was ferocious, just like Marzuka and Teresa. She used to chase big dogs, if one can fathom that. She hissed and took after me as I ran away from her vicious claws. She kept chasing me and forced me to jump over a few terraced landings beneath the house. When the chase was over, I realized that I was in Grandma's vegetable garden, stepping in mud.

Uncle Butros saw me and hurried me and my shoes away before Grandma could see me tracking mud all over her patio. He said to me, "If you don't tell, I won't." I immediately forgot his backgammon rebuff and he became my friend and savior until we left Lebanon in 1948. Years later we used to recall this incident every time I went back to Serhel—before his martyrdom. God rest his soul. He became a saint—even though he loved to eat Teresa's chicken and toss the leftovers to Yousef, Michael, and Bacchus (his great nephews)! He would tell them in jest, "Have a feast! Teresa never gives you any chicken to eat."

The story of the martyrdom of Abbot Butros in 1976 was this. He was left alone in the monastery with another old monk. All the young monks had fled when they saw the rebels coming. A band of Somali mercenaries ordered him to deny Christ. He responded, "I have believed in Jesus Christ for almost a hundred years, why should I change now?" So they cut off his hands, tied his feet to a horse, and whipped the horse away. He died a modern martyr. We know the details from the monastery's cook, who, when he heard the ruckus, hid in a nearby room from where he could hear everything. He subsequently ran and hid in a nearby field, thus living to tell what happened.

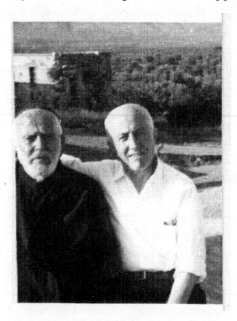

Abbot Abuna Boutros and his nephew, Yousef Zeiter, circa 1972

MUSIC IN SERHEL

On Sundays, after visiting here and there, I would return home for lunch. As soon as lunch was over, relatives, friends, and the village's poor farmers would come up to our house to visit and hear my brother Philip play the violin, with Johnny accompanying him on the mandolin. They used to practice playing etudes written by a certain Jacques Fereol Mazas (1782-1849), an almost forgotten composer who lived at the time of Beethoven and the early Romantics, and was eclipsed by them as time went on. One can find printed music scores for several combinations of instruments written by him. My two brothers became adept at playing Mazas, Vivaldi, and Paganini, the great violin virtuoso, who also wrote some music for violin and mandolin.

I remember the villagers' fascination with my brothers' impromptu concerts. These poor people! All they had ever heard before were their plaintive notes of Arabic songs. They used to look at these young Zeiter musicians with awe and respect because "they could even read notes!"

My brothers used to practice in the lower level of our villa during the week. This room had a beautiful view of the mountains and the valley below, and my brother Philip brought that beauty inside by painting on the walls the wonderful outdoor landscapes. Philip eventually became a great oil painter. He won first prize at the Venezuelan National Painting Exhibition two years in a row (1975 and 1976). In his last years he rarely played the violin and concentrated on painting instead. He became a commercial artist and sold many of his canvasses. His work is now in great demand in South America. He passed away in March, 2005, from stomach cancer following three months of intense suffering.

Following the music sessions on Sunday, the poor farmers would present my parents with produce from their farms—fresh strawberries, figs, all kinds of grapes, feta cheese, and yogurt. Nobody ever brought packaged gifts as we do nowadays. The fruits they brought us as gifts were invariably the produce of their land, and the sweets their wives had made for us kids. Most of them were poor, surviving off what their small parcel of land produced.

Konstantin, my godfather, would always bring mulberries, both red and white. Mulberry trees were abundant in Lebanon because at the time of Emir Fakhreddine in the 17th century (and Emir Bashir in the 19th), Lebanon developed a great silk trade. Silkworms feed on the leaves of the mulberry tree. Once the silk trade had subsided, the trees were used only for the mulberry fruit they produced (which I found to be delicious). I remember the villagers making mulberry juice as a form of refreshing drink in the summer. We would go up to the Convent of St. Simon, high above our house on top of the mountain, and the sisters would serve us refreshing cold mulberry juice after our tiring ascent.

Years later, on one of my return visits, I went up with Dad to the convent after Abbot Butros had died. The sisters had sent Dad a message that they had an old locked trunk that once belonged to his uncle. We went up and, full of emotion, opened the trunk, and found nothing but old shirts, a black cassock, sullied boots, decaying prayer books—the sum total of a saintly old monk's worldly possessions, devoid of material treasures. And yet he was for many years an abbot with absolute sway over the lives of a hundred monks, and had control of the purse besides. His trunk reminded me of these lines from Gray's *Elegy*, which I proceeded to quote for Dad:

> *Can storied urn or animated bust*
> *Back to its mansion call the fleeting breath?*
> *Can Honor's voice provoke the silent dust,*
> *Or Flattery soothe the dull cold ear of Death?*
> —Thomas Gray, Elegy *Written in a Country Church-yard*, (1742)

What was in that trunk made us cry at first because of the memories; but afterwards we were overjoyed, because we remembered that he was now a Christian martyr and saint.

On most Sunday evenings, after the poor villagers had left in the afternoon, the affluent would come to visit. Following pleasantries enjoyed over cups of dark Arabian coffee, the men would invariably switch the discussion to politics and the economy. These well-to-do families were the Raji Daniels, the Yousef (Yamouni) Chalitas, the Mujallis, the Farahs, the Malcouns, and the Abdallah brothers, Sarkis and Tannous. Tannous has lived in Stockton for over thirty years now. I still see him often. When my father came to Stockton to live with us in 1978, Tannous was very good to him; he was his constant companion. As a matter of fact, Dad died in 1986 while reading some Lebanese newspapers that Tannous had brought him that morning. The news from Lebanon was very sad at that time, since the civil war was still raging. Dad loved Lebanon so much it was significant that he died while reading bad news from his homeland. He was a real Lebanese patriot. Lebanon, Poland, and Ireland have been the three unhappiest Catholic countries in the world, and understandibly so, because of their devotion to the Church and the persecutions that that engendered from their neighbouring countries. It is said that puritan Oliver Cromwell killed two million Irishman during his two-year invasion of that hapless country in the mid-17th century.

In 1946, Serhel's evening parties went into high gear for several days one summer. In July of that year the government got wind of a few small farmers planting hashish, instead of their regular red pepper crop. There was obviously more money to be made planting and harvesting hashish than Serhel's customary red pepper crop. So a small detachment of gendarmes was sent up from Zgharta, the county seat, to find the hashish and burn it. Of course, they could not burn the poppy fields until they found out where the poppies were being planted. All week I remember there was one drunken party after another to keep the officers happy and content so they wouldn't find out where the hashish was being grown. This episode reminds me now of the movie *The Secret of Santa Vittoria*, in which Italian peasants are shown hiding a million bottles of wine from the German army for several years during World War II. The villagers, under the leadership of their drunken mayor, hid a million bottles of wine in caves in the nearby Apennine Mountains. Anthony Quinn played the role of the sly mayor who outfoxed the Germans, and his nagging wife was Sylvana Mangano. They were both hilarious in their respective roles.

In Serhel, Sarkis Abdallah was the crafty mayor who kept these parties going to distract the gendarmes. After a week of drunken evenings, the mayor finally took the soldiers to one small field of poppy plants. They set it on fire and went back to headquarters in Zgharta. All the other poppy fields were spared because of the celebrations that the affluent families put on to keep the investigators uninformed. Every time I think of those days I recall the Anthony Quinn movie.

Three summers before (1943), a full regiment of Hindu soldiers came to Serhel to hold maneuvers before going on to the European theater in World War II. The commander was a Hindu major who insisted on sleeping in our house. He told Dad, "This is the nicest house in town, and this is where I want to sleep the next few nights." There was nothing we could do about it, so Dad acquiesced, and fortunately, the officer turned out to be a gentleman from a high caste Hindu family. He plied us with cigarettes, cans of food, and chocolates. But best of all, he introduced Dad to the *Bhagavad-Gita*, the great Hindu mystical poem, in which the reincarnated god Lord Krishna urges Arjuna, the military leader, to do his duty and face the enemy in battle. The Indian major even wanted to marry my sister Mary, but so did everybody else who saw her. She was beautiful. My father, of course, pacified him until the regiment left, and God only knows whether the major survived the war in Europe or not.

WINTER AND SCHOOL AGAIN

Finally, October would come with the mountain fog and cold air—the time we would go down to Tripoli for school and the winter season. Manuel was always the driver and helper. We packed the supplies that were to be carried by donkeys and mules to Karm Sadde, the next town where the asphalted road began. From there, Manuel would load everything in his car and drive us to Tripoli. Imagine, father, mother, and seven kids with all their belongings packed in one "Model T." Mom would hold in her right hand her cut-in-half lemon and smell it along the way, supposedly to keep her from getting carsick, even though the drive was no longer than half an hour! I recall the first time my brothers whistled the tune from Dvořák's *Humoresque*, while the car slowly wound its way towards Tripoli and the Mediterranean. That's how that "Humoresque" became our family tune.

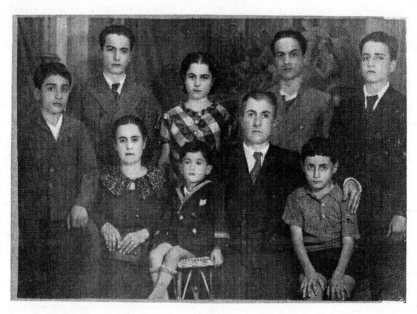

1939 family portrait taken during the school season in Tripoli, Lebanon: seated (l. to r.), Mom (46 years old), Henry (5), Dad (46), Johnny (12); standing (l. to r.), Philip (13), Mike (18), Mary (14), Tony (17), and Edmond (16)

Once in Tripoli, we would unload belongings and supplies too numerous to count (for use during the winter months), and carry them up three flights of stairs to our apartment. For the next several days we would get very busy buying new clothes and shoes before school started. *L'Ecole de la Sainte Famille des Frères Chrétiens*, or the School of the Holy Family run by the Christian Brothers, could be seen two short blocks away from our apartment. One building, which was for the free education of poor children, was kitty corner from our apartment. It was called the *gratuite* because education was free (gratuitous). From the balcony, I would watch the students play volleyball in the schoolyard at break time. One block farther, though, was the huge rectangular colonnade on the interior of the main school building with the school playground in the center. That was where we and the other kids whose parents could afford to pay tuition went. From the inner courtyard the school building looked like a small replica of the inner court of the Louvre Museum in Paris. It had a quadrangular colonnade, with classrooms three stories high surrounding a huge asphalted inner court that served as a playground during recess time. That became my school from second grade to first-year high school.

I had spent kindergarten and first grade at the Italian Carmelite School nearby. That was before the Italians had to close the school and leave Lebanon when Mussolini entered the war on Hitler's side. Lebanon was on the side of the Free French under Charles De Gaulle. Mike and Tony knew only the Italian school, because they were already out of high school when the school had to close. The rest of us (from Edmond down) had to transfer to the French Christian Brothers School. I recall we all had to learn to sing *La Marseillaise* and other French military marching music (the war was raging in France). I liked those tunes then and still hum them to this day. Of course, the Christian Lebanese Maronites have been francophiles since the days of the Crusaders who were their coreligionists and protectors.

I do, however, recall two horrible incidents from this period. Once, when I was nine years old, I was walking home from school one afternoon, a few months before Lebanon was declared an independent state on November 22, 1943. In those days there were a few riots in the streets against the occupying French forces. That afternoon, walking home from school, I saw two French tanks trap several screaming students against a high wall; the tanks did not stop and crushed several of them.

Another time, there was a big commotion across the street from the American girl's school in Tripoli. In full view from our apartment, the traffic had come to a halt and sirens were wailing. A teenage girl from the school was crossing the street when a truck accidently ran over her. My brother Johnny and I ran over. The girl was lying on the pavement, her clothes were crumpled and smeared with soot and blood and her head crushed beyond recognition on the asphalt. She was pronounced dead on the spot. It was a horrible picture. I was only seven years old, and I recall my brother Johnny covering my tearful face with his hands and leading me back home. The grim memory of this incident only slowly lessened with time.

I was glad we were enrolled in the tuition school and not in the free school for the poor, because over there the dean was Frère Ambroise, a strict disciplinarian. He was known for his no-nonsense, tough, almost cruel rule. After all, these kids did not have to pay tuition because it was *gratuite* (gratuitous). So he was not about to allow them indiscretions that wasted his time and theirs. Also, a good number of these students were ruffians from a lower social order. They had to mind, or they would be either punished or thrown out of school. The discipline was strict, and perhaps rightly so.

We, on the other hand, went to the private school campus, which was only one block farther down the road. Dad paid the principal a gold coin a trimester for the education of the remaining four of us. My sister Mary continued her education at an all-girls school run by Sisters.

Mike was already in medical school at the Jesuit-run St. Joseph's University in Beirut. He later went to Italy for one year and did his second year of medicine at the University of Rome. When Mussolini entered the war, Mike, who was a Canadian citizen, was advised by the consul general to leave Italy. So he boarded one of the last trains out of Italy to Istanbul, and from there he was scheduled to transfer to another one that was to bring him to Tripoli. My parents did not hear from him for several days and were very worried. Then Dad had a dream, which he related to us before we had heard from Mike. In the dream, Blessed Joseph, venerated in the village as its native incorruptible saint, appeared to Dad and told him, "Because of your devotion to me, I have saved your son from great harm today." Two days later Mike came home.

As it turned out, the train Mike took from Rome to Istanbul was late. So the next train he was scheduled to be on left Istanbul without him on board. As Mike told us later, that train was passing over a high viaduct in Turkey when it collapsed. Many of the travelers died as several wagons fell about five hundred feet into the ravine below the bridge. Mike took a different route on the next available train and got home safely.

Now, I understand that Rome will soon start the cause for the beatification of Serhel's Father Joseph. Dad would have been delighted if he were still alive. Father Joseph was the village priest when Dad was a child, and he used to compare him to the French Curé d'Ars (St. John Vianney). The great French author Georges Bernanos develops a theme in his novel, *Diary of a Country Priest*, which could have been based on Blessed Joseph's life.

When Mike returned home, he was unable to continue his medical studies. The chancellor of St. Joseph's University in Beirut would not allow him to attend third-year medical school. He was upset that Mike had transferred to a foreign medical school the year before without asking his permission. Mike wanted to work as a clerk at the Iraqi oil pipeline refinery, Tripoli's biggest employer. But Dad insisted on his becoming a medical doctor, as he wanted me to do fifteen years later. Dad was adamant. He had Mike borrow the medical books from another student and had them printed as a single edition at a friend's printing press. Dad said that each book printed cost him several hundred dollars—that's how much he wanted Mike to finish medical school! Mike stayed home that whole year studying the books. Fortunately for him, a year later a new chancellor was installed at the university. He phoned Dad to tell him that the school of medicine would now welcome Mike with open arms for his third year of medicine; and further, he apologized to Dad for what had taken place, because Mike had an excellent record during the year prior to his leaving for Rome.

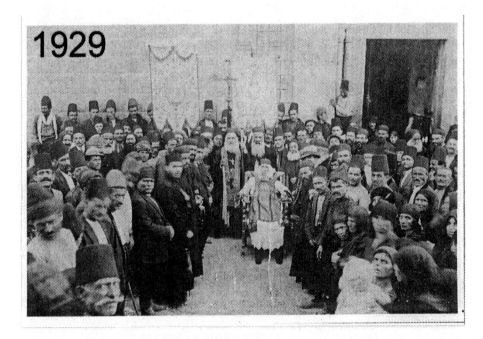

Funeral of Blessed Father Joseph of Serhel (his corpse seen seated in the chair is still incorrupt). The priests can be recognized by the flatter hats, whereas the villagers are wearing either a black fez (*tarboush*) or the conical light-colored *libbadeh* worn by the hardy Lebanese *montagnards*. Grandfather Mikhael Zeiter (second from extreme right above the three rows of ladies dressed in black) is wearing a fez. This picture depicts my ancestors' semi-feudal world full of piety and devotion.

Mike's nemesis, the old chancellor (Père Chanteur), was taken back to France in handcuffs. He was caught using a clandestine telegraphic machine to send secret information to the French "Vichy" forces, which were allied with Germany. The Free French, who controlled Lebanon at the time, immediately took Père Chanteur away and a new French Jesuit chancellor was appointed to take his place. (He learned of Mike's predicament from one of the professors, and knew that an injustice had been committed.) Mike finished Medical School at St. Joseph's at the age of twenty-six, in 1947—after he had lost two years of study. He then interned at the Nini Hospital in Tripoli before he left us to practice medicine in Canada. Dr. Nini was a great surgeon and a professor at the medical school; he administered one of the finest hospitals in the entire Middle East.

My second oldest sibling, Tony, was now in Venezuela, away from the family. One day in 1939, when he was sixteen, he decided to quit school and go to Venezuela against my father's wishes. He emigrated to go work as a merchant with Uncle Paul (Dad's brother) who had immigrated to Venezuela in 1929, one year before Dad's return to Lebanon. Tony stayed in Venezuela for twenty-four years before coming to Stockton in 1963 to live near us. The stories he tells about his life in Turmero, Caracas, and finally Punto Fijo (all in Venezuela), would fill another book. He came to California in 1946 to marry his second cousin Madelyn Barkett, and returned to work in Venezuela for another nineteen years, before returning to California in 1963. Now his children thank him daily for having brought them to California and out of Venezuela. Conditions in Venezuela have become very bad of late. I remember with tenderness Tony's early letters to us in Lebanon. He always ended his letters requesting my parents: *"Busuli Henry bi tizu!"* (Kiss for me little Henry on his butt—In Arabic, a term of endearment).

SCHOOLING AT THE CHRISTIAN BROTHERS

The rest of us stayed in Lebanon and went to the French Christian Brothers school. During the winter school term, I studied much and played little. I was particularly averse to school team sports. In Lebanon, as in most countries outside the United States, it is understood that school sports are not what school is primarily for. To this day, the attitude of most Middle Easterners and Asians is that organized sports (at least, to excess) are "a waste of valuable study time." Unlike Nordic Europeans and Americans, Asians and Middle Easterners generally take sports with a grain of salt. For them, games and circuses have always been the ruling classes' favorite way to keep the rabble occupied, while they pilfer the country. I have maintained this feeling ever since.

The milestones of school life in Lebanon, and other countries under the French system, begin with the *Certificat* (the certification for completing elementary school). The next milestone is the *Brevet* (the brief), which comes at the end of third-year secondary school, and finally the *Bachot* (baccalaureate), which is awarded two years later and means the candidate is ready to enter a university. Graduation, especially the *Bachot*, was by no means a thing to be taken for granted as it is in American high schools. Those who didn't pass were either sent to a vocational school or had to repeat the year. In both private and public schools the final examinations for all three degrees were rigorous and national in scope. Those who passed the *Bachot* would go on to one year of *Philosophie*, during which the liberal arts were studied before entering into the various schools of specialization (medicine, dentistry, law, etc.). I never reached those years in Lebanon because we immigrated to Venezuela one year after I obtained the *Certificat*.

These national exams took several days to complete and several more to review. For the *Certificat*, we were graded on a scale of 1 to 20 or 1 to 10, depending on whether the subject was considered major or minor, respectively. The cumulative mark from all the exams was 170 and all subjects were in French, except Arabic grammar and literature. Since my knowledge of French was thought to be the best in the school, and someone from our school always won the National Award, I was expected to get the highest cumulative grade in the country. But when the results were finally announced, I had gotten 139½ and Shalita (a dark horse) got 141. Ironically, the problem arose in the subject I was best at—French dictation (*orthographie,* in French). I misspelled the French word for rabbit. In my hurry, I spelled it "*lappin,*" instead of *lapin,* with one *p.* That was a costly oversight! The cost was four grade points, and I came in second. I was extremely disappointed, and so were my teachers and my father.

Mom took a different point of view. She took me to the deli for a treat, and told me that in life second is often better than first, because it takes the monkey off one's back and allows one to live a serene and happy life. "*Ya Waladi* (my son), for the moment this may be a humbling experience for you, but in the long run you'll live longer if you accept it gracefully." Quite often, Mom showed more wisdom than did my father with his philosophical bent; her salient virtues were her faith, her love, and her humility—all seldom found in erudite philosophers.

The following year, when we immigrated to Venezuela, I joined the second-year *Bachillerato* (high school) class while it was in progress. I paid attention to Spanish grammar and pronunciation, and remained first in class for the rest of the two years I stayed in Caracas.

While I was preparing for the *Certificat* finals in Lebanon, however, I passed the best spring ever in Lebanon. I recall being very content and happy. I would get up early and walk to school to study when there was nobody in the classrooms. On my way there, myriads of birds would be everywhere announcing the coming of spring. After I got to the classroom, I would open the windows, and the birds would still be singing their merry tunes. It was probably the first time I had paid close attention to birds' songs—a joy that has remained with me all my life. I still listen closely to their variegated tunes during my early morning walks—especially in springtime.

RELIGIOUS PRACTICES IN LEBANON

Some of my fondest memories are of the month of May, Mary's month. Each evening during that month, everyone in the apartment building would go down at seven o'clock to old Ursula's unit on the first floor to say the rosary, followed by the recitation of the "Salve Regina." (All the prayers were recited in Arabic.) Ursula was a very old widow, with the lines of aging all over her face. I recall reading in Will Durant's writings a description of the way Savonarola in his sermons used to admonish the bejeweled ladies of Florence, sitting in the front pew, for their vanity, by pointing out the holy radiance emanating from a scar-faced old widow kneeling in the back of the church, praying with head bent. Ursula's demeanor was like this during the recitation of the rosary. She was very holy—a sort of Juliana of Norwich, the fourteenth century English anchoress and mystic. Ursula was a devout visionary, and would burn incense before the rosary started. Many years later, I remembered Ursula's place when visiting the Trappist Monastery at Oka, near Montreal. The monks would sing the "Salve Regina" to their Queen before going to bed. It was both beautiful and haunting, reminding me of the atmosphere in Ursula's apartment.

At the ages of eleven, twelve, and thirteen, I was an alto in the School Boys' Choir. We would train for Christmas and Easter all year long. On Christmas Eve, we would go caroling in the school neighborhood in front of our teachers' and students' homes. It was innocence itself. Following our caroling rounds, we would end up at the Catholic Latin Rite church, singing the Christmas Midnight Mass.

I also recall the crèche we used to build in the corner of our living room in Tripoli, made out of crumpled brown paper bags. We would crumple the bags to simulate rocky hills and form a cave in the center of the scene; there we would place Mary and Joseph and the animals. Then on Christmas Eve we would put baby Jesus in the crib, followed by the shepherds and their lambs. We would have a miniature tree or two nearby, as part of the décor, but trees never eclipsed the nativity scene.

In walking to our parish Church in Tripoli which was not far from our house, we would pass through a dark, long underpass. St. Michael's Maronite Church was also on the way to the *Tal*, the main city square with its huge clock tower. Next to it was the *Minshie*, the city's park. The park looked huge to little me in those days, but when I returned for a visit, it was no bigger than a city block. I recall having many dreams in Venezuela, Canada, and the United States, having as their background these familiar landmarks in Tripoli.

On rainy winter afternoons, we would often be sent to the corner stand to buy roasted peanuts from "the black man." There were very few black people in Tripoli, no more than I could count on the fingers of both hands. They owned little *fistuk* (nuts) stands here and there with containers full of peanuts, almonds, and chestnuts roasting over hot burning coals to keep them warm and toasty. Just as the Portuguese in Venezuela are mostly bus drivers, or the Palestinians in the United States grocery store owners, so the few African blacks in Tripoli were all peanut vendors. We used to innocently say that it went with the African turf. Now such terms would be considered racial slurs.

One Christmas night we had a rare snowstorm in Tripoli, and when we got up on Christmas Day we walked through snow to go to church. When we returned home, we went up to the flat roof of our apartment building and found it full of fresh snow about four inches deep. While it would often snow in Serhel and higher up in the mountains, we rarely went up there in the winter, so we had little experience with snow. It was unheard of in Tripoli, which sits by the warm waters of the Mediterranean. We made a snowman using charcoals for eyes and ears and a carrot for a nose. My sister, Mary, took a picture of us with it and, for a long time, I didn't know what happened to the picture. I found it recently going through an old drawer and it confirmed my memory that I was wearing a furry white lambskin coat that was brought from Detroit, in 1930, and passed on from Mike to Tony to Edmond to Mary to Philip to Johnny—and finally to me. That coat proved indestructible. Mom insisted that I wear it even on the mildest cool days to prevent me from catching a cold. She thought my sister Mary and I were "delicate." She always recited the Lebanese proverb, "Warmth is good even in the middle of summer."

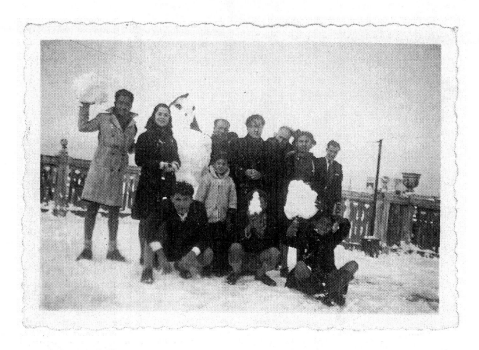

I found this photo only recently; but I have a distinct memory
of when it was taken in 1945 and that I was wearing the
multiple-hand-me-down white lambskin coat at the time. I am
in the center. Members of the Yamouni family, our neighbors,
are with us.

Some evenings Mom would take me to adoration at the Carmelite Latin
Rite church. It was beautiful to tune out the noise of the world outside and
just pray. That was the school church when the Italian Carmelites were still
there. I would pray to God to make me a good boy. I was ten years old then.
By the time I was eighteen, I was asking God (at St. Therese Church in Windsor)
to make me a Catholic philosopher like Jacques Maritain. At age twenty-one
in medical school, I would ask God (at St. Michael's Church in London,
Ontario) to help me become a good doctor, and besides, a mystic and a
philosopher. I would kneel down in the empty church and, with tears in my
eyes and love in my heart, would ask God these things. The memories of the
religious practices I grew up with in Lebanon have stayed with me, as I
continually beg God's help for growth in the spiritual life.

CHAPTER 5

SCHOOL DAYS AND HOLIDAYS

T he most memorable day of my childhood was the day of my First Holy Communion. I was seven years old when Christian Brother Felix undertook our instruction. He was the one who later led us in the boys' choir. On that day, I was dressed all in white, holding a small candle with a white ribbon in my left hand and a small white prayer book in the other. I wore a white armband neatly tied around my right arm. I can still remember how clean and happy I felt. It was the purest, most innocent day of my life.

THOUGHTS ON RECALLING MY FIRST COMMUNION

I realize I have sinned many times since. I have not loved God as much as I ought to, but I have never doubted His existence or His loving power to sanctify us; nor his ability to elevate us to the highest spiritual level we're capable of. The mercy of our Creator and the constant love of our Redeemer are beyond our comprehension. Time and time again, He lifts us up when we have fallen. He cures us when we are sick, through the marvelous working of his own natural laws that allow our complicated bodies to recuperate and heal so consistently. It was the great French physician and biologist Claude Bernard who described the constant return of the body's physiology to its usual and normal state of equilibrium. He coined the term "homeostasis," and wondered how miraculous it all is, in view of the fact that everything else in the universe is in a constant state of breakdown. The Creator forever enlightens our intellect, the part in us that is most divine, like Him. He actively, but slowly, purges us of our vices if we cooperate with His Will, and moves us along the road to spiritual perfection. As Psalm 144 says:

Lord, what is man that you care for him,
Mortal man, that you keep him in mind;
Man, who is merely a breath,
Whose life fades like a passing shadow?

I have never rationalized my shortcomings and sins by using a relativistic amoral stance as an excuse for my behavior. People who find it difficult to believe often look for the things that reinforce their doubt, a practice not too different from the way people of belief act at times. What a loss for the agnostic or self-proclaimed atheist to doubt the evidence presented by the order and harmony found in the universe, the constancy of its natural laws, and the beauty of earth and sky—and above all, God's goodness as He offers Himself to us daily, all over the world in the small, consecrated host! Why put one's faith in something that dehumanizes man and fails to satisfy him?

All you who are thirsty,
Come to the water,
You who have no money,
Come, receive and eat,
Come without paying and without cost,
Drink wine and milk.
Why spend your money for what is not bread,
Your wages for what fails to satisfy?
Heed me and you shall eat well,
You shall delight in rich fare.
Come to me heedfully,
Listen, that you may have life.
                              —Isaiah, 55:1-3

These are the words of eternal life. What a miracle, symbolized by the multiplication of a few loaves and fishes to feed thousands of people. Could that be the significance of the miracle on the shores of the Sea of Galilee? Many theologians have affirmed this to be the case, comparing the thousands of consecrated hosts all over the world to the multiplication of the loaves and fishes. God is among us, not only spiritually, but physically, visibly, and tangibly. How could I forego daily Communion? Why does anybody? It is the daily affirmation of our desire for Truth, Goodness and Beauty. That is the real wealth. True devotion and humility is to feel the need for intimate contact with the Lord, who is Existence (Being) itself. That is the supreme existential experience—the one existentialism worth talking about in this evanescent life.

When the preparations for First Communion were over, school became my primary concern. Even though I didn't like school, I did enjoy most of its benefits. Daily Mass was mandatory for all students at the Christian Brothers School, and there were several daily Masses. It was a school of about two thousand male students, encompassing both elementary and secondary education. I remember seeing the Christian Brothers drinking wine at lunch in their separate refectory. We would spy on them through the glass windows. We were scandalized at first, until Dad told us, "What do you expect? They're French!"

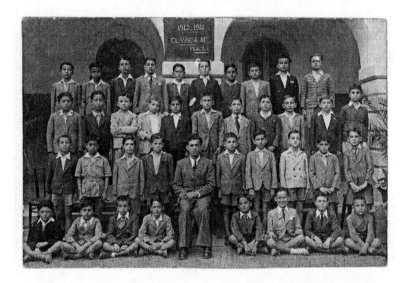

Portrait of third grade at the Christian Brothers school in Tripoli—I am eight years old, in the front row, fourth from the left, next to the teacher's knees. The gregarious smiling boy third from the right must have become a life insurance salesman and for business must have joined all the service clubs in Tripoli!

SWITCHING SCHOOLS, CHRISTIAN TO MOSLEM

All went well at school, until the day my brother Edmond lost his temper and butted heads with a teacher. Edmond was brilliant in school, a scholar and a mathematical genius; but he was also stubborn, or as we say in Arabic *"anid."*

That day Edmond had a spat with one of the Christian Brothers, which was not unusual for him. He tackled one of the smallest Christian Brothers at the school and then lifted him up into the air. He proceeded to run with him held up high through the whole schoolyard, from one side to the other, with the Brother screaming at him the whole time. Edmond did all this in front of the whole school body at recess time. It was obviously very embarrassing to the Christian Brother, so Edmond was punished and ordered to ask his pardon. Edmond wouldn't do it. Consequently, he was thrown out of school, and so were we all, in short order. The principal told Dad that, "Either Edmond apologizes to the Brother in front of his classmates, or all of your sons will have to leave this school along with Edmond."

So, for one whole year we went to the "*Killyeh Al-Islamyeh*," a Moslem *madrasat*, meaning an Arabic Moslem school. The institution was quite well known all over the Arab Middle East, and many of these *madrasats* date back to the time of the Mamelukes (the slaves who revolted against Egypt and ended up ruling that country for several centuries, starting in the twelfth century AD). Salah-ad-Din (Saladin), the vanquisher of the Crusaders, was a Mameluke ruler. When walking with mother into the *souks* of Tripoli shopping, we would encounter various ornate entrances to old buildings, which at one time were the portals to these old *madrasats*, few of which were still functioning as schools in our time. They represented a legacy from eight hundred years ago of advanced Arabic civilization. Tripoli has always been a strong Sunni city.

Now, we had to walk the whole length of the city to go to a Moslem school, rather than to the Christian Brothers' school two blocks away. However, this actually worked out for the best. That year definitely increased our knowledge of classical Arabic. We studied the *Mu'allakats,* the seven famous poems of pre-Islamic Arabia. A poetry contest was held every seven years in pre-Mohammedan days. The poems would be entered in the contest by posting them on the Kaaba, the holy black rock in Mecca. The winner would be crowned with laurel leaves, just as in the days of high Greek and Roman culture. Antar was one of those epic poets; he praised the beauty of Lab'ah (his Beatrice) in his famous poem. Nicolai Rimsky-Korsakov's second symphony is named "Antar," as it describes the poet's life in music form.

In the Islamic school, I would volunteer to read the Holy Koran in Arabic. Everybody knew I was a Christian, but they loved my readings, because they thought they had a potential convert to Islam, or at least a tolerant Christian who respected their Holy Book. *Islam* means "Abandonment to Divine

Providence." Coincidentally that is the title of a classic Catholic book by Father Pierre de Caussade—one of my favorite spiritual books. Many Catholic and Protestant authors have written books on the subject of self-abandonment. All major religions recognize the universal truth that we grow spiritually when we abandon ourselves to the will of God.

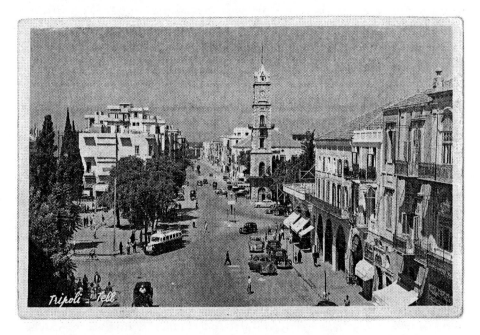

Tripoli, Lebanon, in 1946; to the right of the clock tower is the edge of the *Minshieh*, the city's Public Park and arboretum. Taxis for hire, even up to Serhel, are seen gathered in front center of the photo. Today, most everybody owns a car—*The Economist* in its annual edition (2005) listed Lebanon as possessing the highest number of cars per capita in the whole world—and the new buildings are over twenty stories high; besides, the population is up from 100,000 in my time to a crowded one million now.

We developed new friends at the Moslem School, including the sons of Rachid Karami, the then Prime Minister of Lebanon. We would go and play around the sand dunes next to his home on the shore of the Mediterranean, south of Tripoli. One of his sons who were our classmates was elected prime minister recently, long after his father had passed away. He had to resign recently (May, 2005) because of his close association with the Syrians.

After one year at the Moslem School, the dust settled and we went back to the French Christian Brothers' school. By then, Edmond was studying pharmacy at the American University of Beirut, after he had graduated with honors at the Moslem *Killyeh*. He may have been stubborn, but he was very smart. He was also terrifying. Once he lifted me up above his head and jokingly threatened to throw me down to the street below from the roof of our tall apartment building. I screamed at the top of my lungs until my brother Philip came to my rescue.

RESUMING CHRISTIAN SCHOOL

After we went back to the Christian Brothers, a special event took place at the school through my Brother Philip's efforts—an evening musical performance. For two evenings a small string orchestra was assembled together by my brother and his Russian violinist teacher. They played Rossini's *Barber of Seville* overture, the overture to the *Caliph of Baghdad* by Boieldieu, the *Second Hungarian Rhapsody* of Liszt, and the *Blue Danube Waltz* by Johann Strauss Jr. I still have the program and can picture the whole performance in front of my eyes. On the front page of the program was a photo of me and eleven other classmates, divided into four groups of three, all dressed in "Mozart style" outfits with 18th century three-cornered hats. The program ended with us dancing to Papageno's aria in Mozart's *Magic Flute*, "I am the bird-catcher, ever joyful, hopla, hopsasa!" Needless to say, the memory of that event, so early in my life, did not escape me when fifty years later (2004) I was an ancient Egyptian priest in one scene and the cruel Monastatos' helper in another, in a performance of that same opera in Stockton.

Listening to my brothers play the violin (Philip), the clarinet (Edmond), or the mandolin (Johnny) in those days formed my earliest musical experiences. These memories are as exciting to me as the occasion when I conducted the Stockton Symphony Orchestra twenty-five years later in Beethoven's Eighth Symphony. It is unfortunate that as we age sensations become dull and bland. One day Philip came home with music albums under his arm, just after we had bought a Victrola record player. We went into the living room, closed the door, and listened to a rendition of Beethoven's Pastoral Symphony by Toscanini on five big, thick 78 mm discs. Imagine, in those pre-hi-fi days it took five discs, each one played on both sides, to record a single Beethoven symphony.

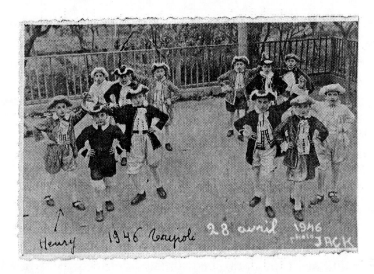

Young dancers, in Mozart's *Magic Flute*, 1946—I am on the extreme left. In front of me, is Sami Zablith, the boy who gave me the little booklet (mentioned later in my story) that served as my travelogue in 1947.

This was the time when the German advance during World War II was at its height. We were all on the side of the Allies, except Edmond. He had a map of Europe and North Africa posted on the wall in his bedroom. He would move colored pins as the German army advanced. He was a partisan of the Axis, even though he was born in Detroit. We would all listen to the Arabic broadcasts of the BBC, or the *Radio Diffusion Française* in Paris, every evening after supper. The whole neighborhood followed the news on our short wave radio. Edmond would rush to his room and move his pins forward or backward on the map depending on the day's battles. When the Axis powers were at the height of their advance, the pins were moved east as far as Alamein in North Africa, and Stalingrad in Russia. Thereafter, as the Axis powers retreated (1944-45), Edmond had to painfully move the pins all the way back inside Germany itself.

When the war ended in the West, on May 6, 1945, Philip painted the flags of all the Allies on two by three-foot sheets of watercolor paper and hung them like laundered towels all along the balconies of our third floor of the building. Everybody said, "Look at these Americans! The Zeiters are celebrating their country's victory!" In those days, the United States was idolized all over the Arab World. America was accepted and loved as the only altruistic power on earth, in sharp contrast to Great Britain and France, who had a long history of plotting and conniving. Their practice was to divide and rule, but not so with the United States of America (at least not in those days).

When President Roosevelt died on April 7, 1945, a few months before the end of the war, all schools in Lebanon and Syria were closed for two days and all flags flew at half-mast. Today, when an American president dies, there are celebrations of joy all over the streets of the Middle East. What has happened? Why the difference in sentiment toward the United States between the years 1945 and 2005?

The adulation of America started to wane with the American government's push for the establishment of Israel in the land which until then was known as Palestine. There was no Israel on world maps before then. Three years after the end of World War II (in 1948) the United Nations, coaxed by the United States, voted to partition Palestine. Since then our foot-dragging (for over fifty years) in solving a problem we helped create in the first place has not endeared us to the people of the Middle East. Still to this day, it is in our best interest, as the only superpower left, to draw up and enforce a just solution on all participants, and to become even-handed in our policy towards the Palestinians vis-a-vis the Israeli State. Israeli technical know-how could improve the whole Middle East if peace ever comes to the region.

An expression often heard, "Oh, they've been fighting since time immemorial," betrays a glaring ignorance of history. Moslems and Jews lived together very amicably—and profitably I might say—for seven centuries in Moorish Spain. Over the centuries Jews were better treated in Arab countries than in the Christian West. Historical examples of this abound. (Islam is derived from both the Old and the New Testament; and Orthodox Jews, Moslems and Christians know that their common enemy is secularism, not each other. John Paul II is one who understood this totally.) Moses Maimonides, the great medieval Jewish philosopher, left Christian Spain and went to teach at Al Azhar University in Cairo during the last years of his life. He is buried in Egypt. Incidently, along with Augustine, Avicenna and Aristotle, he was one of St. Thomas Aquinas' favorite quoted philosophers.

An incisive study of history shows a deep mutual respect between the luminaries in the various religions. There is a continuum of philosophical and theological thought not indigent to any one religion. The wide-spread belief that "religion is the cause of war" is now part of political correctness, but is eminently false. It is, rather, the misinterpretation of the writings of the masters of religion by the rabble, the lower echelons, coupled with the greed of their rulers, that causes animosity and wars. In general, it is the misfortune of present day political correctness to be oftentime historically and philosophically incorrect. If nothing else, it is a confirmation of Alexander Pope's dictum: "A little knowledge is a dangerous thing!"

A STINT IN THE ARMY

Shortly after my brother Philip displayed the Allied flags on our veranda, he was called to serve in the U.S. Seventh Army. Our foreign service knew that he lived in Lebanon and was of age for military service. All of my siblings were registered at the American embassy in Beirut as overseas Americans living in Lebanon. So my brother Philip was called up to serve. He took his traveling bags and reported near Kessel, Germany, where the headquarters of the Seventh Army were located. He spent a few months in training and drilling. Philip had always been the strong, muscleman of the family.

One morning, an Afro-American serviceman in the same platoon asked Philip, "Aren't you tired of this he-man training camp? I see that you know how to play the fiddle. You see that tent over there! They are auditioning musicians to form a band. Why don't you go try out?" Philip took the soldier at his word and went to audition that afternoon. They liked his performance, so they asked him to come back the next morning when the music director would be there.

The next morning, Philip returned to the tent and was ushered in. The music director was a bespectacled, hook-nosed, balding man of about fifty—it was Aaron Copleland. Sitting in his chair, he asked Philip to play any piece he knew by heart. Philip played Dvořák's "Humoresque," the piece we often hummed on our way to the mountains. The director then placed on a music stand the solo violin score of the slow movement of Mendelssohn's E minor Violin Concerto. Philip knew the piece and played the violin part well, so the man told him, "You're on! Report next week! We want you to play in the orchestra."

Little did Philip know at the time that this was the initial attempt to form the Symphony Orchestra of the Seventh Army of the United States. I suppose we wanted to impress upon the Europeans (after the war ended) that Americans had culture. We also wanted to use the army's talent to entertain the troops.

Philip started as lead second violin. The All-American orchestra began touring Europe after the war, playing in Frankfurt, Munich, Strasbourg, and Paris. As time went on, Philip tells me, they played several times at the Paris

Opera House, since Paris was now liberated. After a while, the conductor learned that Philip spoke French perfectly so he took him along in his private army limousine every time they went to play in France.

In time, Philip became first violinist and was of help to all the orchestra members because of the European languages he spoke. He played in the orchestra during his entire two-year stint in the army. One of his original conductors— in fact, Aaron Copeland—spoke some French and enjoyed perfecting that language when directing my brother Philip.

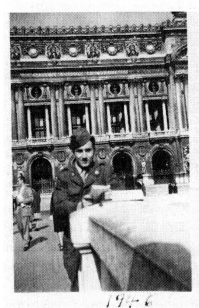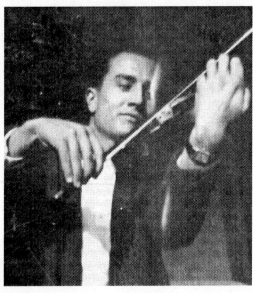

Philip at the Paris Opera House, where he played several times as first violinist of the Army Symphony Orchestra, 1945-47.

When it came time for him to be discharged, the Army offered him a job in the intelligence service, as Philip spoke six languages. But he didn't take the offer. He was homesick, he said to me. He returned to Lebanon and shortly thereafter immigrated to Venezuela. He confessed to me later that his refusal to continue in a very promising army career was unfortunate, because he could have risen much higher in rank; however, he said to me, his artistic bent found the army people to be too brainwashed and straight-jacketed. He returned home in his elegant captain's uniform with presents for all of us. He brought me a miniature electric train (extremely well-built I remember) made in Germany. I was twelve years old then. He also brought

me army binoculars and a sizeable army knife that I thought was fantastic—
I still have them.

A VALUABLE LESSON

During the spring of 1947, just before relatives from America came to
visit us, I learned a lesson I never forgot. On a sunny Friday afternoon just
before the Americans arrived, a few students and I went to the Crusader
Castle by the Mediterranean, built by Richard-the-Lion-Heart during the
second Crusade (he was Richard I of England). I recall running up and down
the medieval stairs. Then we ran up to the top of the tower where we could
see the slits through which arrows were shot at attackers below. On one side
was the deep blue Mediterranean, and on the other side was a view of the
snow-capped Lebanon mountain range. We came home quite late, about
ten in the evening. When I entered through the doorway, I could tell that
Mom and Dad were mad at me. I knew it because of the worried looks on
their faces. Often, I would be out playing with my friends until 8:00 or
9:00 p.m., close to home. But this time, I had not told them that we were
going so far.

Dad, with a stern but worried face, shouted the first question: "Where
were you?"

"Oh, we went to the Crusader's Castle by the sea and loved exploring the
high tower," I responded.

He gave me a backhanded slap on the right side of my face—ouch! That
was the only time in my life that Dad physically punished me. At almost all
other times, I was mindful of him. I think that of all the brothers, I gave him
the least to worry about. That is why I remember that incident so clearly. That
evening he said to me, "I didn't hit you for being late, but for going up the
tower and the turrets of the castle." These outlooks were very high from the
ground below. "What if you had fallen and died? These castles are old and the
stones are all loose. You could have slipped and fallen forty feet below. Never
do this to us again!"

Actually, I have always been averse to taking unnecessary risks—risks just
for the heck of it. I never felt I had to prove my manhood. I went to bed that
night without supper, crying, and mortified. In his wisdom, Dad was always
reminding me that I did not have to make mistakes to learn to avoid them.

"All you have to do," he would often counsel me, "is to watch other people
make mistakes and learn from their behavior what things you ought to avoid.

If you are smart and observant, you'll notice that many people have to repeat the same mistakes again and again to learn from them. Well, with so many fumblers around, just keep your eyes open and you won't have to repeat the same mistakes yourself in order to learn. For that matter, you can attend daily the *school of wisdom* here at home by observing what your brothers have done to get in trouble, and simply don't do it. It's that easy."

This advice was indelibly impressed on my mind one day. When he was a teenager, my brother Philip joined a group of older friends at an idyllic lookout, not far from the village. The young people from the village used to go there for picnics. While the youths were singing along, somebody asked for a guitar or an *Oud* (a popular Arabic large mandolin) to use for accompaniment. So one of the men, Michel Malcoun, asked Philip to go back to town and fetch for him the *oud* he kept at his house. Philip innocently acquiesced and went back to the village to get the instrument. On the way back, he tripped over the edge of a rock and fell on top of the *oud*, breaking it. Everybody was upset and disappointed, especially the owner. I remember Dad giving Philip a good "going over" that evening. He later called me aside and said to me, "Remember, it is never wise to put yourself in a situation where you are responsible for other people's treasured things. Think of what happened to Philip, and learn from it!"

THE AMERICAN VISITORS

During the summer of 1947, we had visitors come from the New World, a visit which changed forever our closely knit family life. From Venezuela came Uncle Paul and his wife Angela. From California, came Cousin Joe Rishwain with his wife Rose and their two children, who were my age. They brought with them aboard the ship a DeSoto limousine which took us all over Lebanon and Syria that summer. My brother Mike and my sister Mary came with us, but the other brothers stayed home because we couldn't possibly all fit in the limousine. I was allowed to come along because I wouldn't occupy much space. Oh, what fun that trip was! We went sightseeing all over. My sister came along because she was like me, petite, and could fit anywhere. Dad came along, too, but as usual Mom stayed home. She would be carsick, she said.

Our Cousin Joe Rishwain's two sons, Joe Jr. and Raymond, traveled with us also. In short, the limousine was packed to the gills. Joe's boys were the first cousins from California I had ever met. I take that back! Peter Rishwain was the first cousin I had seen. He was in the U.S. Army Intelligence Corps stationed in Cairo, Egypt. He came on furlough several times to visit us in Lebanon. He would take me hunting with him and ply me with chocolates and sweets. He wanted to marry my sister Mary but Dad told him she was still too young. (Everybody wanted to marry Mary. She was sweet, petite, educated, and the daughter of Yousef Zeiter.)

So with all of us packed in the eight-passenger DeSoto, we set out to explore Lebanon. Up to that age, I had never been outside of Tripoli or Serhel; I had never even seen Beirut, let alone Baalbeck or Byblos or Sidon or Tyre, all very famous historical places. I was thirteen, all agog to open my eyes to the world.

Thanks to a tiny notebook discovered just a few days ago as I am writing this, I can recall a good part of our travels throughout Lebanon and Syria during that memorable summer of 1947 in the DeSoto with Uncle Paul and Angela, Cousin Joe Rishwain and Rose, and their two young boys, my dad, my brother Mike, my sister Mary, and me—seven adults and three children. How providential, that at this stage of my recollections of the trip of 1947, I found that little notebook! It has both the itinerary of that trip and a few notes regarding my impressions of what we saw. I found it at the bottom of a shoe box of memorabila I kept in the very back of a drawer in my desk at home. And now, after all these years in California, it is smiling at me with details of events that took place fifty-six years ago when I was thirteen (July 31, 1947). The front and back covers of that booklet are made of enamel embedded in silver. I guess that is why it has not rusted through all these years. The front cover lifts up on a hinge, on top. On the inlaid enamel on the front cover is painted a red crusader's cross inside an elaborate crest. The bottom half of that cover shows a building with a small cupola and tiny front doors. On the blue sky above is written in the smallest capital letters the word "JERUSALEM." The front picture embedded in the porcelain looks like the Church of the Holy Sepulchre in Jerusalem. (It is uncanny that on October 9, 2005, I was invested as knight of the Equestrian Order of the Holy Sepulchre of Jerusalem.) On the very first inner page I had written "*Souvenir de Salem Zablith à son cher ami, Henri Zeiter, Le 23 Mars, 1947,* (A Souvenir from S.Z. to his dear friend H.Z.).

I remember us children being sandwiched between the adults in this eight-seat DeSoto limousine. Actually, most of the time the children were pushing each other out of the way, trying to sit by the window. I would mostly sit next to the right rear window with my nose on the glass, trying to see everything and miss nothing. I remember one cool evening writing my name on the inside of the frosted window. Normally, Cousin Joe drove, with Auntie Angela acting as the backseat driver. The only problem was that she screamed every time the car hit a sudden bump. And when Cousin Joe would be backing up with still ten feet left between the rear of our car and another car, Auntie Angela would again scream, "Watch out Joe!" This continued throughout the whole three weeks from July 8 to July 27. Cousin Joe, who has always had a sensitive stomach and suffered from heartburn, would tell Angela, "You keep that up and you're going to perforate my ulcer!"

On July 8, 1947, when I first saw the American relatives, I was on the back balcony of the apartment in Tripoli, holding my iron tripod contraption that I used as a toy machine gun making the sound of "tat-tat-tat-tat," while aiming at the neighborhood kids playing in the field below the veranda. Then, all of a sudden, the porch door opened and I was introduced to cousins Joe and Raymond and their parents from California. I was so embarrassed. My face turned red for looking like a silly child playing with his stupid contraption. Here I was, twelve years old (a supposedly grown-up cousin of theirs), firing away with a make-believe machine gun. I felt like an idiot, but not for long because the minute the parents went back inside, my nine and eleven year-old cousins asked me if they could try out my machine gun. I breathed a deep sigh of relief, realizing that it was okay for boys to be boys.

The cousins wore crew cuts, common in America in those post-World War II days. They were wearing identical shirts lined with alternating stripes of white and black. If they weren't children, I would have imagined they were convicts just out of jail. I still have their photo wearing those shirts—it seems like yesterday. Anyway, we became good friends and still are to this day.

FIRST TRAVELS

Our first voyage was to the monastery of Kus'haya where our Great Uncle Abuna Butros was abbot, as I mentioned earlier. Many of the monks were in the fields harvesting the olives. Later that day we descended to Tripoli and went to see the IPC (the Iraqi petroleum refinery), a large enterprise in those days. It employed many people in Tripoli. That refinery on the Mediterranean Sea was connected to the Iraqi oil fields. It is still there, but, unfortunately, it hasn't been operating for fifteen years because of the American and U.N. embargo on Iraqi oil.

The next day, July 9, we started an auto trip that took us to Beirut, Bikfaya, and Beit-Mery, and the next day we continued to Baskinta, Kfour, Bois de Bologne, and Broummana. All of these places are scenic red-roofed villages, dotting the mountains above Beirut, where the families from the capital city retreat during the summer months in search of the cool breeze gently blowing from the Mediterranean, only a few miles away. Their population triples in the summer months, swelled by the vacationers from Beirut, as well as tourists from Europe and the Arab world. Many rich Saudis and Kuwaitis pass their summers in Lebanon's resorts. These picturesque resorts in Central Mount Lebanon look exactly like the many red-roofed villages one sees in France's Provence or its Dordogne valley, or beyond Fiesole, above Florence, in Italy.

One evening a wonderful chance occurrence took place in Aley, the largest of these popular resort towns. Mike, Mary, Uncle Paul and I were promenading on the main drag when we saw advertised on the marquee Verdi's *La Traviata*. When we approached the cashier, the owner at the door said to us, "No, no! You are our guests tonight. You don't have to pay. The opera is already in the Second Act. Go right in. You'll visit us again, sooner or later, and then you'll pay!"

This wouldn't have happened anywhere else—the Lebanese are known for their generosity and hospitality. Or could it have been that the owner was using his inherited Lebanese business sense in search of future customers? Whatever the case, Uncle Paul invited him to supper with us at a beautiful open-air restaurant the next evening, reciprocating the goodwill he generated. Not to be outdone, the owner invited us all to his home the following day where we were offered *araq* to drink and feasted on delicious *shishkabab* and *kibbe*.

On July 12 we drove to Baskinta. That was Rose Rishwain's parents' village of origin. I recall that visitors could only get to it by a narrow road that hugged the side of an impressive canyon. The valley below was called "The Valley of the Skulls," because every summer a bus or car would fall into it. We were told this fact after we had already arrived at the village, so now we had only to worry about the drive back to Beirut! It was a beautiful village, known for its cherries and apple trees. Rose's relatives who had never emigrated, and had never seen her before, enthusiastically spread a tableful of Lebanese food and pastry, displaying the legendary hospitality of Lebanon. Rose enquired of one of her young relatives if she would want to go back with her to America. The beautiful local girl said, "Here I am the queen of the village, why would I want to go to a big city in America and become an unknown." I thought that was a wise and prudent answer.

The same day we returned to Serhel via Beirut. It was late in the day, but we still stopped, just north of Beirut at the mouth of *Nahr-el-Kalb*, the so-called Dog River. On both sides of the river, etched in rock, are the commemorative plaques of ancient and modern world conquerors. It is sort of a "Kilroy was here" locale, except that these marks were not about private soldiers, but etchings made long ago in the granite cliff commemorating the great conquerors that had crossed that river. One has to be there to feel the awe inspired by such world history. These styli included commemorative plaques of Ramses II, Nebuchadnezzar, Darius I and his Persian army, Roman Emperor Antoninus Pius, the Crusaders, Napoleon III (Louis Napoleon Bonaparte), and more recently Maréchal Foch (Supreme Commander of Allied Forces in World War I), and Général Henri-Honoré Giraud from World War I. The earliest plaque from Ramses II is still there, 3,300 years old, but barely decipherable. Lebanon was the roadway to the Middle East where all conquerors had to pass.

The next day we went to Byblos, now called *Jbail*, probably the oldest continuously inhabited city in the world. This is where the word "Bible" comes from. The Scriptures were written on Egyptian papyrus from Byblos, which was the port of entry of goods from Egypt. Thus the word became "Bible," a derivative of Byblos. The architecture of Byblos has always reminded me of many locations in Rome itself. In Rome, one stands by the Arch of Trajan and overlooks old Roman colonnades, medieval turrets, Renaissance domes, 19th century red-plastered buildings and the 20th century white marble monument to Victor Emmanuel that Mussolini erected for his sovereign. Standing in a single spot, one sees the whole history of European architecture displayed. The same effect strikes one in Byblos. By the seashore and around the well-preserved crusaders' castle, one sees evidence of a myriad of archeological remains: Hittite frescoes, Phoenician sarcophagi, and Greek amphitheaters, where the plays of Aeschylus, Euripides, Sophocles, and Aristophanes must have been performed during the long era of Hellenization that the Phoenicians, Syrians, and Egyptians accepted as a matter of historic evolution; (but which proved so galling to the Hebrews who fought it stubbornly under Judas Maccabaeus and his brothers, winning for a while, but in the long run to no avail). One walks a little bit farther and sees Roman colonnades, Arab *madrasats*, Islamic mosques and Byzantine domed-churches, Renaissance and 18th-century structures. Between the monuments are interspersed many gardens of fruit trees, flowering plants, and the homes of the local inhabitants. The vegetation is lush because of its proximity to the sea. All this made the multiple historical compounds pleasant and cool; (much more appealing than the dry-looking settings at the temple of Baalbeck, the Acropolis in Athens, or the Forum in Rome).

After Byblos we returned to Serhel, high up in the mountains where we stayed for a few days, playing backgammon and eating fresh fruits—it was the season of newly ripe figs and grapes. The villagers were constantly coming up to the house to pay their respects, bringing us fresh fruit and vegetables that they had grown on their farms. The shepherds and their wives brought us eggs, yogurt, and cheese. Supermarkets were unheard of yet.

ZAHLE, THE ADORNED BRIDE OF LEBANON

On July 14, we left for Zahle through Tripoli, Beirut, Aley, Bhamdoon, and Sofar, very well-known summer resorts east of Beirut. Zahle is known as the jewel-adorned bride of Lebanon. It is on the roadway to both Baalbeck to the north and Damascus to the east. In Zahle, we went straight to the Gardens of the Berdaune River, arriving just in time for dinner. "Berdaune" is the collective name given to the many restaurants flanking both sides of the river which comes down from the snow-covered mountains and runs through Zahle.

On both sides of the rushing waters we saw numerous open-air restaurants, one after the other. Where one ended,.the next began, and the owners stood in front, bidding us to come in. Visitors would usually go to a particular restaurant that someone along the way had recommended. Tables with embroidered white covers were already set between streams of running water. The natural beauty of the place was truly spectacular.

The waiters started bringing *Meza* (Lebanese hors d'oeuvres) to our table as soon as we sat down. About thirty dishes of different appetizers normally are brought for the guests to savor before the entrees are served. The *meza* includes *hummus, tabbuli, laban* (plain yogurt), dried *laban* with olive oil, fried eggplant, dishes of all kinds of peanuts, sliced potatoes, tomatoes, and cucumbers. Even offerings of cooked spleen, pancreas, lung, and brain are served as delicacies.

Many friends from Serhel had come from the village to join us that day. So when we sat down to eat, there were twenty four people, twelve of us on each side of a long table. The same dishes full of food were duplicated on both ends of the table so people wouldn't have to reach. The *meza* spread consisted of about sixty dishes stretching from one side of the table to the other. *Araq*, the national liquor, was then served. It was brought in bottles along with many small cocktail glasses half-full of ice. When the clear *araq* is poured into a glass of ice or water, a white emulsion forms making it look like milk. The same reaction occurs with any anis-containing liqueur, including the Greek national drink, *ouzo*.

By the time we had eaten enough *meza*, and had drunk enough *araq*, the entrees were brought to the table: Stuffed grape leaves, stuffed squash prepared with *laban* (yogurt), another kind of squash prepared with tomatoes, *saidalieh* (already de-boned fish on top of a serving of rice,) and always, always, *kibbe*, the national dish. It consisted of lean lamb meat, ground with *burghol* (bulgar) and garnished with specially prepared seasonings. The *kibbe* was brought in many forms: uncooked (*kibbe nayeh*), fried in patties, layered with nuts and filling in between (*kibbe bis-saynieh*), and in large, round balls cooked with filling inside (*'ross kibbe*). Eating at a restaurant in the Berdaune Gardens in Zahle is a veritable feast. People go back there again and again with every visit to Lebanon, or several times during any long visit. Travelers have to pass by it on their way to both Baalbeck and Damascus, both very popular tourist destinations, so the restaurants are constantly full of life and excitement.

On our way to Baalbeck, we passed through Chtaura with its old observatory, then by Ryak, a village lined with Italian cypresses and poplar trees. Chtaura is the wine-making center of the Bekaa Valley, so we saw acres upon acres of vineyards. Back then, I had no idea of how good Chtaura wine was. Wine in Lebanon is usually made by thousands of individual families, all of them owning small vineyards. They all make wine just for their own consumption, and it is usually tolerable at best. But Chtaura was and still is a commercial enterprise.

DAYS OF WINE MAKING

I remember very well our wine-making days in Serhel at the end of every summer. Our family owned vineyards in about five different locations (the plots of land are rather small in Lebanon). At our vineyards, wine making was an experience full of fun. Some of us would be busy harvesting the grapes off the vines, while others would be carrying the baskets full of grapes. At interspersed locations, the baskets would be dumped into larger ones, already secured on each side of a donkey or mule. It was the job of some of us boys to lead these beasts of burden to the yard next to Grandma's house. There, on the patio, some of the grapes would be dumped into great urns for fermentation.

The grapes that were poured in the fermentation urns were already mulch— the end result of our stomping on the grapes with rubber boots. This was done in a rectangular, cemented area that had raised edges which directed the juice to a narrow lip, where it would flow and be collected. The juice was then poured into a copper or crystal distillery boiling over a furnace. After a few repeated distillations, *araq* was produced. Some of the liquid would be distilled again to make rubbing alcohol at seventy percent (140 proof). After more distillations, absolute alcohol would be produced at ninety percent (180 proof). I remember Grandma and Dad would save all of the old bottles for use the next winter. It was unheard of (except for city dwellers) to go to a store to buy wine, *araq* or rubbing alcohol. Like many other families, we produced all of these various forms of liquor ourselves.

I really enjoyed these events during those last summer days in Serhel, before going back to school in Tripoli. The children always begged to help stomp the grapes, and fought to have the next turn. Small rubber boots were provided for us to wear. I remember most of the wine produced was red wine. Dad would give some bottles to the priests as Eucharistic wine, and during our winter stay in Tripoli, both Mom and Dad would distribute bottles of wine as gifts to certain friends in the city.

Our return to Tripoli always took place about two weeks after grape harvesting and wine making. Those days were among my fondest experiences of childhood. They taught us teamwork and brought the family closer together through a common enterprise.

The Chtaura winemaking was much more professional, but I had little knowledge of its scope and quality. I didn't realize how good some of that wine was until recently. Jim Barrett, a close friend of ours who makes some of the best wines in the world—his Chateau Montelena Chardoney won first prize at the Paris wine-tasting in 1974—brought me a bottle of Chtaura red wine as a gift three years ago. Jim took the bottle out of a fancy cylindrical carton and said to me, "Henry, read the label!" It said, "*Chateau Musar, produit de Ghazir, mise en bouteille a Chtaura, Liban.*" Jim told me outright, "This wine is very good, one of the best." After we drank some of it, I dared to ask him if it was expensive. "A few hundred dollars," he said. It's funny how it took me 55 years to learn that there are very good wines produced in Lebanon.

THE TEMPLES OF BAALBECK

After several hours in Chtaura, we continued on to Baalbeck. When it comes to proportion and magnitude, Baalbeck contains the most impressive collection of Roman ruins anywhere in the entire Mediterranean world. Baalbeck, in its way, is as grandiose to the naked eye as is the Grand Canyon. Approaching the city in the DeSoto, we could see the six huge and famous columns of the Temple of Jupiter standing tall from twenty kilometers away. The columns got bigger and bigger as we drove closer. As we closed in on them they were monstrous, the largest columns of antiquity anywhere, each consisting of three gigantic individual drums of Egyptian red granite placed on top of each other for a total height of about eighty feet. The usual size of Greek or Roman columns, even the very big ones, is only about twenty to forty feet of height.

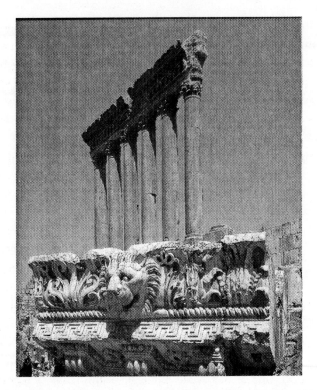

Of the original 58 huge columns of the temple of Jupiter (Baal), only six remain standing. Each column consists of three cylindrical drums of granite that were brought up the Nile in Egypt and transported by sea to Byblos, then carted over Mount Lebanon to be positioned in place at Baalbeck (the city of Baal) in the central Bekaa Valley of Lebanon. No one knows how these superhuman feats were accomplished. Notice, the large section of freeze with the lion head, seen in the foreground, and compare it size-wise with the tiny section of missing freeze on top of the columns. That's where it fell from. That gives a sense of how huge those columns are.

We learned from our guide that Baalbeck was built by Roman emperors as a complex of several temples dedicated to honor the various gods of the ancient world. In the second century AD, Christianity was gaining a foothold in the Roman world. The so-called Antonine emperors of AD 138-180 (Antoninus Pius, 138-61, and his adopted son Marcus Aurelius, the stoic emperor-philosopher, 161-180) wanted to affirm the relevance of the pagan gods in order to counteract the rapid spread of Christianity. It was as if they suspected that Christians were fast increasing in numbers, while the Roman world (along with its various gods) was coming to an end. The Antonine emperors never dreamt that their suspicion would be fulfilled, so they wanted to visibly affirm to the whole pagan world that their ancient gods were still relevant. They undertook the construction at Baalbeck, because it was centrally located between three continents. The whole enterprise was meant to be a visual testament to their ancient rites, which in time became obsolete with the spread of Christianity.

We first visited the temple of Jupiter. Its six gigantic columns were part of an original fifty-eight surrounding the quadrangle-shaped structure. Then we were taken to the intact temple of Bacchus, with all its columns well preserved. After that, we visited what remains of the temples of Venus, Neptune, and Baal himself, the chief Middle Eastern god—the equivalent of the Greek Zeus, the Roman Jupiter, or the Nordic Woden (Wotan). The assembly of all these temples was what gave the city the name of Baalbeck (the City of Baal).

In AD 313, when Constantine declared (through the Edict of Milan) Christianity as the religion of the empire, he ordered the work at Baalbeck to stop. The guide showed us, pointing to some of the bas-relief ornaments, where the work stopped after almost 200 years of construction. One frieze looked perfectly finished on one side of a huge portal, while its mirror-image sister on the other side was partially sculpted, but never finished. The guide was very knowledgeable and decribed to us the history of the temple in great detail. He told us that the temples and the habitations of the priests, priestesses, and pilgrims were air-conditioned by ingenious systems of cisterns and aqueducts. "They brought the water in aqueducts," he informed us, "from the melting snows of Mount Lebanon. The water was allowed to flow down in between the double-thick walls of all the temples to cool the interior by a process of evaporation." He showed us the double walls and the spaces where the water flowed.

I have returned to Baalbeck on several occasions; once with my wife and in-laws; next with our two sons; another time with my brother Edmond; and lately with Dr. Bill Latham, a well-seasoned traveler friend from Stockton. I have visited these places with my father, my brothers, and acquaintances from Serhel, always with a view to showing them this grandiose temple. Every time I visit I learn something new. Baalbeck is majestic, rather like seeing the Grand Canyon in Arizona for the first time. Things of that magnitude are scarce, so when a person encounters them for the first time, they are rarely, if ever, lost to memory, even down to their minute details.

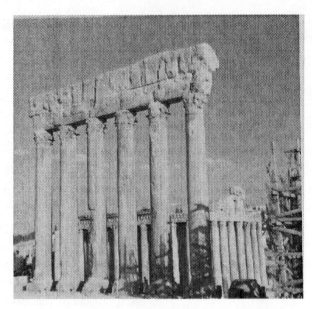

The complex of Roman temples at Baalbeck, Lebanon, built AD 150-313. The backside (interior) view of the six columns of the temple of Jupiter are seen hiding part of the smaller temple of Bacchus with its colonnade intact. A summer music festival takes place under the larger columns, with the temple colonnades lit up with various colored hues. In 1968, I saw Herbert von Karajan conduct the Berlin Philharmonic in Mozart and Brahms, beneath the gigantic columns. They are the largest columns in the world, the remains of the 58 columns that once surrounded the Temple of Jupiter. What looks like clouds in the backround are the snow-capped crests of Lebanon's mountains.

ANCIENT DAMASCUS

On Tuesday, July 15, we drove to Damascus, one of the most ancient cities in the world. It was full of hustle and bustle, with many narrow streets going in and out of a multitude of bazaars or *souks*. We saw the Mosque of the Ommiads (aka Ummyyads). Between AD 700 and 800, Damascus was the capital of the Moslem Empire under the Ommiads, the caliphs who ruled before the center of the Caliphate moved to Baghdad under the Abbasids (Harun-al-Rashid, Al Ma'mun and others). We saw what was purported to be the tomb of St. John the Baptist. We also visited the *Château des Arabes*, where is buried Salah-ed-Din or Saladin, the famous Moslem antagonist of the Crusaders. One of the more interesting spots in Damascus (which I have since visited on several trips to that city) is the house that St. Paul went to after being blinded by the light of Christ's apparition. The guide even pointed out the opening between the house and the city wall, where St. Paul escaped by being lowered down in a basket into the street below, as described in the Acts of the Apostles. He had to run away when the Damascene Jews heard of his sudden conversion to Christ and were intent on killing him. I recall that Joe Rishwain, as well as Uncle Paul, each bought one of those elaborate backgammon tables, beautifully inlaid with mosaics. There is actually a style of laying mosaics called *damascene* inlay. Forty years later, Cousin Connie Rishwain bought me one while on a visit to Damascus. It embellishes our living room.

On July 17 we drove back to Zahle, and from there through Beirut to Tripoli, finally arriving in Serhel on July 20, 1947. July 17 was actually the night we stayed at a hotel in Aley where we saw *La Traviata,* as I mentioned earlier. After resting for a few days in the village, admiring the awe-inspiring scenery, the visiting relatives returned to America with all of my brothers and one sister. I was left alone in Lebanon with Mom and Dad, and it would be another year before we immigrated to Venezuela. Before the relatives left we visited Kos'haya Monastery to see Uncle Butros once more. The American relatives said goodbye to him and continued on to Beirut, where they boarded a plane and took off for New York.

CHAPTER 6

THE FAMILY DISPERSES

While they were in Lebanon, the American relatives had convinced my brother Mike to go to Windsor, Canada (where he was born), to set up a medical practice there. My sister, Mary, accompanied him to consult other doctors in America. She had contracted tuberculosis, just as her mother had some twenty years earlier. It was fortunate that she had traveled with my brother because he was instrumental in making the diagnosis and immediately had her admitted to Herman Kiefer Hospital in Detroit (which was then the Detroit Sanatorium). They treated her for six months with isoniazid and streptomycin. She was in the hospital for a whole year before she was released in healthy condition. How sad it is that the wonder drugs that could have cured Aunt Ramza, Gibran, Chopin, Keats, Chekov, the whole Bronte family, and many others, had not been discovered yet!

From there, Mary went to Venezuela to join Uncle Paul and our brother Tony. She has never had a recurrence of the disease, and at the age of 80 she is still alive and well. She eventually married Michel Braiz (Breis), a distant cousin who is a descendent from the original Mukari family. He was the caretaker of our mountain home in Serhel in the winter, when we were at school in Tripoli. After their marriage Mary and Michel stayed in Venezuela, and they remain there to this day. They have a daughter, whom they named Ramza, after my aunt.

Philip and Johnny went back with Uncle Paul to Venezuela, where he and our brother Tony needed help to run their business enterprises. In the meantime, Edmond got a call from the American Consulate in Beirut advising him to return to reinstate residence in the United States, even if for a short visit, so that legally he would not lose his American citizenship due to being out of the country for so long. Fortunately, he was already in pharmacy school at the American University of Beirut, so he easily transferred to the University of California at Berkeley—from one American pharmacy school to another.

At that time, there was a group of Christian Palestinians from Jaffa (now Tel Aviv) attending the university with whom Edmond became good friends. In 1948, however, they had to quit school because their middle-class parents in Palestine were dispossessed of their homes and land, by the onslaught of European Jewish immigrants—who in turn, had been dispossessed by Hitler and his cruel anti-semitic Holocaust in Europe. "It is unfortunate that those who were sinned against in Europe had in turn become the dispossessors of yet a third party who was innocent of what had gone on in Europe before" (Arnold Toynbee). The parents of Edmond's schoolmates had thus become destitute refugees during the 1948 Israeli-Arab War, and had finally, lost all hope of recovering what was theirs with the de facto establishment of the state of Israel. Edmond stopped attending classes when his friends did, even though he did not have the same reason to do so, because Dad was constantly sending him money to pay for his schooling; yet Edmond left school just the same and began using his stipends to help his Palestinian friends. They were all out of school now and had nothing better to do than to party with Edmond's money. Eventually, these antics came to the attention of Cousin Joe Rishwain Sr. in nearby Stockton. He immediately reported the circumstances to Dad in Caracas, who alerted Mike of the situation. Edmond was induced to leave Berkeley and was enrolled in pharmacy school at Wayne State University, close to big brother Mike. He graduated with honors a few years later and all ended up well for him. To all of us, this incident confirmed the importance of the close relationship that exists within our extended family.

LIFE WITH MOM AND DAD

After all the siblings had left, autumn came upon us with lightning storms and rain. The three of us were all that was left of the original family of nine. We descended to Tripoli for the winter season. Little did we realize (or so much as think) that an epoch was ending. The twenty-eight years of the Yousef, Ramza, and Badwyeh family were ending, having lasted from the beginning of the ten years spent in Detroit to the end of the eighteenth year of living in the Lebanese mountains and on the shores of the Mediterranean. Those years of my elementary and secondary education in several languages, as well as the years of World War II when Lebanon remained untouched by the destruction taking place in Europe, were fading away. All the years of intact family cohesion, finally fell to the sword of Damocles. This happened when the American visitors returned to America and took with them my brothers and sisters—away from us forever.

The memories of those years have proven to be long-lasting. The written word can never fully capture the deep experiences of our childhood days, but our hearts will always contain their sweet fragrance. The original aura of my fourteen years spent in Lebanon cannot be conveyed adequately, because it has been told in segments here and there. It is difficult to paint adequately the entire picture, the true gestalt, so to speak, of those wonderful, beautiful, tender years of childhood, when affection was plentiful and the disappointments of adult life had not yet been encountered.

When we came down from our dear village to the vast Tripoli apartment that fall, it appeared larger than it really was, because of its emptiness. We also felt a vacuum in our hearts. There was less laughter and less *joie de vivre* because there were fewer loved ones around. My mother felt all this the most. She would reminisce about her previous constant companion, my sister Mary, and cry. What could she say to Dad, who like most men was not used to discussing or savoring the small talk, the little details of daily life? I was even less talkative with her, having left the hustle and bustle of our former life and settled into a quiet aloneness.

Having admired Dad to the point of emulation, I became like him, more concerned with my own thoughts, my own solitude, my own questions about life and death—I was contemplative by nature, even at that tender age. I was a serious young man. I would read the international front page of a newspaper long before I would look at the inner pages concerned with sports or local happenings. Even now I hardly read newspapers, except for the major headlines. In some ways, Mother was no different from her son, and she felt sad and alone. Dad would go downtown and discuss a million wonderful things with friends: politics, wars, or philosophy. Is beauty akin to truth? Is goodness ultimately rewarding? Does the apparent success of dishonest people make them happy, or are they really miserable inside? His philosophic mind was always working, and yet he was practical enough to realize the evanescence of the daily chores he performed, even though he did them responsibly and ably every day. He would go downtown to visit his Greek Orthodox friend, Saba Arab, and they would discuss religion and politics for hours on end. I remember

Dad telling him, "All of you *Rum* (Greek Orthodox) are stubborn and full of false pride. We all have the same dogma and rituals. So why don't you all join the larger Catholic Church and get the centuries-old schism over with, anyway? But no! Your false pride won't let you!" And they would both laugh and hug each other just the same as before.

Mom found it strange that men would spend so much time discussing life or the afterlife. She knew instinctively that life was benevolent everywhere, and because of her deep faith, she trusted that the coming of an afterlife is a foregone conclusion. She would often say to my sister Mary, "Why try to reinvent the wheel when the Church has perfected its design over two thousand years?" Actually, she was right. I liked her approach more than Dad's, even though I was analytical like him. What was all that mind work of Dad to Mom? It all meant nothing! It wasn't even interesting; it wasn't close to her heart; in fact, it was totally impersonal. That's how she approached Dad's philosophizing, since she could neither fathom his abstract mind nor out-argue him logically. That's why she missed her daily talks with Mary. She knew that Mary was gone, but did not realize at that early stage that the pieces of our closely-knit family would never again be put back together. It was the end of an era, which had consisted of daily contact, a lifetime of closeness, laughing and crying together—the termination of a certain lifestyle of intimacy.

I was also affected by this sudden loss of loved ones, but much less than Mom. I was still quite young, younger than my nearest sibling by seven years. I never expected to be the only child at home. Nonetheless, I continued playing my solitary games, not caring whether I played with other classmates or not. I could still do what I loved to do most: read, play music, listen to my elders' political discussions, and retreat into my own world of introspection and imagination. I loved to read historical novels then. I guess that's when I started getting interested in history. It seems to me now that I was on the verge of turning into an old man at the age of thirteen. Oh, I would talk to Mom and go with her to the delicatessen—we both loved sweets—or she would take me to the movies—she loved the panache of Esther Williams' films. I would also pray with her, for we both enjoyed praying together. Yet she was as dear to my siblings (her sister's children) as she was to me. I still hear accolades from my siblings and their wives, constantly given in memory of her. They all testify to her unselfishness and her devotion to husband and family.

Mom was a sincere and humble woman. Even though she spoke several languages, she was simple in taste and desires. She never expected much out of life. She led a somewhat joyless life, but full of selfless love. She never fully experienced pleasure or luxury, and she wore little or no makeup. She would always try to catch up with Dad when walking down the street, begging him to slow down as she had callused feet for as long as I can remember, and could never keep up with his pace. She would ask him for money, not for herself, but to buy the children new shoes or clothes. She had dark hair, big dark eyes and a slightly crooked right middle toe (which I inherited from her). Mom liked almanacs that had a page of explanations for each day. On each page were printed the daily horoscope, a proverb, and the name of the saint of that day. She would use certain Italian expressions that, to this day, I don't have a clue what they meant. She would say, for instance, "*Mister Conte con la brague onte.*" I know this was not Italian. It may have been Romanian or even Basque. I don't know—only she knew!

Early, during the winter of that year, Mom started nagging Dad to take us to America where *her* children were. He would tell her, "They're not *your* children! They're your sister's children. Your child is here with us!" "Joe, let's go and visit the children even if only for a few months," she would coax. "It will only be like a pleasant short vacation for the three of us." Little did she realize that once she had left she would never return to Lebanon—that she would die in America. In subsequent years, we have all gone back and forth to Lebanon several times, but not Mom. She had a fear of flying and that fear stayed with her to the end of her life.

When people heard Dad tell her, "They're not your children," they would always argue with him. "Yes they are," they would say. "She treated and cared for them better than their mother would have, and she never thought of them as *not* her very own." Dad would admonish everybody saying, "We're not going back to America! I'm retired and over there I would have to start working for a living all over again!" He would tell me how he left America before the depression and preserved his life savings, whereas his brothers and their progeny lost most of what they had in the crash of the 1930s and had to start working even harder than before. He taught me to work *for a living*—and he emphasized that—only until I had saved enough to live comfortably. He said that enough meant; "far less than what most people think they will need to live on." "Work for a few years," he would say "and then enjoy the leisure of intellectual and spiritual pursuits." "Leisure," he said, "means reading, writing and perhaps gentleman farming and educating your children and grandchildren." It was the kind of thing that George Washington and Thomas Jefferson, our founding fathers, would have said. I am certain Dad never read Joseph Pieper's excellent treatise, *Leisure, the Basis of Culture.* Such thoughts were intuitive to him, the sort of wisdom formed by the experience of a lifetime. He was already fifty-three when I was thirteen, so I learned much home-grown wisdom from him.

I was the youngest child of seven—and by seven years at that—so I had the good fortune to live with my parents as they aged.

I suppose I could write a book on the advantages of still living with older parents after all the other siblings have left the nest. Even though he never specifically said it, Dad lived preparing himself for the final exit from this world—eternal life. "The driving force behind those who work into old age is usually the desire to accumulate possessions," he would often tell me, and then add, "That's what is called greed." Like a true philosopher, he had no use for luxurious living. I guess, deep down, he remained a pensive "monk" to the end. Mom's worries were terrestrial, closer to home, and yet her aversion to financial greed, when she noticed it in friends and relatives, was as strong as Dad's. She had worked as hard as he had when they were in Detroit, and considerably harder later on at home (while the seven children were growing up) and yet she knew when enough was enough. After they came back to America, she was worried about my working too hard or studying too much.

In those days, nobody had yet used the terms type A or B. Neither Mom nor Dad realized that my very admission to medical school would ensure that I would become a Type A, whether I was one before or not. Come to think of it, I was quite laid back in college. I enjoyed those years and didn't work so hard at living or labor so much at my studies—most of it came to me naturally. But in medical school, we all became driven, and the competition to get good grades was furious. High grades were needed for acceptance into good internships and residency programs. "Son," Mom would say to me, "rest a little while— you're going to wear yourself thin."

Oh, how much she worried about me being physically thin. When I was ten, some doctor told her to grind eggshells and put them in orange juice or lemonade, and make me drink it because I needed calcium. In the old world, the parents used to be proud when they had an obese child. "*Smallah*! Look how fat and healthy he is," they would say. As a matter of fact, my parents had brought back from Detroit this saying, "Eat fat to be fat!" Or was it, "Eat fat to stay warm," during the freezing Detroit winters. They used to say it in English, which we never spoke at home in those days. We spoke either Arabic or French. I guess back then in cold Detroit an extra layer of fat didn't hurt; and in former times parents wanted their children to be fat so that, when the cholera or yellow fever came, the fat ones would survive longer by using up their body fat, even though these diseases had long become a thing of the past in America, Lebanon, and most of the Middle East.

During the latter half of 1947 and all of 1948, Mom missed the rest of the family very much. As for me, I was enjoying a great deal of attention, with or without my siblings. Ever since birth (so I was told), my birthdays had been celebrated with gusto. On July 31 the fattened calf was regularly slaughtered. Normally, in Lebanon in those days, the feast of the name-saint was a more important date than the birthday. In my case, that would have fallen on July 13, the feast of St. Henry (the beatified Holy Roman emperor who lived around AD 1010). Nowadays, birthdays are celebrated with fanfare all over the world just as they are in America. I am sure that celebrating my birthdays in those days was a carryover from when my parents were in Detroit in the 1920s. I recall a photo of myself holding a round chiffon cake on a platter with thirteen birthday candles on it in front of the Serhel house. In the photo, I had thin legs and a thin face dwarfed by large glasses.

DR. 'EIN AND HINTS OF THINGS TO COME

The glasses put me in mind of my second visit to an ophthalmologist, a Dr. 'Ein in Tripoli. My visit to Dr. 'Ein's office was occasioned by myopia. While waiting for him, patiently sitting in the examining chair, I noticed the rows upon rows of clear lenses arranged in tidy order in a compact transparent case to my right. I was attracted even further by the cleanliness and order in which every instrument was placed on the table to my left. That particular picture must have remained in the back of my mind till the day I decided to become an eye doctor. The name 'Ein, oddly enough, means eye, in Arabic. That was his real family name!

Earlier, I had to pay Dr. 'Ein a visit because of hay fever. My eyes first started itching on a beautiful, sunny day when Dad and I went hiking in a field full of spring flowers. I remember looking at a highway far away, and at that distance the automobiles looked like little toy cars. I recall wanting Dad to buy me one of those toys. The memory is amazingly vivid. I can still picture the cars far beyond the field of flowers. The first car was red, the second blue, and the third brown—a station wagon. I recall a wonderful fragrance of blooming flowers, and suddenly I began to rub my eyes to alleviate a mild itch. Little did I know then that the rubbing would increase the itch and discomfort. It felt as though needles were piercing my eyes. So Dad took me to Dr. 'Ein's office. He prescribed estivin, a solution made of flower petals, one of the early anti-itch medications. Antihistamines and cortisone were not discovered until the late 1940s and early '50s. It did help lessen the itch a little. Dr. 'Ein also prescribed cold compresses.

I remember lying in bed for two days, feeling as if I had pins and sand in my eyes. While I kept my eyes closed (they felt better that way) I kept thinking of the little cars across the beautiful field of flowers. The whole image has stayed in my imaginative recall as one of the clearest memories of my childhood, in spite of the annoying itch and discomfort of allergic reaction. On my last visit to Lebanon, in 2000, Dr. 'Ein's son, a physician himself, told me that his father often talked about his friendship with the Zeiter family. The old doctor had passed away a few years before.

Later, in Windsor, I used to go for eye checkups to Dr. Beuglet's office. He was a French-Canadian ophthalmologist, who found a change in my myopic condition every year. Myopia increases rapidly at the age of greatest growth, teenage years. The eye gets longer as the body gets taller, and that requires constantly stronger concave lenses. Again in Dr Beuglet's examining room, as in Dr 'Ein's, I found myself fascinated by the shining clear trial lenses arranged in rows, and would wish that I was the eye doctor who was using them to help people see.

Ten years later in medical school in London, Canada, I again became fascinated with the instruments that were used in the eye department. Dr. Tyson, the head of the eye service, took me up to the third floor one afternoon, to show me the binocular microscope that magnifies the retina, optic disc, and the other inner structures of the eye. What a sight of colors that was! Looking through the pupil, I could see clearly the yellow optic disc, the orange retina, and the reddish macula with a yellowish spot in the center, the *lutea*. The red arteries and the bluish veins crisscrossed each other feeding the retina. The whole spectacle reminded me of the biblical story of Joseph's multicolored robe. It was a Monet, a Renoir, or rather a J.M.W. Turner, with his wild swirls of warm earth colors. I thought it would be good to become an eye specialist, just to enjoy these colors every day, even though psychiatry was in the back of my mind as another possible specialty. (I thought psychiatry would help me explain my dreams and my pressing desires.) What contrasting specialties these two are! Why, of all the fields I could have chosen, did I consider entering one of these two dissimilar specialties? It would be a few years before I would find out the answer to that question.

MY FATHER'S DREAM

One cool summer morning in Serhel, I recall dad relating to us a dream he experienced the night before. He had dreamt about the mayor of the town, Sarkis Abdallah. In the dream, Sarkis ran up from the village with urgency, jumped on the high rock that stood behind our house (Dad pointed to the rock) and shouted at the top of his voice, "Fire! Fire! The forest is on fire!"

Dad continued, "Then I looked up at the mountain, over there, and saw fire and smoke rising above the forest." (This part of the dream was in color, he told us.) "Within seconds I saw, now in black and white, the villagers in tattered clothes rushing up the road right here," he continued, pointing to the dirt road next to our house. "They were followed by their wives and children, all with buckets of water, moving en masse towards the forest to put out the fire."

If Dad had told us about this dream an hour later, we wouldn't have believed it. But he mentioned it about thirty minutes before we saw the mayor of the town running up from the village, almost out of breath; he jumped on the same rock that Dad had pointed to earlier, shouting "Fire! Fire! The forest is on fire! Help! Help! We need water to put it out." When Dad was telling us about his dream earlier, we were all sitting outside on the porch around a table we always used for breakfast. We were still there, mesmerized, when we saw the villagers rushing up toward the forest with their buckets of water, babbling and shouting instructions to one another. We were stupefied! Dad's dream and that whole scene around were like a fairy tale. We didn't want to believe any of it, but it was all true, happening before our very eyes.

I had always been impressed by Dad's wise, prudent, and prophetic nature. But this, now! This was an entirely different thing. It was a scene out of the Old Testament. I was shaken to my depths, to say the least, and so were my mother, my siblings and our two maids. As I recall that event of my childhood, I can understand why I always valued Dad's counsel above anybody else's.

The other day I glanced at some small photos that I've had inside a desk drawer for many years. One was of Dad pruning vines behind the house in Serhel. In the photo, he had the pruning shears in his hand and was looking at the camera. He was happy, leading a simple life, pruning his vines.

Another photograph I found in my drawer displays a little boy, about seven or eight years old, wearing summer shorts and a pair of worn-out sandals. That was me, crouching on the side of a "bir," a small dug out, cemented cistern we had on the patio just below the house. In the photo, I am seen turning a faucet to let water out of the house's main water reservoir into the smaller cistern. It was my job to scoop up the water with a small bucket and irrigate the pots of multicolored flowers we kept on the patio in front of the eight Greek columns that gave our white house such an elegant look (in a village with many simple adobe houses). I look like an innocent, poorly dressed street urchin, half smiling, half sad—like the painting by Ribera entitled *The Boy with the Clubfoot* in 17th century Spain.

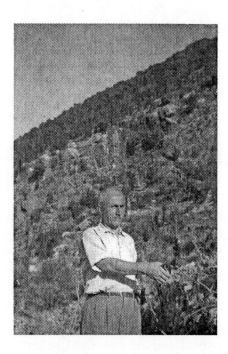

Dad seen pruning the vines in our Serhel vineyards,
November, 1947, his favorite hobby

Ever since my siblings left for America, Mom had continued to plead with Dad about joining them. In the meantime, I was in my first year of high school in Lebanon, *le cinquième*, "the fifth year," counting backwards from the day of high school graduation, a reverse nomenclature compared to ours. Here, in America, we number the grades from first to twelfth in order of ascendancy. In Europe and the Middle East, the first grade is numbered twelfth and the final high school year is number one. I was good at school, but foreseeing that sooner or later we were going to leave for America, I began to slack off and live on my past glory. I tried to get away with many things, and I did. Once teachers know you are a good student, they will let slide stupid mistakes. From my experience, I was also aware that some teachers would often just scan a top student's exam papers or homework and still give him an "A", without thoroughly analyzing the work presented. I used to test them by writing something quite outrageous in the middle of a book report or an exam, and would find out later that it was rarely corrected or commented upon.

TILL EULENSPIEGEL'S MERRY PRANKS

In contrast to the conservative bent I acquired as I got older, I showed the exact opposite attitude early in life. I used to love being close to the edge, but, when it came down to it, would never go over the brink. So in class, just out of boredom and for diversion, I taught three or four boys in the back row how to make coffee inside the classroom by using a homemade contraption. The process centered on a small metallic container that one of the Armenian boys brought us from his father's dental practice. We would fill the little container with water and a pinch of coffee, add a little sugar, and place it over an alcohol-containing syringe-sterilizer that once belonged to my doctor brother. We would then ignite the alcohol with a match to heat the improvised coffeepot. We would always place the contraption inside a folding desk, beneath the inkwell (with the inkbottle removed). There was only one problem, which we eventually solved. A little smoke would spiral out of the inkwell hole. So to hide the smoke from view, we made use of the big boy who sat in front of our "coffee house." He would lean back and sit tall so that neither the teacher nor anyone in the front rows could see the smoke. We would drink the coffee in the back row, and then get ready to make another batch. To pass the coffee around, we poured it in small "thimbles," (which the dentist father of our classmate used to mix his dental filling paste).

The teacher and the boys in the first row didn't catch on for several weeks. But one day we passed a few thimbles full of hot coffee to the rows ahead of us. It was an unnecessary risk, and we were caught. When the teacher's attention was drawn to what was happening, he got worried because he saw smoke spiraling out of the desk's inkwell. He thought that it was on fire and ran out of the classroom to the hallway to fetch a fire extinguisher. Before he returned (a matter of seconds) I had extinguished the fire and put everything in my school satchel. When he returned and saw no fire, he blamed the boys in the row ahead of us for rowdiness. They never told on the rest of us, deeming that among schoolmates it would have amounted to snitching, a dishonorable thing to do.

Even if I were to be punished, I had the magic "booklet," and two good marks would have been erased as payoff for my bad behavior. Now the booklet that would have saved me was called *le livre des bons points*, or the book of good marks given for good behavior. It was a small booklet that contained about twenty little pages of blotter-like paper. For every good performance in class or on exams, the school seal would be stamped on one page. Sometimes for an exceptionally good essay or model behavior, two *bons points* would be stamped in the booklet. The Christian Brothers (emulating God's last judgment when sins would be weighed against good deeds on a scale) decided that these good marks could be erased as punishment for bad behavior. When that occurred, the stamp would be voided by crossing it with a large "X", using "indelible" ink from the teacher's inkwell.

Nobody in class could figure out why I never ran out of good marks. But that only lasted for about four months. Then, I gave one of my friends my secret recipe for "reincarnating" good points, and he got caught. He never confessed that I was the instigator, but the jig was up.

It so happened that several months before, when I was being castigated, the teacher asked me for the booklet and then crossed out the good mark on the very first page. I couldn't believe my eyes. I knew for a fact that I had at least the first ten pages crossed out for bad behavior (all within the past two months). When the teacher handed me back the booklet, I quietly went back to my desk. I opened the booklet and noticed that all the ink "X's" that I had gotten over the past two weeks had disappeared, except for the one the teacher had just crossed out on the first page. I couldn't believe it! I knew that it wasn't a miracle, because God doesn't reward bad behavior. Something else had taken place resulting in the disappearance of the ink from these pages.

After searching and searching, I realized that two nights before, I had forgotten the booklet in the back pocket of my school uniform when I handed it over to the maid to wash. When I got home I asked her if she had washed or pressed that particular pair of pants. Mariam said, "Yes, two or three days ago I did both. Why do you ask?" We put our two heads together and figured out that wetting the pages and pressing them with a warm iron washes away the supposedly indelible ink marks. We further found that if the pressing iron was too hot, it would singe the small pages and ruin them altogether. In this manner, we found a valuable system for erasing the Xs of bad behavior.

Mariam got the biggest kick out of the whole thing. She became my accomplice over the next few months. So, from then on we started to wet the page that was crossed off and then gently apply the iron on the book as a whole. Presto, the mark would be gone. This trick worked for almost four months, but then I learned the hard way that one must never teach another one's crimes, because sooner or later both will get caught. My behavior in class, however, improved markedly from then on. I did not want to be executed like that irrespectful prankster Till Eulenspiegel in Richard Strauss' famous tone poem *Till Eulenspiegel's Merry Pranks*.

By the time I reached my final year of school in Lebanon, I had gotten over these antics. However, I knew that I was soon to leave that school, probably forever, so I ceased applying myself academically. At that point, Dad took me out of the school altogether (Easter 1948) and thought it more worthwhile to hire a tutor to teach me the Spanish language, since we knew we would soon emigrate and go to Venezuela.

UNKNOWN FUTURE

One of the memorable events from those days was when one of my best friends, Antoine Yamouni, told me his family was leaving for Venezuela. We were standing on the patio of an old uninhabited house whose original owners must have emigrated long ago. The house overlooked the Mediterranean to the right, the village below, and the Kadisha Canyon to the left. There are many of these abandoned houses in the mountain villages of Lebanon. Most of them become dilapidated, after the owners and their families emigrate to more prosperous countries in search of work and a better existence—just like the house ruins one finds all over the countryside in Ireland. This emigration continues to this day among the Christian population of the entire Middle East, but particularly among those who had lived in the Holy Land for centuries, because they find themselves pressured by both the Moslems and the Israeli Jews.

The sun was setting on the Mediterranean Sea and I remember the whole episode with great nostalgia. Antoine, my friend, was telling me, "Henry! Our whole family is leaving for the New World and my Dad thinks we're going to do very well because we have relatives there who will help us get started with our own business." "It's going to be great," he said. "It will open the door to success and happiness." After he finished enumerating the advantages, I told him, "Antoine, in this life happiness alternates with disappointment and sadness, no matter where you find yourself. You have high expectations of the New World that may or may not pan out." Years later I read a similar thought in this passage from Hilaire Belloc's *The Four Men,*

> *What are you doing? You [and your parents] are upon some business that takes you far, [far away from this blessed land of your birth], not even for ambition or for adventure, but only to earn. And you will cross the sea and earn your money, and you will come back and spend more than you have earned. But all the while your life runs past you like a river, and the things that are of moment to men you do not heed.*
>
> —Hilaire Belloc, *The Four Men* (1910)

I hated to lose such a good friend. His family took him to Venezuela and after working there assiduously for many years he immigrated to California this time around, and settled in Stockton, with only a modest lifestyle to show for it. For several years, after we left Lebanon, I would dream that I was walking on the same path that led to the uninhabited house that must have belonged to somebody who had left for the New World long before and would never return. In those dreams, Antoine and I would be going down the hillside to his house where his mother, Josephine, would offer us tea and cookies.

A TAPESTRY OF IMAGES

Our memories are often a conglomerate of visual perceptions, maybe from occasions when we have had several encounters with someone or something at different times. I would call this phenomenon "involuntary memory" made up of images like a collage.

One of my most vivid early memories was a sad one. It occurred during the summer when we were in Serhel. I saw several men bring George Mansour down from the pine forest, after a tree trunk had fallen on his head. George was working as a lumberman for a construction firm. I recall George's wife, Maria, my dad's first cousin, and her mother Msahieh, weeping and wailing. George's daughter Yvonne, one of our closest friends in Stockton now, was two years old then. Yvonne and her sister Isabel subsequently grew up fatherless, so the whole family depended on my father for direction and sustenance. When George Mansour died, Yvonne's mother was pregnant. She named the child George. He also died prematurely in an auto accident in Venezuela fifty years later.

Maria, the widow, eventually lost her sight from glaucoma. I recall operating on her with Dr. Roger Sayegh in Tripoli, thirty years ago. The members of that family had a miserable life indeed. Dad eventually placed the children in a grammar school run by the Sisters of Charity in Tripoli, and that was their only chance to receive an education. I also remember Dad and Mom taking in the Jacobs children to live with us for over a year, when Dad found them one day homeless, wandering in the Souks of Tripoli. Peter lives now in Stockton and has done very well for himself. I recall the times Dad would send Peter down to the village spring to bring us fresh drinking water. He would dash down the dirt road with such speed that pebbles would fly behind his heels like shots from a machine gun. When we see each other now in Stockton, we reminisce about these wonderful scenes of childhood.

Again memories and images flood into my mind from the times when we came up to Serhel for our annual summer vacations. Maria and her mother would be waiting for us at the back door of our house. I vividly recall how Mom and I would descend to our villa, from where the main road ended, two hundred feet from the house. We would then see Msahiah (the widow) and Maria (her equally widowed daughter), crouched on a low wooden bank, with their backs resting on the rear wall of the house, always dressed in black, still mourning their dead husbands. In the Mideast black is the sign of grieving, of widowhood and of poverty, and once a woman had started wearing black, she rarely, if ever, went back to brighter colors. Showing faithfulness to the memory of one's beloved—forever—was an unwritten code in that society. It was a scene straight out of the Anthony Quinn movie *Zorba the Greek*.

Upon arrival at the back door of the house, Maria and Msahieh would kiss us three times on both sides of our cheeks before we went in. Inside, we usually found fruit and freshly squeezed lemonade prepared by them a few minutes earlier. They were part of the family, very dear to my parents, and they would often help around the house and at the time of the grape harvest. They were rarely far from us, even overseas. In the old country there were Msahieh, Maria, Yvonne, and Isabel. Later in Venezuela there were Maria, Yvonne and Isabel—Msahieh having died back in Lebanon, shortly before her daughter's emigration. Now in California, Yvonne and her husband, Charlie Zaiter, live not far from us. Maria and Isabel both passed away in Venezuela. The only one of the group who ever owned a house was Yvonne, together with her husband Charlie, one of my closest friends. Yvonne now wears black clothes forever mourning the passing away of Msahieh, Maria and Isabel. Charlie maintains day in and day out a calm and humble demeanor. He is happy and satisfied with life without many expectations. I see him frequently, whenever I need a silent listening partner. We both belong to the Secular Carmelite Order and always go to the monthly meetings together. May God keep him happy and content!

Another scene involved Yousef Abi-Samra, a descendant from one of the original branches of the Mukari family. He used to help Dad make huge amounts of burghol (bulgar, or cracked wheat) from wheat grain. I can still see him standing on a flat wooden thrasher pulled by a bull, going round and round over the recently harvested wheat shaff, trashing it to release the grain. Another thing I recall was the night Dad shot the shepherd dog lurking outside the house thinking he was a wolf. The next day we had to bury him in the field because we never found the owner.

When everyone was having a siesta in the afternoon, I would imagine myself to be a great sculptor and would dig deeper and deeper into a rock behind the house under the pine trees. The hole was about two inches wide. I had started the project a few summers before, using the tip of a Swiss army knife that was given to me as a present. Every time I return to Lebanon, I look for that same hole in that same rock behind the house to see if I'm still alive and the world is still the same; and when I find it, memories of those days cascade out of me like a waterfall. Then I am assured that yes, there is something permanent left from our past. It's like in this small hole in the rock, "I find the character of enduring things" (Hilaire Belloc).

After supper the family would take a walk on the road above our house. As the family walked in tandem, I would lag behind, fascinated by a little anthill, with the ants coming and going with a load quadruple their size. We would come back from the walk and go up to the roof, just in time to see the silvery moon rising over the high mountains to the east. It seems to me that the moon was always full—at least that's how I remember it. I also recall attending Mass on Sundays and still see in my mind's eye the curious glances of the humble villagers riveted towards any visitor present whom they hadn't seen before. They would all look sideways without turning their faces, trying to figure out whether the visitor was someone's relative returned from America or just an occasional guest from a neighboring village.

The best evening of all, though, was when my brother Johnny and I ate dinner on the flat roof of the house, after having been starved almost to death during a four-day bout of malaria. We were famished waiting for Mom or the maid to bring up our food, looking at the surrounding forests and mountains nearby. For four days they gave us nothing substantial to eat, except purée, as this was the old way to "starve out the fever." How cruel and ridiculous was medical treatment in pre-antibiotic days! Then Mom and the maid came up to the roof carrying various dishes of fried eggs and sausage, potatoes and salad. That was the most delicious meal we had ever eaten; it was a feast never to be forgotten. After 60 years, the taste of every morsel is still fresh on my palate.

As described in Aristotle's *De Anima*, *imagination* consists of the perceived sensual *images* as stored in our mind, while *memory* itself is only the recall of *the time* when these perceptions took place. That being so, I can understand why I feel the texture of the warm Lebanese bread, and the lemony, salty taste of the salad every time I recall the event. Even the crispiness of the fried potatoes and the viscous yellow yolk of the "over-easy" eggs, comes to my recall now.

Also in front of me now is the image of Mom's happiness at seeing us feeling better and eating with gusto all the food in front of us down to the last morsel. In contrast, I recall now the extreme bitterness of the anti-malarial quinine tablets we were forced to take for four days prior to that fine meal. As a young boy I could never swallow medicine tablets, so I would keep the quinine tablets in my mouth for a few minutes, actually chewing them, before I was able to swallow the horribly bitter substance. I didn't know then that quinine is one of the most bitter things on earth. The taste lasted for days and comes back to me every time I think of that unforgettable evening meal.

These images, and many more, remained the subject of my dreams at night for several years after we had emigrated from Lebanon, both in Caracas and in Canada, and they are alive at this very instant, as I am writing about them.

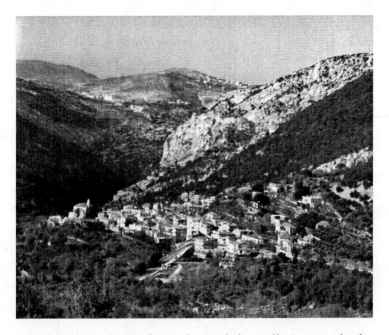

Serhel looking (away from the Kadisha Valley) towards the Mediterranean; the steepled St. Michael's Church is to the left; our summer villa is the flat-roofed white house to the right—on the same eye level as the church.

CHAPTER 7

EMIGRATION

On a fall day in October 1948, the expected moment finally arrived. We drove to Tripoli, then to Beirut, where we were going to board a ship called the "Marine Carp" (a refurbished navy transport). It was to sail to New York via Piraeus in Greece, Palermo in Sicily, the Azores in the middle of the Atlantic, and then New York harbor, our final destination. On our last day in Beirut there was a parade that we watched from the seventh-floor veranda of our hotel. It was held in honor of fourteen-year-old King Feisal II of Iraq, who was visiting Lebanon that day. I started identifying with him from that day on because he was exactly my age. I recall my sadness ten years later in Canada, when I heard of his assassination. That was the end of the monarchy in Iraq and the beginning of the rule of a series of military dictators, the last one being Saddam Hussein.

The Mediterranean was very calm as we left the port of Beirut. We were up on the sunny deck looking back at the coastline and the mountains. Beirut, with its tall buildings, could be seen well from out at sea. As the ship moved away from the port we were able to distinguish myriads of red-roofed villages higher up on Mount Lebanon, dotting the hills all the way up to the snow-covered mountain crests. With the ship yet farther out at sea, an array of Lebanese coastal cities began to appear on the horizon: Beirut, Jounieh, Byblos, Batrun, Saida (Sidon) and Sur (Tyre) to name a few. Behind the coastal cities, the mountains of Lebanon rose majestically. It was quite a sight—not to be forgotten, but to be enjoyed again and again on every subsequent return to Lebanon.

The chain of mountains in Lebanon rises rapidly from the Mediterranean. Within a mere twenty miles from the coast, the altitude is over 10,000 feet.

The steep rise was like Mona Kea and Mona Loa on the big island of Hawaii, except that in Lebanon the mountains are populated with hundreds of picturesque villages, dating back to the times when Egyptians, Assyrians, Babylonians, Greeks, Romans, Crusaders, and French and British troops passed by conquering the land, interbreeding with the local population, and leaving behind them the stamp of their architecture and culture, one civilization after another. This may originally have been a reason why so many Lebanese think it necessary to speak several languages. It is a natural gift after centuries of intermingling with every empire and civilization that took its turn in conquering the Mediterranean basin.

There are Lebanese physiognomies that look European and others that look Middle Eastern. The Lebanese insist that they are Phoenician stock, not Arab. Recent research by National Geographic archeologists, showed that over 80% of the Lebanese population, both in the mountains and the coastland, both Christian and Moslem, have the same DNA as that found in Phoenician bones found in sarcophagi. All of these conquering cultures would rise to a golden age and then decline and disappear, or be absorbed by the religious fervor of the next civilization. In *A Study of History*, Arnold Toynbee studied the rise and fall of twenty-two civilizations. He describes the natural lifespan of civilizations as always beginning with newly found religious vigor, followed by a golden age in governance, literature and the arts, and then declining into a long period of overstretched empire, overspent economies and final moral and physical decay.

As the ship was sailing away from the Lebanese coast, my thoughts went to the Phoenician cities of Sidon and Tyre, where our alphabet was first developed and then passed on to the Greeks and hence to the Romans. From these two cities the Phoenicians, boasting the greatest navigational skills of ancient times, established and colonized Carthage in North Africa, Valencia and Barcelona in Spain, and Marseilles in France before they were conquered in turn by the Greeks and the Romans. The Phoenicians traded their wares and those of others in all of these cities: spices, olive oil, wine, and, best of all, the majestic colored robes which later became known as the "Royal Purple." The purple dye was extracted from a mollusk that inhabited the waters, off the coast of the Eastern Mediterranean. It was also to Tyre and Sidon that Christ and the apostles often went to preach.

As the ship sailed farther into the Mediterranean Sea, we could see the city of Byblos to the North, an ancient port through which marble from Egypt was brought to build the temples of Baalbeck. It was through Byblos that

Egyptian papyrus and other writing parchments were imported. As mentioned already, they were then used to write the holy books, thus the term Bible (from Byblos). The coast of Lebanon is not only a beautiful meeting of land and sea like the California and Oregon coasts, but it bears testimony to the long history of many civilizations.

It was only fitting that the ship was sailing in the direction of Piraeus, the Greek port of Athens—that city of ancient culture, art, and philosophy that outshone the Phoenician culture in brilliance and gave humanity the great gifts of its civilization. Those gifts included the philosophers: Thales, Heraclitus, Parmenides, Socrates, Plato, and Aristotle. They also included the tragedians: Aeschylus, Euripides and Sophocles, together with Aristophanes and Aesop, the satirists of human foibles. That same culture produced Myron, Praxiteles, and Phidias, sculptors whose works we admire in the world's museums.

The civilization that Greece bequeathed is testimony to the fact that the formative elements of history are basically cultural and intellectual rather than economic. History is guided over the centuries by the ideas and beliefs of select luminaries, by the cultural waves they produce with their notions of what is good, true and beautiful, and through the disciplines they employ to propagate these beliefs such as philosophy, religion, literature and art. A secular society, like the one ours is becoming, attempts to build a culture devoid of its origins. That has always pointed to the slow, but inevitable death of the civilization. It has been almost a century (1922), since T.S. Eliot foresaw the horrors of a godless, secular society just around the corner (Hitler, Stalin, Mao), and warned in *The Wasteland*, "I think we are in rat's alley / Where the dead men lost their bones . . . We who were living are now dying." And again, in *The Hollow Men*, "We are the hollow men / We are the stuffed men / Leaning together / Headpiece filled with straw." The traditions that have propped up our culture over the past two millenia have deteriorated considerably since Eliot's dire warnings. Have we become a slowly expiring civilization?

Our ship slid gracefully into the port of Piraeus, but we never disembarked to visit Athens—that beautiful city which I was to visit many times later in my life. However, it was at Piraeus that about two dozen girls of marriageable age boarded the ship to come to the United States. They were traveling to join their fiancés or husbands in the U.S. military whom they had met probably close to the end of World War II. They were a wild and boisterous bunch in the prime of their life. American soldiers on oversees duty had probably met them on the beaches or in the villages or perhaps in the bars and alleys of Piraeus or Athens. The girls were mostly young and beautiful of face and body, and they paraded their assets on the ship decks every chance they got. I was in the midst of my puberty and didn't fail to admire those gifts of God to which poets dedicate their lyrics and composers their music.

After Piraeus, we stopped in Palermo to pick up more of those war brides going to New York. The Italian girls who came on board were Sicilians, no more or less beautiful than the Greeks, but considerably more modest in dress and behavior and appearing to be more serious about the promises they had made. There were no Sophia Lorens or Gina Lollobrigidas, yet they were quite pretty.

AMERICA

As we passed the Strait of Gibraltar and entered the Atlantic, the sea became tempestuous and unruly—sea-sickness set in. We were told that the turbulence was due to the Gulf Stream current and it was normal in that area of the Atlantic. The ship was swaying sideways and back and forth; and the nice spread of food on the dining table appeared to us unappetizing. We ate little for two days in a row. As we approached mid-Atlantic, the ship stopped at São Miguel in the Azores. The islands were lush green with abundant vegetation. Dad bought a Madeira hat and we ate lots of pineapples, the main produce of the island, and by the time the ship sailed toward New York, everybody had become more serene and tranquil. We had passed the stormy currents of the Gulf Stream and had recovered from our seasickness.

Three days later, when the Statue of Liberty came into view, we knew that we were about to enter New York Harbor. We disembarked with the rest of the passengers and were immediately taken to Ellis Island. All immigrants were taken there, even though in our case we were just passing through the United States on our way to Venezuela. It was my first contact with territorial America, and I found it disappointing to be corralled on that forsaken island. After all, we were known as "the Americans" in Lebanon, and my parents had already lived in Detroit, and had six American-born children. While still on board, we could see the New York City skyline, with the Chrysler and Empire State Buildings towering into the sky. There were no cubes (Twin Towers) then, and there aren't any now. Yet the original skyscrapers formed a magnificent sight, the likes of which I had never seen before. At last we had reached America, the continent my grandmother described as "the land of milk and honey" and "the land of plenty."

The two-day experience at Ellis Island brings to mind the many immigrant jokes I was to hear years later.

Q.: "Why are there so many Italians in New York named TONY?"
A.: "Because when they get on the boat in Genoa, so they won't get lost, they stamp on their forehead "TO N.Y.""

I heard this next one, years later in San Francisco: There lived a Chinese man in San Francisco's Chinatown called Isaac Greenberg. He got the name standing in the immigration line, waiting to be admitted. The officer asked the man ahead of him his name, and that man answered: "Isaac Greenberg." So, when the Chinese man moved up the line and the officer asked him his name, he simply replied, "Sam Ting." The officer heard "same thing," and registered him as "Isaac Greenberg."

But life was not so funny on Ellis Island. We were enclosed, so my first impression of the United States was that of a concentration camp. I had to sleep on a cot in the middle of a huge dormitory. There was lots of snoring, and some people would be talking aloud in their foreign tongues until midnight. On the positive side, I marveled at the plethora of American products in the canteen: Coca Cola, Pepsi Cola, Kraft Cheese, Kellogg's Corn Flakes, Raisin Bran, Philip Morris, Lucky Strike, the magazines *Time* and *Life, Fortune* and *Newsweek*. Such abundance of goods was mind-boggling. Products of various brands were piled up on the shelves everywhere, as high as the ceiling. I recalled what my grandmother Marzuka used to tell me about the prosperity and abundance in America. As a matter of fact, every time Tannous Farah (our neighbor in Serhel who had lived in Canada) would say "Vive le Canada!" Grandma would counter with "God Bless America!"

I remember in particular the many immigrants of varied features, colors, and costumes crowded in the Great Hall at Ellis Island. I said to myself, "What a mixture of people. Does this make up America?" And that was in the days when mostly Europeans came here, before the great influx of Southeast Asians, Latinos, Russian Jews, Yemeni Arabs, and various others.

There were a few permanent residents on the Island, working in the dining room or in the canteen. Most of these people had no country and no citizenship, and they were not wanted anywhere—neither back in their country of origin nor in America—so they were allowed to stay and work and live on Ellis Island. One man in particular, who worked the coffee stand, was from somewhere in Yugoslavia. I was told he spoke fourteen languages; I learned later that it was not unusual for Croats, Serbs, Lebanese, Jews, and Armenians to speak several languages. But fourteen languages! That was extraordinary. (It is said that James Joyce had some knowledge of seventeen languages; he included expressions from many of them in *Ulysses* and *Finnegan's Wake*, helping to make these books almost indecipherable.)

After three days on Ellis Island, we were shipped to New York. Mr. George Farah, a friend of Dad's and a long-time New York City resident, met us. For many years, his kind heart made him a one-man welcoming committee for the people coming from Serhel to New York. He was sincere in his concern, having experienced first hand the loneliness and bewilderment of arriving for the first time in a huge city. I remember Anis Simon (an elderly friend of ours in Stockton) telling us how upon arrival at Ellis Island he saw a shiny silver dollar on the sidewalk. He didn't pick it up, however. Instead, he kicked it in the gutter saying to himself, "I don't want anyone to think that I am in dire need. Besides, I'll find many more of these; they say the streets in America are lined with silver and gold." He then told me, "Unfortunately, it took me several weeks to find a job and earn my first silver dollar."

DETROIT

The next day, Mr. Farah took us to La Guardia Airport, from where we flew to Detroit to visit my brother Mike, my ailing sister Mary, and the many relatives from Serhel who were living there. It was an American Airlines silver plane that took us on a two-hour flight to Detroit. What a thrill it was to fly in an airplane for the first time!

The plane landed at Willow Run Airport in Detroit, where my eldest brother Mike met us with open arms. He immediately informed us that Mary was in the hospital with tuberculosis. He never informed us of this before hand, wanting to spare us the agony of worry. "Fortunately, they have just discovered a drug (streptomycin)," he said, "and after a regimen of shots of the miracle antibiotic, she is recovering now." She eventually survived the disease that had killed Khalil Gibran, his mother, and three of his siblings. (It had killed Chopin, Alfred de Musset, John Keats, Anton Chekov, Robert Louis Stevenson, Franz Kafka, the whole Bronte family, and many other great poets and artists in the prime of their creative life. In the nineteenth century it was known as the "romantic disease," but there was nothing romantic about it.)

We went straight from the airport to see Mary at Herman Kiefer Hospital. She was sitting in bed and looked as beautiful as ever. She not only survived, but went on to marry in Venezuela, and is still alive at the age of eighty. Yet Mary has always complained of having a "delicate" body—it was a term Mom often used when referring to both Mary and me. I've lived long enough in health and vigor to be able to laugh off Mom's description, thank God. I participate vigorously in athletic activities. Mary, on the other hand, has been unable to shake off those parental admonitions. In fact, she has never weighed over one hundred pounds. She is petite (five feet in height) and is always worried about her health, even though she is determined and capable in all other respects. Perhaps she never got over those dire warnings of childhood.

After going to the hospital, we went to stay with Shiben Courey, a cousin who owned a grocery store on Congress Street, not far from where Dad's grocery store was located in the 1920s. From there, Shiben took us to his new home in Grosse Pointe, an upscale suburb of Detroit. We stayed with the Coureys because Mike was dating their daughter, Irene, at that time. She was Mike's third cousin and future wife. The Coureys had a big house, and for two weeks we slept in what was formerly their daughters' room. Of their five daughters (Mae, Julia, Mabel, Irene, and Sharon), only the last two were still living at home at that time. All the others were already married and gone from the house. It was unbearably humid and hot that week, even though it was October. I didn't know yet about the extreme summer and winter temperatures prevalent in the continental climate of the Midwest. It was stifling, and it never cooled off at night. I disliked that climate for the whole twelve years I lived there (1950-62).

During the two weeks we stayed in the Detroit-Windsor area we visited my brother in his office several times. Dr. Michael Ziter is the name my brother uses. It was an erroneous spelling of Zeiter that was written on his original Canadian birth certificate. No one in the family paid attention to it until he returned to Canada; he became stuck with that registration and spelling. Marriage-wise, Mike was quite a catch. He was the golden boy of the Zeiter family. He was a shining light: well educated, impressively handsome, and he spoke several languages. And yet, he still had to court Irene for some time before winning her over. She was originally dating an accountant, she told me. I'm glad she never married him. She and I have become very close friends over the years.

I learned to respect my sister-in-law as a capable and honest you get-what-you-see person. She has mothered five excellent children. The whole younger generation of our family looks up to them as an example of well-brought-up progeny. The same could be said of Madelyn, my Brother Tony's wife, and Yvonne, Edmond's wife. Back in 1948, when I first met Irene, I knew very little about her. But her younger sister Sharon caught my eye. As Mike and Irene's marriage became a reality, everybody's eyes were on Sharon and me. But nothing ever came of it.

STAMP COLLECTING

At the Courey's grocery store on Congress Street. Irene gave me a gift for which I was very grateful. As the Coureys were still cleaning the attic of their previous house on Congress and Larned Streets (next to the store), she led me to a large box that contained thousands of stamped letters. I had told her the day before that I collected stamps. That gift was the start of my extensive collection of United States stamps. The letters belonged to her family from way back, but they were going to the dumpster now. I guess, a part of me was following in the footsteps of my mother's uncle, Philippe, who was the stamp dealer back in El Mina, Lebanon. I have continued collecting stamps to the present day.

With the newly found stamped letters to which Irene led me, I practiced a time-tested method of removing stamps from mailed envelopes without damaging them. I had learned from Uncle Philippe how to cut that part of the envelope surrounding the stamp; how to place the cut-off part in a flat water basin; and how long to wait before peeling the stamps from the envelope. Some of the stamps would separate themselves from the underlying paper and be floating on top of the water while still in the container. Sometimes the original glue on the back of a stamp would be saved if it was not left in the water too long. It was delightful to collect the stamps off envelopes. It is an accomplishment that is not enjoyed by those who routinely buy all their stamps from a dealer. To me, that is like shooting fish in a barrel; somehow devoid of the original fun of fishing.

II

EDUCATION AND CULTURE

CHAPTER 8

CARACAS

After visiting with Mary in the Detroit sanatorium, we boarded a plane that took us to Caracas—and two years of living in a semi-tropical, third-world country. It was a time when I grew mentally and emotionally as well as physically. Two years of experiences at school, coupled with daily interactions with newly found friends and a growing sense of personal self-esteem, led me to a higher awareness of myself and everything around me.

We were met at the airport by my brother Tony, who came with a chauffeur to take us to Caracas, higher up in the mountains via a treacherous road. The tropical vegetation was overwhelming in its vivid colors. As we ascended, we noticed the barrios of Venezuela's poor on the hills on both sides of the road. The situation of the poor has not changed in fifty years since then, except that the road from the airport is now a major eight-lane highway of which the affluent Venezuelans are proud. However, under the present ruler, Hugo Chavez, the squalor of the barrios and the misery of the poor are becoming a more pressing reality for the survival of the rich.

The school term had just started in Caracas, and I was enrolled in second-year *Bachillerato* (high school) at an elite academy run by the same order of Christian Brothers I had just left in Lebanon, except that here the school was called simply, "La Salle," after St. Jean Baptiste de La Salle, the order's French founder.

I soaked up knowledge and the new culture like a sponge. I soon learned that Spanish literature was just as varied and impressive as was France's or the Arab World's, which I had studied earlier. This realization did not stop there, for when I was studying in Canada two years later, I learned that English literature had as much right to that claim. I was becoming aware of the richness of all the world's literatures. In my Spanish literature class, I read Cervantes (*Don Quixote*), Tirso de Molina (the original creator of the universal character

Don Juan—the story of Mozart's *Don Giovanni*), Lope de Vega (the most prodigious dramatist ever, with 800 plays to his name), Calderon de la Barca (*La Vida es Sueno*, or "Life is a Dream"), Quevedo, and Gongora to name but a few. It helped that my father expected it from me. He didn't mistakenly feel as many parents do—that he was asking too much. He figured it would make a man out of me, a man who would have a universal knowledge and thus be better able to deal with adversity. He did it all with encouragement and sympathy, and he was right.

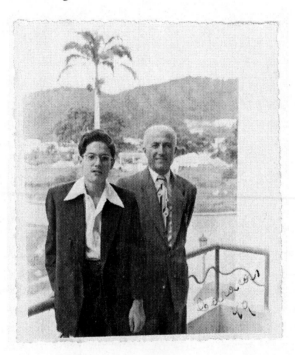

That's me, the studious, bespectacled one, with Dad, standing on the balcony of Tony's condo in Los Chaguaramos, Caracas. We had come from Lebanon five months before (in 1948), and I was in my fifth month of second-year *Bachillerato* with the Christian Brothers in Caracas.

Earlier, after we landed at Maiquetia, Caracas' airport, my brother Tony and his chauffeur drove us to Uncle Paul and Aunt Angela's house in an upscale area of Caracas. For eight months we lived all together in that house, until we moved from Uncle Paul's house to an apartment on the outskirts of town that Brother Tony had rented. My cousins Renee and Paulette were still quite young, ten and eleven respectively. I became their older friend and helped them learn how to ride a bicycle, even though I had trouble riding one myself.

Madelyn, my sister-in-law, was my second cousin. She was in the flower of youth, statuesque with bronze skin and an elegant posture. Her friendliness and her beauty warmed my heart. The last time I had seen her was when the Barkett family had left Lebanon for California ten years before. I was five and she was fifteen at that time.

Angela (Uncle Paul's wife) had come from a very large family. Her father was a kind, elderly man whom I got to know well. He had a small clothing store next to Uncle Paul's and my Brother Tony's large general store. I used to walk from school to Uncle Paul's store when classes were over in the afternoon. On the way I always passed through Plaza Bolívar which had a towering statue of Simón Bolívar, the Liberator, riding a huge horse in the middle of the square—every town or village in Venezuela is built around a square that has either a bust or an equestrian statue of *El Libertador*. I would stay around the store until my brother closed shop. Then he would drive me home allowing just enough time for supper and for me to finish my homework before bedtime.

I would often go next door to visit Angela's dad in his tiny store (an eight by twelve-foot cubicle). Years before, he and his brother were partners in a very successful wholesale business, Kimos Brothers. The firm was well known in Caracas. There were disagreements over running the business, however, after which my adopted older friend had a falling-out with his brother. He ended up with nothing to show for his share of the partnership. Tony told me that the older brother took advantage of Angela's father's kind nature and actually ripped him off, ending up with everything. The story impressed itself on my mind so much that later on in life, I never went into business with siblings or close relatives.

Angela had four sisters, all from Mr. Kimos's first marriage. His wife died when the children were young; so Mr. Kimos went back to Becharre, Lebanon, where he met a younger woman and got married a second time. In certain ways the story is similar to that of Dad marrying my mother after her sister had died. Mr. Kimos came back with his young wife to Caracas where she bore him six children of her own and took care of his five older children, besides.

This old man was trying to feed a dozen people from the meager profits of his small shop. Eventually, all of the children grew up and married well. When I was in Venezuela, his grandchildren would always be around Uncle Paul's family and we were all playmates. It is amazing how often I have met older men married to younger women. These marriages were quite successful because of the devotion and sacrifice of the younger spouse.

Mr. Kimos's marriage to Adele lasted until his death. As he got older, she cared for him; it was the one satisfaction in his life that gave him true happiness. He confided all this to me as we became close friends. It was a practice of mine to befriend older people ever since I was a child.

We stayed at Uncle Paul's house for about eight months. One Sunday morning in 1950, I was listening to music on the radio when, suddenly, the program was interrupted with an announcement that North Korea had just invaded South Korea. I remember that my brother Johnny was visiting us from Punto Fijo, where he worked with our other brother, Philip. The news and commentary about the conflict were followed by a memorable recording of the Tchaikovsky Violin Concerto. That was the first time I heard this musical jewel. I recall that my brother Johnny, who loved Tchaikovsky, made me kneel down on the floor as he raised his hand on top of my head, and made me swear that I would always consider Tchaikovsky the greatest composer who ever lived; and further, that if Tchaikovsky was a Communist in his day, so would I be one too! We both laughed at his enthusiasm. Thankfully for me, Tchaikovsky died of typhoid fever in 1893, twenty-four years before the Communist Revolution took place in 1917; so I didn't have to become a Communist.

ENCULTURATION

The Monday morning after our arrival to Caracas, my brother Tony took me to the school to register. The principal wanted to put me in first year. I said to Tony, "I've been in first year in Lebanon already; tell him to put me in second, and if I don't keep up with the class, he can always take me back to first." The principal smiled and I entered second year *Bachillerato*. It took me three weeks to be at the head of the class. We were handed report cards every week that had to be signed by the parents. Uncle Paul got the honor of signing them for the whole two years I was in Caracas. He was delighted to peruse my grades every week. He told me it gave him a lift. He had little formal education himself.

Going to school at the Christian Brothers' "Colegio de la Salle" was challenging. Two courses in particular impressed culture upon me. In second-year high school, we took World Literature, starting with the epics *Ramayana* and *Mahabarata* (including the *Bhagavad Gita*), the *Iliad* and the *Odyssey*, Virgil's *Aeneid*, Dante's *Divine Comedy*, and Camões *Lusiads*. We read Tasso and Ariosto, Milton, Goethe, Tolstoy, Tagore and others. The professor who taught this class was Rafael Caldera, a devout Catholic attorney in Caracas who volunteered his services and taught gratis. He eventually became Venezuela's president in the 1970s. The following year we took the History of Art, touching on Phidias, Praxiteles, Myron and Greek sculpture in general, and we continued our learning about the master painters all the way through the Renaissance and up to the Impressionists. I enjoyed the history and the illustrations the teacher showed us. That course gave me a permanent interest and love for painting, sculpture, and architecture.

Tony was very kind to me. He would give me a five-bolivar silver coin every now and then. I would put it in my pocket and treat all my schoolmates to sweets. La Salle was a big school of two thousand students, with a huge central courtyard surrounded by Ionic columns. In architectural design, it was similar to the Christian Brothers School I had attended in Tripoli.

I soon discovered that I was using the knowledge and courses of my first-year high school in Lebanon to a distinct advantage in my second-year high in Venezuela. As it turned out, the process continued when I came to North America two years later: I found out that what I had learned in my second and third year of high school in Caracas was being taught in fourth-year high school in the United States and Canada.

It was then that I realized that elementary and high school education in Canada and the United States was relatively poor at that time. But I found out later that undergraduate and post-graduate education in college in these countries rival the best in the world. The discrepancy between the poverty of primary and secondary education in North America, and the preeminence of university education in the same region, was puzzling to me. I could see that many students had difficulty when they reached college because they were poorly prepared in elementary and high school. (That is not always the case as I have grandchildren in high school right now taking college courses in their honor classes. Obviously, much depends on the individual student's motivation and on the interest that responsible parents take in their children's education.)

I already knew from personal experience what Allan Bloom of the University of Chicago was to write about many years later in his best seller *The Closing of the American Mind.* Bloom's thesis regarding the inadequacy of education in public schools in America documents the ignorance of incoming students, not only of basic grammar and math, but of the values of Western culture and art in general. Bloom particularly lamented the fact that in the last decade of his teaching career, (as opposed to prior decades), he could no longer find any students who had an ear for good music, having devoted their hearing exclusively to noisy trash and the screaming voices of untrained singers, devoid of any claim to good taste or musical talent.

I never had that problem thanks to the courses I took in high school in Lebanon and Venezuela, and to the great music I constantly listened to on cultural radio stations. Once I was given a taste of Western Civilization's history and culture in high school, I was spurred on to continue learning on my own. That kind of personal learning has cultivated in me a love for music, art, philosophy, history, and religion which have remained over the years a source of inspiration and joy in my life. It was such depth of culture and resulting artistic sensitivities that Allan Bloom was referring to in *The Closing of the American Mind.* In contrast, he referred to the students who entered his classes in the 1970s and 80s as either "business aspirants," or "technology automatons," describing at length their cultural ignorance and their undeveloped tastes. A love of excellence in life or in art had not been inculcated in them at an early age, neither at home nor at school.

As early as 1932, Jose Ortega y Gasset in his *Revolt of the Masses* and in his *Dehumanization of Art* treated in depth of the *mass man*'s brutish interests and emotions. He compared the common man to "a buoy, floating on the surface of the current," without a mind or will of his own, with the result that he is easily manipulated by propaganda, slogans, and suggestions coming from outside of himself (radio, TV, movies, editorials, and the rest).

Earlier yet, Alexis de Tocqueville predicted that all this would probably come to be the ultimate result of republican democracy— what we see now as a sort of dumbing down of the citizens' minds into a pseudo-democratic, multicultural, technological model, devoid of higher spiritual aspirations. He wrote, in 1831,

> I see an innumerable multitude of men [the masses], alike and equal, constantly circling in pursuit of the petty and banal pleasures with which they glut their souls . . . Subjection to petty affairs is manifest daily and touches all citizens indiscriminately . . . This continuously thwarts them, and leads them to give up using their free will . . . Over these kinds of men stands an immense, protective power which is alone responsible for securing their enjoyment, and, fatherlike, tries to keep them in perpetual childhood. It aims to see the citizens enjoy themselves, provided they think of nothing else but enjoyment [fun!] . . . Why should it not entirely relieve them from the trouble of thinking at all?

The philosophical and social essays of Hilaire Belloc, G.K. Chesterton, Christopher Dawson, T.S. Eliot, Berdeyev, Santayana, C.S. Lewis, and many, many others in the past century, have also treated amply of this same subject, and all of these authors came to Allan Bloom's conclusions, long before him. I thank God for the teachers, the books, and the traditional style of education that taught me the philosophy of history and culture. In addition, traditional education taught me respect for my elders and the great achievements of the past.

In those days in Caracas, access to serious music was mostly through radio broadcasts. Television and its hoopla had not yet entered the culture of the West. Television in its early days, though, was a great sponsor of live classical concerts and other culturally informative programs. In those early days of TV, it appeared as though the new medium would be used for education, and for improving the *mass man's* taste. Alas, that was before commercialism and advertising drowned the preeminence of culture during television's broadcasting hours! Once the masses were targeted for exploitation, all hope for the role of television in inculcating education or culture was lost. The masses clamor for instant gratification and for what is lowest in human aspirations, and television's commercial sponsors flooded them with their hearts' desires.

Fortunately, what added to my acute awareness of beauty and art while I was reaching maturity was the accessibility of Radio Diffusion Nacional de Venezuela, the public education station in Caracas. I constantly had that station on at home, whether I was studying or resting. These stations are still on the air in every city in America, under the aegis of Public Education radio or television. In Caracas, I would also hear my brother Philip play the violin, and the whole family's interest in art and serious music influenced me in those early years of my life. I learned about Mozart, Haydn, and Beethoven. I went to free concerts on Sunday mornings at the "Teatro Municipal" in the "Centro" (downtown). I remember particularly hearing Sergiu Celibidache conduct a vibrant Beethoven Fifth Symphony, and I heard Nicanor Zabaleta, the greatest harpist of his time, and Pablo Casals, the "poet of the cello." Celibidache passed away in 2003 at the ripe old age of 98. The longevity of conductors and soloists is legendary. I was still listening to Toscanini conduct when he was eighty-five and Arthur Rubinstein, the pianist, lived into his nineties. The few symphony conductors, who die early, such as Guido Cantelli or Giuseppe Sinopoli, die in an accident. Maybe all the waving of the arms by conductors, or the pounding on the piano by powerful pianists, is good cardiac exercise?

MY FRIEND, BRAHMS

I remember Venezuela mostly for my incipient love of Johannes Brahms. I can still picture the evening when I first heard his Second Symphony. The windows of our apartment were wide open, since the weather is so beautiful in Caracas all year. Hannah, our teenage maid from Lebanon, was playing the coquette. We would chat and tease each other when Tony and Madelyn and Mom and Dad were gone visiting in the evenings, which was often.

I was trading remarks with Hannah when twenty minutes into Brahms' Second Symphony on the radio, I was struck by the main theme at the beginning of the second movement. I stopped everything and asked Hannah to listen attentively to the music with me. I slowly began to realize how opulent and majestic, and full of substance Brahms's music is. It is more melodious than Haydn's, has longer passages for the strings than Mozart's, and is more subdued than Beethoven's. I tried to explain all this to poor Hannah, who understood nothing of my excitement.

As time went on I started paying closer attention to Brahms. Next, I heard the Second Piano Concerto. Many years later, my wife and I, and all four of our children adopted the melody of the initial call of the French horns as "our song." I heard, in turn, the Violin Concerto, the Fourth and—oh!—finally, the First Symphony entered my life. What majestic, ponderous, noble and purely abstract artistry. Twenty years of working on it elapsed before Brahms was satisfied enough to publish it, because he lived in the shadow of Beethoven and didn't want to publish anything less worthy than the master's Ninth Symphony.

Three years passed before I first heard Brahms' Third Symphony. I was already in Canada. I recall vividly that I was sitting in my Brother Mike's car, waiting for him to return from a house call. We were parked next to a wheat field close to San Joaquin, a little town in Essex County, Ontario, Canada. It was the Sunday New York Philharmonic broadcast at 3:00 P.M. which I listened to religiously every week. The conductor was the fabled Dimitri Mitropoulos. I almost swooned on hearing the second movement with its long, soaring string passages. I kept looking at the wheat field flailing in the wind under the clear blue sky as the music was going on. Mike was still inside the patient's house finishing his call when the final movement came, with the passage that sounds like the opening four notes of Beethoven's Fifth. I fell in love with that Brahms symphony more than any other.

In my imaginative recall, I have combined the memory of the field of wheat flailing in the wind and the white sun-drenched steeple of the San Joaquin church across the field with the beauty of the music. The joy of that particular group of events, years ago, still reverberates in my heart whenever I listen to that symphony or think of it. We describe Beethoven's music as titanic, Bach's as devoutly religious, Mozart's as simultaneously tragic and comic, superficial and deep, Schubert's as melodious, Tchaikovsky's as sad and Russian, and Wagner's as epic and German. But the term for Brahms's music is majestic.

It was a term I got exposed to many years later when I was attending a rehearsal of the Stockton Symphony Orchestra. Peter Jaffe, the conductor, was having the orchestra go over (again and again) a delicate passage of Brahms' Second Piano Concerto, when suddenly, Audrey Andrist, a former Conservatory of the Pacific professor of piano, sitting next to me exclaimed, "How majestic!" "Eureka!" I said to Audrey in response. "That's the term I've been looking for, for over forty years!"

And yet, it is Haydn and Mozart who remind me of Venezuela, because the radio station played these two composers the most. To this day, certain pieces of music have the stamp of places I've been to in my life. Haydn's "Surprise Symphony," the "Military" and the "Drum Roll," bring various Caracas scenes back to mind. In Lebanon, Arabic music is almost always sung, far from the abstract and well-developed music of Mozart or Brahms, to say nothing of Bruckner or Mahler. All in all, Venezuela was a fruitful experience for me, musically and culturally. ·

I have always proselytized on behalf of classical music, just as a religious missionary would preach the good news, because I firmly believe that great art and sublime music are divinely inspired and spiritually uplifting. For this reason, I find great satisfaction in sharing artistic and musical experiences. They lead to the love of Beauty and, as a consequence, to the love of God.

A NATION RELAXED

While we lived in Caracas, my sister Mary and my brother Philip lived in Punto Fijo, a city of several oil refineries built in the 1940s when oil was discovered in Venezuela. They owned a general store there and lived in the American compound run by one of the oil companies. I visited them several times there. Life in Punto Fijo was akin to life in the Old West. It was a wild place with immigrants from all nations, particularly Portuguese, Lebanese, Columbians, and Italians. The discovery of petroleum attracted many adventurers and seekers of fortune, just as gold did in California in 1849, a hundred years before. We drank beer and "Green Spot," an orange drink, because the water was undrinkable. The weather was hot, but dry, and we would go swimming in the afternoons in the Caribbean. It was eternal summer and sunshine.

Madelyn and Tony went to California that summer to visit Madelyn's family, so I stayed in Caracas with Mom and Dad and the young maid. I was carefree at play, but intense in my studies.

Living in a subtropical country was exciting. I used to travel inland with Uncle Paul or with other relatives who went there to collect money owed them from previous sales. The interior, called *llano*, was unspoiled and sparsely populated at that time, with hot days and humid nights. The vegetation was lush everywhere with myriads of flowering trees and all kinds of insects and creeping things. The people were down to earth and unspoiled. I have always wondered on those trips to the llanos, the hinterland—what Australians would have called the *outback*—whether the inhabitants ever worked at all.

From the windows of our traveling wagon, we would see them sitting around in front of their humble adobe homes, watching the people and the traffic go by. Many could be seen sleeping in their hammocks in mid-afternoon as if the heat and humidity had sucked out of them all their energy. Once or twice I have actually seen a person sleeping on his belly on the horizontal branch of a tropical tree, with arms and legs hanging limp on either side of the branch, in total languor—just as in a jungle movie the lions, panthers, and other big cats are seen sleeping on a tree branch in the oppressive heat, with listless paws hanging on either side of them.

In the Venezuelan interior there was no formal education for the young in those villages and everyone wore simple clothes—no coats, no fancy shoes, and never any ties. Even in the capital, shirts were invariably white and sleeveless, rarely colored as seen in Hawaii or South East Asia. As a matter of fact, I still keep a school yearbook from my Caracas days. It contains a 1949 photo that shows all of the students in the class picture wearing dark jackets over white shirts; quite a few (12 out of 32) are wearing the lapels wide open. The dark jackets and the ties were worn by a number of the classmates only for the occasion of the class photo. During regular class, it was an open white shirt and dark pants. Indeed, Venezuela had a relaxed way of life.

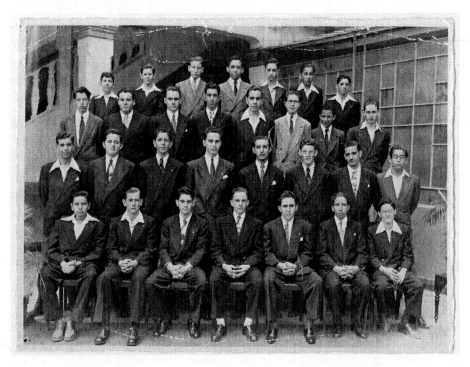

1950 Portrait of the honor students in second year *Bachillerato*, at the *Colegio de la Salle,* in Caracas—I am seated in the front row on the extreme right.

CHAPTER 9

CANADA

After two years in Venezuela, Dad decided that we should go to Canada to be next to my brother Dr. Mike. For one thing, he missed the absence of seasons. The weather in Caracas itself was much milder than that in the interior of Venezuela. Caracas was built high on a plateau, surrounded by high mountains, with spring-like weather all year. The Spanish Conquistadores built their capitals in the Americas on high plateaus, thus compensating for the semitropical latitude by high altitude. Mexico City was built 7,500 feet above sea level; Caracas, 3,000; Bogotá, 8,500; Quito, 10,500; and La Paz, an incredible 12,000 feet above sea level, making it the highest large city in the world. After a few years in Caracas, one got tired of this unchangeable weather and lost track of the seasons. It was a beautiful climate, but the same all year round. Like happiness and peace, unless they occasionally alternate with a little turmoil and vexation, one grows tired of them. Variety is the spice of life. Thus, in spite of the weekend birthday parties with piñatas and the multiple weddings and anniversaries we were invited to, Dad got tired of all the fanfare and the unchangeable weather. The same social whirl went on and on, with no variation to excite his mind. Mom, on the other hand, was always happy living in warm and sunny climates.

After the summer break, following two years of restless social activity, Dad said to me, "How would you like to go to your brother Mike in Canada, since the school year is about to begin over there." It was September 1950. Dad reassured Mom and me by promising, "We will follow you there soon." He bought me a Pan American Airways one-way ticket to Windsor, Ontario, with transit through New York City.

These were the days of paranoid McCarthyism in the States, when the McCarran Immigration Act, named after the Senator from Nevada, was passed by Congress. It was named the Internal Security Act of 1950. This act effectively changed the four-hundred-year policy of almost unlimited immigration to the United States. No more, "Send to my shores your poor and persecuted, and I will care for them." The implications were severe even in the area of transit through the Continental United States. Everybody was considered a Communist until proven otherwise, including a sixteen-year-old youth who was merely passing through New York.

I had been ticketed to fly to Windsor after landing in New York, all arranged by Pan American Airlines. I was to depart New York within one hour after arrival there, without having to leave the same wing of La Guardia International Airport. But, U.S. immigration would not let me pass in transit without a U.S. visa stamped on my passport. "But I am not even staying here," I said. "Sorry, it's the law," I was told. So, Mr. Lombardi, Vice President of Pan American Airlines at the time, came to the airport from the head office of PAA in Manhattan to see what could be done to allow this frightened youngster to go through. It was actually embarrassing to Pan Am because their ticket office in Caracas was the agency that told my father that an American visa was not required for passing through the USA in transit.

While Mr. Lombardi was investigating what could be done, the Immigration Service kept my passport as security and gave me free rein to visit Manhattan for five days. How odd! I could not go through in transit, and yet they let me stay in New York City itself. I visited the Metropolitan Museum of Art and I attended a New York Philharmonic concert with Dimitri Mitropoulos, conductor, and another one with the NBC Symphony (the fabled Toscanini conducting). I could go anywhere I wanted without an escort or guard. A contradiction! A paradox! An oxymoron! Call it what you will, the whole thing didn't make any sense. But staying in a large hotel paid for by Pan American and frolicking around in the "World's Biggest City" in those days was the most fun I had ever had.

I attended a Robert Taylor and Orson Welles movie called *The Fox*, or something of the sort. Welles' played Cesare Borgia, portraying him as a capable, but sly and ruthless, prince. In those days, I had not yet read Machiavelli's *The Prince*, a political analysis based on the rule of Cesare Borgia. When we analyzed *The Prince* three years later in a college history class in Canada, I kept on thinking of the Orson Welles movie and of all my adventures in New York City.

On the fifth day, Mr. Lombardi gave me the bad news: U.S. Immigration would not let me continue to Canada without a visa, no matter what! Their whole position was rigid and illogical and left me with a permanent distaste for the U.S. Immigration Service. What risk would there have been from a sixteen-year-old youth who was not staying in the country, only passing through, not even leaving the airport? In those days, international terrorism and/or plane hijacking was unheard of. Their attitude could not have been blamed on that, as it might be today.

Thus, when my problem proved insoluble, I was put on a Pan American flight and sent back to Caracas. I recall having an overnight stop in Curaçao, in the Dutch Antilles, where again I passed the evening at the movies. When I arrived in Caracas, Mom told Dad, "You see, God does not want Henry to be away from us." Dad's reply was, "He is going out of this country, regardless of all these impediments. There is no future for him here. Over there in Canada, he will study and look to a bright future alongside his oldest brother Mike, who will take care of him until we get there."

Dad solved the impasse by purchasing a one-way ticket for a flight on KLM from Caracas directly to Montreal, bypassing the United States altogether. Pan Am begged him to get a visa and send me back the same way, through New York, but to no avail. Dad told them, "No way! The American authorities will probably find something wrong with the visa; so we can't trust their motives anymore, can we?"

He forced Pan Am to pay for the KLM flight when they initially didn't want to. He was tough and would not yield. He was my hero! I arrived in Montreal and took an Air Canada flight from Montreal to Kingston, to Toronto, to London, Ontario, and finally to Windsor. I guess this must have been that airline's milk route. But when I arrived nobody was waiting for me at the Windsor Airport. Edmond and Mike had waited for three hours the prior week, when I was flying on Pan Am, but I never arrived. I guess once was enough for them.

Promptly, I took a taxi to Mike and Irene's house on Rossini Avenue in East Windsor. Edmond was alone at the house—our first reunion after several years. The taxi driver blew the horn in front of the house to see if we were in the right place, and Edmond came out of the front door wearing a sleeveless undershirt and shorts; he always wore those undershirts on hot summer days. After the usual hugs and kisses, Edmond uttered a phrase that I was to hear again and again every hot summer day for the next forty years. "Henry," he said, "it is so hot, you could fry a pair of eggs on the sidewalk."

I was to hear him repeat that expression with gusto on hot days over the next four decades that we lived near each other, first in Windsor and later in Stockton. Edmond paid special attention to the breaking of records, whether they were baseball records, football records, high or low temperature records or any others. When we went into the house he asked me, "What are you going to do in Windsor?"

I said, "I'm going to be a student, of course" pronouncing the *u* as in "stud" or "mud" (as an "*a*" is pronounced in Latin or the Romance languages).

He corrected me, "You don't pronounce the *u* in student like a Latin *a*. You pronounce it as a Latin *i* followed by a Latin *u*, like in 'mule' or 'mutant,' but you could also pronounce it like a simple Latin *u*, as in 'rule.'"

"But why isn't *student* pronounced like stud or mud," I complained to him.

"Who knows?" he said to me, "It's a crazy language! But be patient, you'll learn it." *Que locura!* (Good grief!) I said to him in Spanish and continued for a while speaking to him in the Spanish and Arabic languages where vowels are always pronounced the same way, no matter where they occur in a word. And yet, in spite of that, I proceeded to learn English in short order, eventually majoring in Honors English and History in College. Yet after fifty years, I still have a slight accent when speaking English, whereas in Spanish, French, Italian, Latin or Arabic, I don't have one.

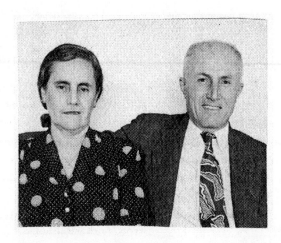

Badwyeh and Yousef Zeiter (Mom and Dad) both aged 57 in 1950.

ASSUMPTION HIGH SCHOOL

After I put my bags away, Edmond told me that Mike was visiting Hosen and Mary, his wife's uncle and aunt. We got in the car and drove two miles, so I could see Mike, Irene, and their first baby Michael, who was three months old at the time. The next day, Mike took me to Assumption High School to help me register in fourth-year, even though classes had already started the previous week—my delay by U.S. Immigration made sure of that. We met

Father Brown, the principal, and the same thing that happened in Venezuela took place here. He wanted to place me in third year, which he thought would be easier, to give me a chance to learn English. It was *déjà vu* all over again. I whispered to Mike in French, "They wanted to do the same thing to me in Venezuela but I didn't let them. Please tell him to put me in fourth, and if in one month I'm not keeping up with the class he can take me back to third year."

The priest smiled and said, "Okay." He understood French. Within a month, I was the top student in a fourth year class of about 200 male students. The school was run by the Basilian order, so it was the first time since first grade that I was not in a Christian Brothers school.

My parents were still in Venezuela living with Tony and Madelyn, and they were close to where Uncle Paul lived. (To this day, Uncle's progeny are still in Venezuela, except for his oldest son, Pablo, who lives in Stockton, California.) My first eight months in Canada were spent with Edmond at Mike and Irene's on Rossini Avenue, Windsor.

A novel sight to me was the Corner Soda Fountain about three houses away from Mike's. I would go there after school, sit on one of the high stools, and order a chocolate sundae just like the one my mother used to buy me after school in Lebanon. The minute I tasted the first bite, I would picture myself with Mom at the deli we used to go to in Tripoli. To this day, chocolate sundaes remind me of Mom picking me up from school and taking me to the deli to have ice cream. I am even reminded of the route we used to take back home, passing by Aunt Philomena's apartment on a sunny Mediterranean afternoon and the sweet smell of the orange blossoms in Mr. Harb's backyard by the alley we took as a shortcut. At times (during such recalls), I can even smell the perfume Mom used to wear.

School was going well at Assumption High during my first year in Canada. I found the Canadian students kind, caring, and *polite*—a word hardly mentioned nowadays. There was a world of difference in their attitude (from that of the native-born Venezuelans) towards immigrants. In Venezuela the natives disdained the recently arrived by calling them "Musiu," a derogative term derived from the French "Monsieur," which to them meant "foreigner." As a matter of fact, because of the preponderance of mestizos and mulattos in the general population, they called anyone who was clearly white-skinned a "Musiu." In Windsor, I would take the bus from the corner of Rossini and transfer at Pilette Avenue (next to the Chrysler plant with the smoke stacks) to a bus that would take me the rest of the way to school. Edmond would take the same first bus and then transfer to one going to the Windsor Detroit Tunnel. There he would board the Tunnel bus and then transfer to one that would take him to Wayne State University in downtown Detroit, where he was finishing his studies in pharmacy.

BROTHER EDMOND

Edmond was friendly with everybody, a trait his sons Eddie and André inherited. Eddie, in particular, has taken this trait to perfection. After studying chiropractic in the Bay Area, he came back to Stockton and befriended both the relatives and, literally, the rest of the city. His gregarious personality has propelled him to great success both financially and socially in his chosen field. He even inherited my brother Edmond's philosophic bent and his passionate love for serious music. I treasure that in him. Often when I see him, I see my brother in him. The power of genetics never ceases to amaze me.

My brother Edmond always befriended the bus drivers while in Windsor. He would chat with them while riding along. I was surprised one day when Cliff, one of the drivers, loudly called Edmond from the bus stop across the street: "Hey! Edmond! Thanks for the tip on the Brahms First Piano Concerto," he shouted. "The first beat of the orchestra threw me for a loop. I almost fell from my chair. It was glorious! Thanks again!"

I thought to myself "Wow! I'll have to hear this First Concerto. Good for you Edmond," I thought, "for trying to help people become cultured." Both of us were forever proselytizing for converts to classical music, much more than we were doing it for our church. We believed that the appreciation and enjoyment of sublime music was one of the shortest ways to God. After school, I would reverse the bus route on the way back home. I would have for companions Charlie Parent, Ed Browell, or Bob Kennedy, since we all lived around the same area of town. We had all become close friends. During the spring of 1951 our discussions were reaching such an elevated cultural level— so we thought, full of youthful zest—that we decided to hold regular meetings and called ourselves "The New Renaissance Club!" Youthful enthusiasm has no bounds! We kept that name for several years. Literature, philosophy, history, and politics were discussed into the wee hours of the morning. What would I give for those carefree days to return!

Late one afternoon, Bob Kennedy introduced me to Barbara Craig. It was a beautiful spring evening, and we were getting tired of our "New Renaissance" talk, so Bob suggested we go to the Craig home. I had not met Barbara, but I knew her brother Bill, who eventually went on to Ottawa Medical School. On entering I was introduced to the father, who was sitting in the family room drinking a beer. We sat down with him to visit. While we were talking we could hear the notes of Brahms's Second Piano Concerto (my favorite) coming from the adjoining room. The father informed us that his daughter was practicing for a concert she was performing the following week with the Windsor Symphony Orchestra. Wow! I thought to myself. I had not expected such an advanced level of piano playing. I didn't even know that Bill had a sister, let alone one who could tackle such an extraordinarily difficult piano work with such expertise.

We moved over to the other room and watched her play for a while. Her hair was flaming red, shining in the setting sunlight coming from the open window, and she had freckles on her face, like a true redhead. She was kind enough to let us stay in the room while she was practicing, and soon we all became friends. There was no private dating within that group, so I never took her out as such. But I was attracted to her looks and saw her often since she liked playing the piano for me. We were about the same age, and she came once or twice to our "New Renaissance Club" discussions. However, shortly after the summer passed, she left town to study in some conservatory and our paths never crossed again. I'll always remember her long, natural red hair moving to and fro as she furiously played the piano.

While at Assumption, I would come home from school in the afternoon and find my sister-in-law Irene at home. We would sit in the small breakfast nook with one or two of her neighbors who were in the habit of visiting in late afternoon. One of my strongest memories from those days was sipping coffee with the ladies in the dinette and gazing at our backyard and the yard beyond, a distance of about three hundred feet. The exact image has persisted in my memory—an ordinary scene but for the extraordinary light. It was afternoon in autumn, and the orange rays of the setting sun were gloriously reflected on the leafless tree trunks and their naked branches in the yard. The long shadows of the tree trunks stretched over the multicolored fallen leaves. I would be making a few comments to the ladies now and then, yet hardly listening to their small talk, my eyes fixed on the *chiaroscuro* scene outside the kitchen window. The aura of the setting sun has always been for me the loveliest part of the whole day.

That ordinary scene transports me back to my childhood in Lebanon, when I would be fascinated with the colors of sunset—not only those in the sky over the setting sun, but also the alpenglow on the mountain crests, even the gold on the wall of my bedroom in Serhel, where the sunlight would be reflected pinkish-orange, and then would move higher and higher on the wall until it disappeared. The lingering and yet fast disappearing final sunrays have always symbolized for me the autumn of life. O, the romantically sweet melancholy of it all! I was an inveterate romantic, and now I find myself exactly in those sunset years! I still appreciate the fading sunlight on the wall of my room at home—perhaps even more than before. And during the fall and spring seasons, I often focus my eyes on the rising reflection of the last sunrays on the mountains around Lake Tahoe, half in a dream world, mesmerized, until the final pink of the alpenglow disappears over the crests of the Sierra Nevada. The conjunction of all these beloved symbols over time has preserved, in a special romantic place in my imagination, that otherwise particularly common scene of Irene's sunlit backyard.

Irene would send the ladies home and start supper before Dr. Mike came home. In those days, I had little Michael to play with. One evening, Mike and Irene went to the movies and Edmond was studying at the pharmacy school library, so I stayed home to baby-sit little Michael. He woke up and started crying and he wouldn't stop nor go back to sleep. I was desperately trying to calm him down, so I wrapped a towel over my head and made it look like a babushka. He thought I was his mother and peacefully went back to sleep. As life would have it, at that very moment Mike and Irene returned, and were puzzled to see me looking like an old woman with the pseudo-babushka around my head and neck.

Big brother Edmond, the future pharmacist, I remember, would use me to quiz him from a prepared list of definitions of medicines and herbs, for his pharmacognosy tests (the course that dealt with the origins of natural drugs). I would ask him from a list he gave me: "What is ipecac? What is morphine? What is heroin?"

Edmond would reply, "It is the dried powdered extract of the red root of this or that plant," or "It is an extract of the opium plant," or "It is a derivative (digitalis) from the foxglove plant and improves the contraction of the heart muscle."

Edmond was very good at school, especially after he had left behind his playboy years at the University of California in Berkeley. Here he was under the watchful eye of his older brother, Mike—the doctor who was respected by the whole extended family. Years later, my mother-in-law Harriet informed us that she learned at the bridge table, from one of Edmond's pharmacy professors, that he was "the brightest student that Wayne Pharmacy School had seen in years."

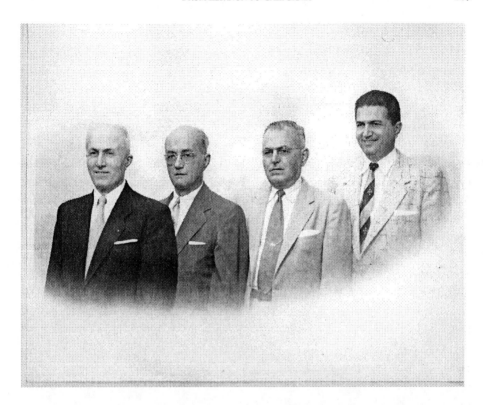

Dad and his brothers circa 1954 (l. to r.): Yousef (Joe), Ass'ad (Mike), Tannous (Anthony) and Boulos (Paul, later Pablo)

DR. MIKE

My other brother, Dr. Mike, was a sterling example to follow for his children, all of whom became physicians or specialists in medicine and other paramedical professions. He was always thought of as the golden boy, particularly by Dad. Mike practiced family medicine, which in those days meant general practice, obstetrics, and all kinds of common surgeries like tonsillectomies, appendectomies, hernia repair, and so on. He wanted to specialize in general surgery when he came to Canada after World War II, but all the veterans returning from the war had the first pick of the available fellowships. So, after two years of training in medicine and surgery, he settled into practice with a Dr. George G. George.

Three years later Mike left Dr. George and started his own practice. When I lived with him and Irene, he was frequently out of the house making night calls and late hospital rounds and would often come home quite late. Edmond and I would baby-sit little Michael whenever Irene went out shopping or visiting neighbors. Little Michael grew up to become a surgeon, along with Mike's two other sons, Paul and Dale. I once asked Mike how was it that all his children ended up with a medical career, including the two daughters, one a pharmacist and the other a physiotherapist? He told me that, as they were growing up, he would take them with him to the hospital on Saturday and Sunday morning rounds, and during summer vacation he had them answer the phone in his office. Besides, he told me that he would often challenge them to name any profession which was nobler, more satisfying, or more helpful to their fellow human beings than medicine, and their answer was always in favor of medicine.

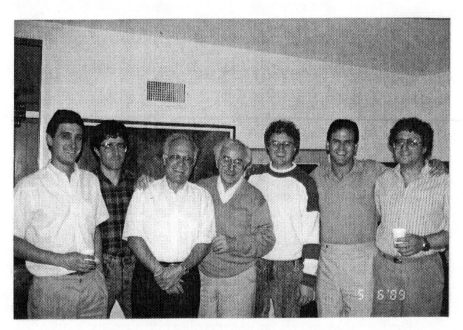

The seven MDs (so far!) among the progeny of Yousef Zeiter: (l. to r.), Drs. John Henry, Dale, Henry, Mike, Paul, Joe, and Michael. Dr. Joe's son is presently at Wayne State Medical School and John Henry Jr. is certain that he too will become an ophthalmologist to keep Zeiter Eye going.

Twenty years before his children were old enough to decide on medicine, Mike had me work in his office every summer, answering the phone or doing errands. It provided me with pocket money, even though he told me later in life that he would have given me the spending money anyway, since I was his "youngest brother," whom he "loved dearly;" he wanted to make sure I emulated him and went into medicine by having had the experience of working in a medical office. Mike was always kind to me, and after my internship he advised me to specialize (so as not to have too many night calls), even though he had a busy practice and was in need of a younger partner at the time. Many times he told me, "My dear little brother, you have the grades to go on and specialize, and the four years you'll spend doing that will pass in the blink of an eye, before you know what's happened." Mike had Dad's wisdom drilled into him, and this made it easier for me to listen to him and heed his advice.

STUDIES AND DATING

Seven months after I arrived in Windsor, Mom and Dad came from Caracas to Canada. That was in May of 1951, just before I graduated from high school. I remember explaining to Dad why I had to take a girl to the prom. He was set against it. "You're not old enough; you're not prepared," he said.

He was right about the preparation. I had never dated before; it was simply not done in Lebanon or Venezuela. I had never danced before, either, but one could learn how to dance. I insisted on going—not that I cared about the prom, but because I was going to take beautiful Beverly Malach, the daughter of one of the women who used to sit with me and Irene at the kitchen table in the late afternoons.

Well, Beverly was beautiful. Besides, she was tall for her age; she looked sixteen or seventeen, when she was only thirteen. She was still in eighth grade. No other high school graduate would take such a young girl to the prom. But Beverly was physically mature and looked older.

My brother Mike finally convinced Dad to let me take Beverly to the prom. Actually, he got mad at him for being so old-fashioned. So I went to the prom and Beverly was a knockout. We never revealed her age. She had the looks of Virginia Mayo, the Hollywood actress who was in several movies with Ronald Reagan. Ever since my Caracas days, I loved Virginia Mayo movies. I went to most of them. To me, she was better looking than Betty Grable. She was, in fact, my all-American girl: blonde and blue-eyed with a fair complexion and sparkling eyes.

UNCLE PAUL'S DAUGHTERS

In those days, dating patterns were different in various countries. I have an article in front of me from the March 21, 1962, edition of the *Windsor Daily Star*, courtesy of my brother Tony who saves these things. It describes an interview with four South American girls who were attending Windsor's Saint Mary's Academy in 1962; that was eleven years after I had asked Dad to let me go to the prom with Beverly. Interestingly enough, the article included the photos of two of the young ladies interviewed; they were my two cousins Renée and Paulette Zeiter (daughters of Uncle Paul). The interview will save me a lot of explaining about the dating habits that we were brought up with, and the social and cultural mores in those days. The article also contains references about education overseas which parallel my experience while in Lebanese and Venezuelan schools. Here are selected parts of the interview, including the short introduction by the reporter:

Windsor Daily Star, March 21, 1962

In Mexico and Venezuela a girl does not go to a dance until she is at least 15. And from then until the day she marries she never has a date without being accompanied by a third person or another couple. No matter how strict this may appear, four Latin American girls interviewed recently would not have it otherwise. The four, now students at St. Mary's Academy, were asked their opinions of Canadian and American girls. Two of the girls are of Lebanese parentage but were born and raised in Caracas. They are Renée Zeiter, 18, and her sister Paulette, 16. The others, Claudia Escalante, 15, and Alicia Pineda, 14, are from Mexico City. Here are the questions they were asked and the answers they gave.

Q— What do you think of Canadian education and students?
Claudia: "We learn more in our schools in one or two years than you do in all four. We have as many as thirteen subjects in any one year."
Paulette: "Students here know very little about painting, sculpture and music. You mention J. S. Bach or Leonardo da Vinci and they don't know what you're talking about.

	To make things worse, they are even more ignorant of world geography and history."
Q—	What surprised you most in the way teenagers live in Canada?
Claudia:	"Teenagers have too much freedom here."
Renée:	"I find there is not enough childhood and I see a crazy adolescence. A 13-year-old girl in Caracas is still a child. She wouldn't think of twisting, having a steady boyfriend or even curling her hair. A girl that age would be home studying, for one thing. There is too much of a rush for everything here."
Alicia:	"Many girls here are already bored with life when they reach 19 or 20."
Q—	What customs are followed among girls in Latin America?
Renée:	"A girl goes to her first dance when she is 15 or over. The first dance always goes to her father."
Paulette:	"A girl is never alone with her boy friend until the day they walk out of the church as husband and wife."
Claudia:	"And the boys prefer it that way. When they marry they know the girl has not been lewd and experimented with everybody in school. We usually double date, or several couples go out together."

These remarks, coming from Renée, Paulette, and Claudia in 1957, describe the way we were all brought up, and explain why it is that I mention time and again that free and easy dating was not a common practice where I grew up. This may also explain, in part, my timidity at being forward with Beverly, Barbara, Penny, or any other girl I met or liked.

WINDSOR BREEZE

Graduation was the day after the prom. Father Brown, the principal, singled me out for a special prize. He told the assembled crowd, "This student next to me came from South America while fourth year was already in progress; his first exposure to the English language, which he barely knew, was Shakespeare's *Romeo and Juliet*; and later in the year *Hamlet*; would you believe he ended up first in his English literature class?" . . . Applause . . . My father and my brother

Mike were sitting high in their chairs like two peacocks. Father Brown had stood up in front of all our Windsor and Detroit acquaintances announcing this—a big, big thing for a proud Lebanese immigrant family. Father Brown went on to mention how he wanted to put me in third year but I insisted on entering fourth year. He said that he was glad I didn't ask him to be in first-year College, because he would have missed "the opportunity to meet such an outstanding student who was able to adjust so rapidly and assimilate a different culture than his own." When he said that, Dad puffed up even more as he sat in the front row of the guests. I was afraid he was going to burst like the bullfrog that wanted to be as big as a bull in Aesop's fable.

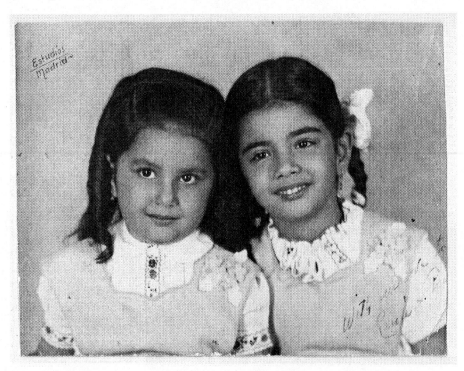

Photo of Cousins Paulette and Renée Zeiter taken when I first arrived in Caracas in 1948

Those four years separating elementary school in Lebanon from high school graduation in Canada seem to me now like an eternity; I had lived in three countries and learned their languages in those four years. This is another example of how slowly time grinds on in our youth, and how fast it seems to pass as we get older. Someone has claimed that we compare present lapses of time with the years of our life that have gone by; in other words, relatively speaking, a lapse of one year is like an eternity to a one-year-old infant, because he can only compare it to his life of one year. To a ten-year-old, one year seems shorter than it does to the one-year-old infant, because it is only one tenth of the duration of his life of ten years so far; and so on, until we get to say seventy, when one year is only one-seventieth of the years that we have already lived. An interesting psychological explanation of time perception—indeed, one I can relate to. For me, it seemed like eons had transpired in the four-year span between living in Lebanon and now in Canada. Yet deep down, I was still the same Henry Zeiter.

When my parents finally came to Windsor, they bought a house downtown on Gladstone Avenue, but soon after, we moved permanently to a house on Reginald Street, farther out of town and closer to Mike's house on Rossini. The first abode was a yellow brick house two stories high on the west side of Gladstone Avenue, with a tiny backyard. One Saturday morning, while I was assembling stamps for my collection in my room upstairs, I noticed an exceedingly beautiful girl sitting on the porch in front of her house across the street. I began to watch her coming and going, but never had the nerve to approach her. Several years later I read in the papers that she was Miss Canada and runner up in the Miss Universe contest. I knew who she was from the name and birthplace mentioned, but when I saw her photograph following the article I knew for sure.

We stayed only six months in the yellow brick house, before we bought a larger one on Reginald Street, closer to my brother Mike. I recall listening to Cesar Frank's D minor Symphony and two of Schumann's symphonies (no 1, the *Spring*, and no 3, the *Rhenich*) in the backyard of the first house, where I had hooked up the phonograph to an electric plug outside the house. That was my first exposure to these composers, and I fell in love with their music.

I passed a pleasant summer working in Mike's office in the morning and spending leisurely afternoons and evenings reading or listening to music. When autumn arrived I entered Assumption College, run by the same Basilian order of priests as the high school. The first year was uneventful—I took the usual introductory courses. I remember we had a student in class, big and tall, who played hockey with the Windsor Spitfires. Father Armstrong who taught the chemistry class would often ask me to lend him my lecture notes so he could study from them, since he missed so many classes because of hockey practice. Father Armstrong was also director of athletics at Assumption so he encouraged the hockey player to practice his sport and wanted me to help him all I could in his studies.

In chemistry lab, which was in the afternoon, I sat next to Georgina Sikish, who struck me as a nice girl. I got to like her; so one afternoon, thinking I was paying her a compliment, I told her that she would make a very *homely* wife some day. What I actually meant to tell her is that I thought she would be a good *home*-maker some day. She was furious and abruptly walked away from me. Father Armstrong came over and asked me, "What did you tell her?" After I told him, he took me aside and explained to me that in English, "homely" means ugly. I never knew that. I was shocked by what I had said and immediately apologized to the girl, explaining to her what I had meant to say. After that episode we became good friends.

At the end of the school year, Father Armstrong asked me if I would let him stencil the lecture notes I had taken, so he can use them for the following year's class. He was very nice to me because I had helped his hockey player, Al Arbor (the "Red Head"). Al eventually played for the famous Detroit Red Wings during several championship years, and finally became the coach of the New York Islanders. Thinking of Al reminds me of another sportsman who was my classmate, Reno Bertoia. Two years after we began college, he was called up from their farm team by the Detroit Tigers and became their regular third baseman. For the first three months of the season, he accumulated a .415 batting average, which was as high as Ty Cobb or Ted Williams ever had during their prime. Then, the *Detroit Free Press* had an article on him which hinted that he was taking tranquilizers. After the article came out there was a big fuss about it in the press. Reno's batting average started going down until it dipped below .200 and he was sent back to the minors. He was never heard from again. The newspaper reporter, however, had failed to mention in his original article that both of Reno's parents had been killed in a car crash six months before, and that his doctor had put him on tranquilizers because of the resulting acute depression. I have questioned the veracity of news reports ever since.

CHAPTER 10

LEARNING TO LOVE LEARNING

In the summer of 1951 (at the age of seventeen), I registered for a six-week summer session and took two courses I knew I would eventually need to complete the requirements for my Bachelor of Liberal Arts Degree: philosophy and psychology. Those six weeks changed my life forever. Once I had a taste of philosophy, I became entranced with the subject. I decided to study it and practice it as a lifetime pursuit. I have never lost interest in philosophy and psychology, even though I went on to medical school and entered ophthalmology residency. Philosophy was to be my avocation, and it blended well with serious music and with my love of beauty in nature and art, and in lasting friendships.

Father Dwyer was the teacher of both courses. He was an Aristotelian Thomist and taught what is called the *perennial philosophy*, that is, the enduring philosophy for all seasons. As he put it, the philosophy that came down to us from the Greeks (Socrates, Plato and Aristotle) to Augustine, Thomas Aquinas and Duns Scotus; then on to Bossuet, Lacordaire, Newman, Chesterton, C.S.Lewis, Maritain and Gilson—that was the philosophy for all ages. That is why it had lasted 2,500 years. It was the way of thought finally adopted by the Universal Church, and praised by Leo XIII, Pius X, and Pius XI for being the most consistent and perennial exposition of reality for over two millennia.

That summer was the first time I realized that philosophy is a protean discipline comprising *many branches of inquiry*. My old notion was that it dealt just with *morals* as Confucius did, or the existentialism that Sartre expounded, or the political philosophy that Ayn Rand wrote novels about, or philosophical poetry like Gibran's. I began to realize now that philosophical discipline had little to do with those who claim to be philosophers by including some philosophical or moral injunctions in their literary works. I learned from what I read, but particularly from a short and concise textbook, *Maritain's Introduction to Philosophy,* that to learn philosophy one has to recognize that the discipline contains many levels of inquiry. Thus, to be a professional philosopher one has to study logic, epistemology (the study of knowledge itself), natural philosophy (the natural sciences), taxonomy (the classification of things into categories), astronomy, mathematics in all its branches, metaphysics (the study of being itself), theodicy (natural theology without revelation), psychology, the philosophy of history, ethics, politics, and, finally, aesthetics. What a list of disciplines, I said to myself, all wrapped up in one field, philosophy.

To understand that this field consists of the knowledge of all these varied disciplines and to have a grasp of the fundamental rules of thought and those of logical investigation is to be a true philosopher, a full-fledged lover of wisdom (*philo-sophia*)—not just a specialist in one's own field of expertise. I learned that writing a novel or two with philosophical themes, being a preacher or an orator, being a statesman or an intuitive poet, does not make one a philosopher in the true sense of the word. After I learned all that, it was what I wanted to become. I wanted to have an intimate acquaintance with metaphysics, psychology, theology and the theories of art.

I discovered that a whole world of significant concepts and universal ideas existed out there. I also realized that in my previous education it had been kept a secret from me. In Thomas Hardy's novel *The Return of the Native* the protagonist, Clem, returns to his village on the English heath, armed with such fundamental knowledge that he finds it necessary to completely empty his students' minds (unlearn them) of all the trifles they had been taught before his return, if he was to succeed in exposing them to learn how to think. That was a fair description of my sudden realization that up to that time I had not been taught the "one thing" that my mind was craving for. I also found out that there were objective, universally applicable principles and conclusions that went beyond the subjective, relativistic, and "one-thought-is-as-good-as-another" concept that was the prevalent view in most universities. I also learned that the tenets of a perennial philosophy traveled a moderate middle of the way course between utter materialism and total idealism; that Aristotle and Thomas Aquinas were the philosophers of common sense, never straying out to extremes in their ideas or postulates. They made sense to me since they elevated to a higher plane what I knew already from basic unadorned common sense.

I also became quite aware that simply teaching the history of philosophy and of the various philosophers—as is routinely done in most university courses on this subject—leads to skepticism at best, and to despair and relativistic agnosticism at worst. That method is quite inferior to teaching first the tenets of philosophy itself as an objective discipline with its proper rules and parameters— long before attempting to dazzle the young students with the various theories of this or that philosopher. A student's mind, if not armed first with the habit of logical thought and the rules of objective inquiry, invariably becomes confused and is unable to separate the ideas of the philosopher being studied from the personal opinions and prejudices of the teacher.

A CLASSICAL EDUCATION

It was this interest in philosophy that propelled me, years later, to investigate a small and relatively new liberal arts college devoted uniquely to classical education: Thomas Aquinas College, in Santa Paula, California. The College's curriculum is based exclusively on the Great Books of Western Civilization and the Socratic seminar method of instruction. In classes of about 16 students, a "tutor" (what their professors are called) leads students in discussions of the basic ideas found in the greatest works ever written.

This approach is remarkable, as students are led to think for themselves by being grounded in fundamental principles of philosophy, handed down from the greatest thinkers of all time. Students learn to distinguish between opinion and principle and can dissect the writings of any philosopher, ancient or modern. They learn to separate the chaff from the wheat, whether they are reading St. Thomas's *Summa Theologica*, Descartes' *Discourses*, or Hegel's *Philosophy of History*. I am happy to have served on the Board of Governors of Thomas Aquinas College for over twenty years, and it was thanks to my exposure to philosophy at Assumption College that I was able to recognize the value of this kind of education.

Thus, when Father Dwyer handed us a list of Twenty-Four Philosophical Theses of Thomas Aquinas to study during the last week of his philosophy course, I had no idea it would change my life. Father Dwyer showed us, through Aristotelian and Thomistic philosophy that there are certain premises and conclusions that are objectively true. These twenty-four sharp arrows have withstood the test of time and are far removed from the skeptical approaches of Hume, Schopenhauer, Nietzsche, Sartre, and many others. He led us to see that philosophy is not a helter-skelter, "any-theory-will-do", kind of discipline, but the royal road to understanding.

Several years ago, when the British thinker Christopher Derrick wrote his critique of modern college education, *Escape from Skepticism,* he subtitled it,

"Education as if Truth Mattered." It was a comparative analysis of methods of liberal arts education. He found that the system used at Thomas Aquinas College (like the system I was exposed to at Assumption) was the ideal way for students to learn first how to understand, analyze, and dissect what has been handed down to us through the Great Books and then to accept or reject the ideas. He explained there is no sense in teaching comparative philosophy without grounding students first in logic, epistemology, mathematics, and natural science. Then, and only then, is a student able to distinguish between tested laws, theories, and pure opinions; between right and wrong, truth and error. He observed first hand—as I have done over the past twenty years—the students at Thomas Aquinas College in tutorials, studying their subjects in the Socratic tradition of dialogue between each other and the tutor; and the professors querying students on their positions and expecting them to cite passages from the work under study to support their positions. Derrick called that kind of education "a bulwark against skepticism," especially in its virulent "modernistic" form.

Derrick found out, in contrast, that students at the run-of-the-mill university begin as confused stoics, progress to confirmed cynics, and end up as educated skeptics. But not so at the colleges based on the Great Books using the Socratic Method, where the student acquires the fundamental rules of thought and conversation. I have visited these campuses and have attended their tutorials, and I know for a fact that Derrick was correct.

I wanted to go into philosophy after graduation, but Dad suggested that I go into medicine like my brother Mike. He said to me, "You'll live comfortably—most philosophers die poor." He encouraged me, though, to keep up my interest in philosophy as an avocation, since the pursuit of the great truths was also dear to his heart.

He told me, "If it turns out that after becoming a physician you don't enjoy the practice of medicine, you can always go back into philosophy; but then you'll have your M.D. degree hanging on the wall as a distinguished prize. You'll be the only professor at your college with such an honorable degree, beyond your diploma in philosophy or history or whatever."

FROM PHILOSOPHY TO LITERATURE AND HISTORY

After having acquired the bare essentials of philosophical theory, I developed a deeper view of history, which was of great help to me when we took History 360 (Modern European History, Honors Course). Father Mulvihill, the professor, insisted on several essays during the year. I still have my fifty-page dissertation on "The Golden Age of Spanish Literature." He was shocked when I handed it to him. He had asked for essays of ten pages.

He then directed me to the right historical materials and got the whole class interested in searching for the philosophical meaning of the course of history. (He advised us to read R. H. Tawney's *Religion and the Rise of Capitalism*, Max Weber's *Capitalism and the Protestant Revolution*, Berdeyev's *The Meaning of History*, Ortega y Gassett's *The Revolt of the Masses*, C.E.M. Joad's *Guide to Modern Thought*, Arnold Toynbee's ten-volume *A Study of History*, and works by H.G. Wells, Belloc and Christopher Dawson—the latter being his favorite historian.) On my own, I started reading Will Durant's social and anecdotal treatment of history in his multi-volume *Story of Civilization*. What a refreshing way this was to learn the meaning of history, in place of the usual chronological recitation of dates and events! We also delved into the philosophical interpretation of the why and why not of historical events and read Mommsen, von Ranke and Hegel. It was an "honors class" and Father Mulvihill treated it as such. I had studied the rudiments of world history in both Lebanon and Venezuela, but now I was deepening that historical knowledge and applying philosophical insight as to "why" history proceeds the way it does.

It was while writing my thesis on Spanish literature that I first ran into the mystical poetry of St. John of the Cross, and, through the recommended bibliography, decided to read Jacques Maritain's seminal work, *Les Degrés du Savoir* (The Degrees of Knowledge). After tracing the various levels of knowledge, from opinion and whim, to scientific and mathematical theory, to psychological, philosophical, and theological fundamental ideas, Maritain finally arrives at St. John of the Cross and the mystical experience. He places it within the realm of the highest type of intuitive knowledge. I was fascinated by the approach developed in Maritain's book. As I became busier later in life, I would go back again and again in my spare moments to the lyrical and literally divine poetry of St. John of the Cross. The writing of the thesis on Spanish literature gave me a special appreciation for all the wonderful works of the Spanish literary giants.

I also enjoyed the English honors courses. One course was designed to touch on Shakespeare, the Elizabethans, and the Stuart era of mystic poetry; the other encompassed the 18th, 19th, and 20th centuries. I particularly loved the mock-heroic style of Alexander Pope. *The Rape of the Lock* was delightful. Pope could also write very serious poems, to wit, *An Essay on Man*, from which we get the expression "A little knowledge is a dangerous thing." For an asthmatic, small, deformed man, he was a most elegant writer of epic poetry.

I fell in love with his translations of Homer's *Iliad* and *Odyssey*. We also studied a good deal of Keats, Shelley, and the Romantics. What beautiful poetry! Years later, in conjunction with reading a biography of Gibran, I decided to look into the mystical poetry of William Blake whose symbolic sketches were a model for Gibran's paintings.

In those days, Assumption College had a tradition of awarding a prize once a year to a notable exponent of Christian thought. The founder, Father Murphy, named the annual lectures, "The Christian Culture Series," modeled after the Gifford lectures at Edinburgh. Some of the early recipients were Sigrid Undset, Evelyn Waugh, Christopher Dawson, Gilson, Maritain, Bishop Sheen, Philip Murray, Frank Sheed, William Fulbright, Marshall McLuhan, Muggeridge, and Charles Malik.

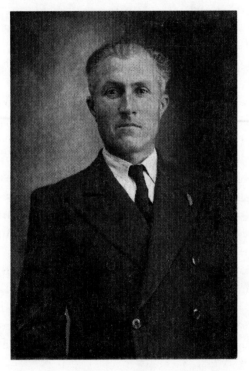

Yousef Zeiter, circa 1945: the heyday of his poetic and
literary production

The last one, Dr. Malik, was the drafter of the "Human Rights Bill" of the original Charter of the United Nations (1945-50) when he was the Lebanese ambassador to the UN. He was also a trained mathematician, a philosopher, and an Arabic literature scholar, for whom Dad was to give a rousing recitation of one of his poems in Arabic. I recall telling Dad to keep in his pocket a copy of the poem that he was going to recite from memory, just in case he forgot a line. He sent me out of the room, as he was memorizing it, and told me not to worry. Nevertheless, I sneaked a copy of the poem into the right pocket of the coat he was going to wear. When we got to the reception at the auditorium, I told him smiling: "Dad, the poem is in your right pocket, just in case."

He said to me, "Thank you son, I'll remember that." And sure enough in the middle of the long poem, he lost his way for a few seconds, but immediately pulled the written poem from his right pocket and read for a second or two. After a few verses he put the paper back in his right pocket, and finished the recitation in blazing oratory. I was proud of him, and he was smiling at me, as if to thank me. When we returned home he said to me, "Thank you son. The pupil has become the teacher."

MORE SCHOOLING

In second-year College, I attended zoology, physics, and chemistry labs, since I was preparing to enter medical school. I found the complexity of chemistry, physics, and biology a great contrast to the fundamental simplicity of philosophical concepts. During those years, I was living at home eating Mom's great Lebanese food and talking with Dad about his readings and writings and about my future. We regularly visited family and friends and were often visited by my oldest brother, Dr. Mike, and his family. We also saw much of his wife Irene's family. Shiben, her father, would come over to Mike's to play poker with the men once a week. This was always preceded by a big Lebanese dinner prepared by Mom or Irene, or Irene's mother, Mary. The Sunday get-togethers alternated between Mike and Irene's house in Windsor and the Coureys' house in Grosse Pointe, near Detroit. It was around that time that Mike bought his cottage in Belle River Township on Lake St. Clair. The Coureys had a cottage on the Michigan side of the lake, for several years before Mike bought one. They sold it when their son-in-law, Mike, bought his. These cottages were for summer living, as proximity to the lake ensured a cooler, more tolerable summer than the stifling hot weather of the inner city.

Mike's cottage became a fixture in my memory. It has always reminded me of good food, good times, and family fun. The weekends were best of all. There would be over fifty people at any one time, eating, drinking, swimming, boating, and talking. Mike and Irene's hospitality became legendary among the Lebanese colony in the Detroit-Windsor area. Recently, Irene told me that one day a lady drove into the driveway with a carful of kids, and asked her if the place was a public beach.

Just before summer began, I successfully completed second-year College. It was during that year that I dreamt that I was sitting in a huge hall for an analytical geometry final exam, anxious and frustrated, because I found myself unable to solve a single problem in the three hours allotted. As time passed within the dream, I started to panic, and when I reached an intolerable level of discomfort I woke up, just as one always wakes up from a dream in which he is about to die. My brother Mike told me that for many years after his graduation he would have the same kind of dream. One of his most persistent dreams was repeating medical school.

Years later, after graduating in medicine *cum laude*, I would often dream that I had gone back to medical school to repeat all four years. I knew within those dreams that I already had an M.D. degree, but for some compulsive reason I wanted to get another one. Except that this second time around, school appeared to be more difficult. Oh! The dreams of success are paradoxically dreams of the fears of failure. Thus, Mike was repeating medical school in his dreams and I was doing the same, even after having been in a successful practice for a long time. I subsequently learned that this type of dream is not uncommon in people whose life has been rewarded with success. After marriage, I was told by my wife Carol, that her, and all her family members, all university graduates, have experienced different variations of the same dream at one time or another.

I knew that I would be transferring to my third year of pre-med at the University of Western Ontario with which Assumption was affiliated. I took several additional courses that year, intending to get my bachelor's degree in three years instead of four. The summer of 1953 was memorable because I started dating Beverly Malach again. She was older, a more opulently endowed sixteen-year-old now, and in second-year high school. It was still a ridiculous match between a petulant high school teenager and a third-year college student. However, I have to remind myself that I was still an eighteen-year-old teenager myself. Beverly was prettier now, in the full bloom of youth, and the crush I had on her wasn't going away. We had our ups and downs, even though we saw each other no more than once or twice a week.

I recall taking her to see a movie entitled *Born Yesterday* with Judy Holliday and William Holden. We held hands when they held hands. We hugged when they hugged. There was a scene in the movie in which the lovers were reclining on the lawn at a pop concert in Washington, D.C., listening to the National Symphony Orchestra play part of Beethoven's Second Symphony. So I asked

Beverly if she would like to go to an opera or a symphony concert with me. That was a dumb thing to ask a pretty teenage girl. She wasn't awfully interested. So I wrote a mock-heroic poem à la Alexander Pope and sent it to her. But when I realized that she didn't pick up the satire, I wrote her a second poem that was more romantic in style. That poem revived the relationship for a few more weeks, but it was fated to die by the end of summer.

Philip and Mary and their families came from Venezuela to see us that summer and we had a pleasant visit for several weeks. However, my unavoidable hay fever hit me strongly that year. (The pollen count was said to be higher than usual in mid-August, the date when the Eastern-ragweed starts flowering every year.) Dad and Michel, my brother-in-law, and his brother Antonio, drove me up to the small town of North Bay, Ontario, which was an area above the hay fever zone. I roomed at the house of a Lebanese lady whose son managed a local summer baseball team. I was thus introduced to baseball under the lights. I had a lot of fun watching all the night games because there was nothing else to do after sunset there. I met and became friends with many of the fans.

One free afternoon I was trying to introduce my landlady to the pleasures of classical music and was having a tough time getting through to her. After she told me to turn the music off because it was bothering her ears, she bent down, picked up one of the tops her grandson was playing with, and began spinning it on the floor, listening joyfully to the humming sound it was making. She raised her head, looked at me and said, "Listen to the wonderful music the top makes." I guess she was trying in turn to instill in me the love of the monotone music she liked! I figured *Chacun à son gout!* Literally, French for each to his own taste!

It was a good vacation, nonetheless. It lasted until I was to start my third year of college. I transferred to the University of Western Ontario's pre-med final year. Dad drove me to London, Ontario, and sure enough, he found Mrs. Aziz, another old Lebanese widow where I could board. Her house was not far from school. She treated me like her own son and I became friends with her son Mitch who was still living at home. Her other son, Victor, was a professional photographer who, through my efforts, ended up doing all the official photos of the school's graduating students for the next five years.

Tom Poisson (a French-Canadian classmate) was also in premed rooming at the same lady's house and we became longtime friends. Each weeknight Tom and I would take a break from evening studies around 8:00, and while walking to the ice cream parlor four blocks away, we would discuss whether our strong attraction to women was aesthetic appreciation of their beauty or whether the whole attraction was nothing more than sexual desire. We never solved that problem, but I think we were rationalizing quite a bit in the process.

HUMANITIES IN PREMED?

Early in the school year, the university registrar, Ms. Ellison, approached me with an unusual proposal. She had noticed from my transfer records that I had all A's in my humanities courses. This was uncommon for a premed student. She further noted that the grades in my science courses were equally high. She advised me to take more humanities at Western and fewer of the required science courses. She said she would waive the requirement for some of the science courses and would guarantee me admission to the university's medical school. I was both surprised and delighted. I could have my cake and eat it too. Normally, all pre-med students, everywhere, had to apply to almost twenty medical schools to make sure that they would get accepted into at least one of them. Besides, premed students had to take all of the required premed courses. Here was the registrar herself asking me to apply only to her medical school, and guaranteeing me admission. But why was she doing this?

When I dared to ask her the reason behind her unusual request, she informed me that McGill University in Montreal (a more prestigious medical school) had been experimenting with admitting a few humanities students for the past several years, and now Western Ontario wanted to try the same thing. To her, I was the perfect candidate. The purpose of all this was to find out if students versed equally in the sciences and the humanities would make good doctors. McGill's experience had been very encouraging, she told me, and she had been thinking that I might be a good candidate for the experiment.

Years later, medical schools across the country began to experiment with this approach. My wife's nephews, Drew, Jeff and Brad, and her niece Mary, were accepted into medical school after majoring in economics, engineering, psychology and English literature, respectively. But that was thirty years after my experience.

It ended up that Western was the only medical school I applied to, knowing that I was accepted prior to the application. A most unusual arrangement, it allowed me to take, within the required science courses, only organic chemistry, physical chemistry, and comparative anatomy. This allowed me time to take honors courses in English drama, modern English literature, and honors history. I was allowed to skip premed embryology, biochemistry, and bacteriology since, as she said, I would be taking them in medical school anyway. The next year in medical school I enjoyed these courses immeasurably; and as I found out a year later, I did not miss anything by not taking these courses in premed, mainly because they were taught in greater depth in medical school anyway.

The two honors English courses I took were the most fun. Dr. John Graham, a very polished writer and poet, taught both English literature honors courses. In one course we studied the English novel from its inception in the seventeenth century to the present. The second course was contemporary English literature, mostly poetry. I became acquainted with James Joyce, T.S. Eliot, W.H. Auden, W.B. Yeats, Robert Frost, Allen Tate, and Ernest Hemingway. Incredibly, many of these authors were actually my contemporaries, still alive in the mid-twentieth century!

I was thoroughly enjoying myself and soaking up tons of new knowledge besides. All this increased my confidence in writing both prose and poetry. It led me later in the year to tackle what Dr. Graham thought would be a very tough subject for a thesis, "Alienation in Modern Society and Literature, as exemplified by James Joyce, T.S. Eliot, and Ernest Hemingway." That was in 1953-54, my last year of college, when I was nineteen years old.

The dissertation of the thesis began with a history of the lives of the authors, with an emphasis on their progress or regress from their beliefs. T.S. Eliot, progressed from being an agnostic American author to belief in the traditional tenets of Anglo-Catholicism, and, he became a prophetic poet, the most celebrated of the first half of the twentieth century. Joyce left his traditional country and faith for a life of restless wandering in continental Europe. He was a linguist of the first order and established a new style of writing, but he lost his bearings and his soul in the process. Hemingway, never had a faith to start with, and after several adventures he turned morose and ended up committing a skeptic's suicide (he may have been bipolar).

Then I searched for the reasons why these authors alienated themselves from the modern world. I used these three authors as examples of the many other sensitive artists who also found solitude to be necessary for their survival. I ended the thesis with a historical analysis of the genesis of modern times and the sources of widespread *angst* and subsequent alienation.

Now "all study and no play" makes for a dull student life, but we had our share of fun in Dr. Graham's class. Often, he would ask us to sit in a circle around him and discuss the books that were on the course. The class was really a tutorial, with him as the leader of some of the brightest students in the school. That was an unusual class procedure at Western. Now many years later, that's how all courses are taught at Thomas Aquinas College. It is called the Socratic Method.

ULYSSES AND PENELOPE

Across from me sat a beautiful red-head from Hamilton, Ontario, who became the subject of many of my dreams. Her name was Penelope. It took me several months to ask her to go out with me. I was shy and inexperienced when it came to the fair sex; my innocence was in fact exasperating. I've mentioned before that in my upbringing dating was not an item on the agenda. I guess this kept me out of trouble; but it also denied me much youthful fun. I would arrange to sit close to Penny at football games. I would sit near her in the dining hall. I would admire her while sitting across from her in class. (We sat in a circle for the tutorials.) Dr. Graham would often ask someone in class to read poetry or prose from the books we were studying. One day, he simply looked at me and nodded, meaning it was my turn to read. In the honors class on 18th-century England, we were studying Alexander Pope's peerless iambic pentameter translation of Homer's *Odyssey*. It so happened that I had read that chapter the night before, which described in heroic verse Penelope's meeting with Ulysses on his return home. Pope's translation does justice to Homer's original "heroic verse." I had memorized some of the verses, since they referred to Penelope. She was now sitting across from me in class. I stood up, looked into her eyes for about five seconds, and then started to read:

> *First from her eye descends the rolling tear:*
> *"Say, once more say, is my Ulysses here?*
> *How could that numerous and outrageous band*
> *By one man be slain, though by a hero's hand?"*

The passage was referring to the slaying of all Penelope's suitors by Ulysses. My! O my! I was trying to think of it as referring to what I would do if anyone dared touch my Penelope. I continued:

> *"Ah, no! (With sighs Penelope rejoined)*
> *Excess of joy disturbs thy wondering mind;*
> *How blest this happy hour, should he appear,*
> *Dear to us all, to me supremely dear."*

I looked up; her eyes were fixed on me and puzzled. Going on, I read:

> At length Telemachus: "Oh, who can find
> A woman like Penelope, unkind?
> Why thus in silence? Why with winning charms
> Thus slow to fly with rapture to [my] arms?"

There, I made a Freudian slip; the text actually said "to *his* arms."

> "Canst thou, Penelope, when Heaven restores
> Thy lost Ulysses to his native shores;
> Canst thou, O cruel, unconcern'd, survey
> Thy lost Ulysses, on his signal day?"

She started blushing, lowered her skirt, and bent forward to give me her full attention as I kept on reading.

> While yet he speaks, her powers of life decay.
> She sickens, trembles, falls and faints away.
> At length recovering, to his arms she flew,
> And strain'd him close, as to his breast she drew.

With everyone intensely looking at me, I kept reading the "heroic" verse. Knowing full well that Penelope was starting to understand, I recited the next six verses from memory, as I had learned them because the subject was Ulysses' wife as well as my Penelope.

> "Since when no eye hath seen thy tongue reveal'd,
> Hard and distrustful as I am, I yield."

I stared at her with longing, and Penny was smiling now. I continued, as Dr. Graham was enjoying it too.

> The ravished Queen with equal rapture glows,
> Clasps her loved lord, and to his bosom grows,
> Nor had they ended till the morning ray,
> But Pallas [Athena] backward held the rising day.

The class roared as I finished reading. Poor Penelope—she was crimson red. Several days went by and I finally got enough nerve to ask her out. Tom Poisson had given me his tickets to the University Mustangs Saturday football game, so I asked her to go with me. It is difficult for me now to figure out why I was afraid she would refuse me (it was an intuitive premonition as I soon found out). That same unwillingness to take a chance, essentially, the fear of being rejected, plagued me even in medical school. But to my surprise, Penny accepted my invitation with a smile, and we sat close to each other during the game. Suffice it to say that I paid scant attention to the game. We talked for a while about Dr. Graham and the honors class. As we warmed up to each other, I began to get cozier, but not for long.

"I am engaged to Bob Murray," she said to me, "but I accepted your invitation because you have always been so nice to me in class. Do you remember when you read me that poem? It felt good to be the center of attention, but Bob is a very jealous fiancé."

She knew that I knew Bob. He was in my pre-med group at school. Well, that information kind of spoiled the fun and crushed my hopes. How often is it that we wake up from an interval of fantasy, as from a dream, to find that fantasy is not reality? That was it! But I always admired Penny and we remained friends for the rest of that year at Western.

I loved the academic life at college, a hundred times more than I cared for either elementary school or high school. I enjoyed all the courses, both the sciences and the humanities. I loved the intricacy of physics, chemistry, biology, and mathematics (I was in my second year of calculus), and I found myself equally fascinated by the thoughts and creativity of the poets, the writers, and the philosophers. I was developing a Renaissance man's outlook on life.

Later in medical school, I would enter the church, kneel before the altar and beg God to let me become a Catholic philosopher. It's a petition I had started earlier, in fact, when I began earnestly reading some of the Great Books as part of the program at Assumption College. I was reading a lot on my own also, and I especially remember enjoying Thomas Merton's conversion autobiography, *The Seven Story Mountain.*

VISITS HOME

I remember often hitch-hiking a ride home to Windsor. That was safe to do in those days, and fortunately drivers were unafraid and willing to help. Times have changed. I had no car until I was an intern. Sometimes, I would go home to Windsor with Tom Poisson, who was driving his old car. In the winter, I would leave London behind with four feet of snow and get to Windsor to find hardly any. London was in the snow-belt, like Northern Ohio and up-state New York, whereas Windsor, surrounded by three lakes, was in the Carolingian zone of flora and fauna, quite warm in comparison. That was one of the trivial facts I learned in my course on municipal affairs that year. Windsor and London, Ontario, were examples of severe climactic difference within a circumscribed area.

Windsor's warmer weather was a good reason to go home once or twice a month during the cold Canadian winter. Mom always welcomed me with open arms. I was her only child and she missed me, but she always wanted what was best for me, even though that meant being away from home. Our second and more permanent home in Windsor had two stories in the form of a duplex. It also had the customary Midwest basement. We rented the upstairs and lived below on the first floor, where we had three bedrooms, a living-family room open to the dining room and kitchen. We had only one full bathroom. Our quarters had enough large windows that the sun shone inside all the time. That's how I remember it. But I know that it could not have been so nice, since Windsor got a lot of precipitation, winter and summer. But memory is selective; we bury the unpleasant and easily recall the pleasant—I remember the sunshine of those days but I have forgotten the dark clouds and the frequent rain and snow of the Midwest.

At college in London, I had to take a night class to get enough credits to complete my Bachelor of Arts degree in three years. It was the most boring course I ever took: Municipal Affairs. Then on graduation day, I sat next to a music major, whose name started with a Z like mine. Brahms' Academic Festival Overture was being played by the school's marching band—a piece played regularly (like Elgar's *Pomp and Circumstance*) at graduations all over the world. I asked the music major if she knew what they were playing. She didn't have a clue. Apparently, even in the arts, great technicians often do not have general knowledge even within their chosen profession.

BRIEF RESPITE

Graduation was the first week in May and medical school wasn't starting till early October. My grades were good enough that I didn't have to write finals, and so vacation for me started two weeks before graduation. I ended up having five months of vacation that summer, the longest such stretch I ever had. My brother Mike suggested that I work for the summer. He got me a job in a printing shop. My duty was to gather the lead letter-types and melt them in a furnace so as to preserve the lead for re-use. The heat and the smoke were suffocating. I came home twelve hours later dirty from head to toe with grime and soot all over me. Mother was furious with Mike. That was the same mother who had dressed me in white as a child and expected me to stay spotless. I stripped off my filthy clothes and took a one-hour bath.

The next day, she told Mike to use me in his office, and I worked for him off and on for the next few summers when I was still in medical school. I enjoyed the mornings when I worked with his Swedish nurse, Dorothy, while Mike was at the hospital performing surgery. Dorothy, a blue-eyed blonde of the Virginia Mayo variety, was very pleasant to me since I was the boss's brother and I had the possibility of becoming her boss one day; the family thought that following medical school and internship, I would come back and practice with my brother some day. Dorothy and I would schedule the afternoons full of patients, but I rarely stayed in the office after one o'clock. I used to leave early and had the rest of the day to read or to drive Dad's new Pontiac up and down Lakeshore Drive and admire the girls promenading on the lakeshore. As evening approached I would meet with my "New Renaissance Club" friends, Bob Kennedy, Ed Browell, Charlie Parent, and Jacques Gauthier.

Uncle Paul and my brother Tony came with their families from Venezuela to Windsor that summer and stayed with us and with brother Mike for about four months, before they all departed to Italy and Lebanon, along with Irene's parents. Tony and Madelyn stayed in Lebanon for almost two years; they then returned to Caracas with a butler and two maids. The butler also became Tony's chauffer driving him around in his DeSoto. Of course, one could afford a butler and two maids when Venezuela was awash with income from oil, iron, and copper exports. But now the days of prosperity, like everything else in life, are gone and Tony and Madelyn live unobtrusively in Stockton across the street from the city's Catholic high school. Tony has gifted the school with an eighteen-foot marble Madonna and child erected across the street from his bedroom window, so he could see Our Lady "from the bedroom on first arising in the morning," he told me. My partner Joe, Tony's son, has sure picked up these Venezuelan high-life habits. He lives alone in a six-thousand-square-foot home and keeps a husband-and-wife combo as his personal gardener and maid. He owns two limousines and has hired a retired minister, Carl Coleman, to drive him around. I wonder who influenced Joe to adopt this life style. Carl, the man of the cloth, tells me that he's always preaching the advantages of a chaste and simple life to Joe, with little success so far.

MUSICAL INTERLUDE

That summer I stayed home spending my time at Mike's office in the mornings and mostly reading the Great Books and listening to classical music in the afternoons. I knew when the various broadcasts of concerts and operas would be on radio or TV. For several years I was a constant listener to the Sunday radio broadcasts of the New York Philharmonic, with Dimitri Mitropoulos as conductor, the Boston Symphony Saturday morning rehearsal broadcasts with Serge Koussevitzky, and the Saturday evening broadcasts of Arturo Toscanini's NBC Symphony Orchestra. Also on Saturday afternoons there were the Metropolitan Opera broadcasts with Milton Cross as narrator. I even used to write down the weekly concert programs of the New York and NBC orchestras in a little booklet that I still have. In fact, many years later, my daughter Suzie sent me a book of musical anecdotes by a certain Hans Heinsheimer. He was apparently an Austrian musician who became an impresario in New York at the time I was hearing those concerts on the radio. He claims in his book that he helped assemble the NBC Symphony for Toscanini. He mentioned in the same book many of the concert programs I had listened to. As I was reading his book, I went back and unearthed my booklet and, sure enough, every concert he mentioned was annotated in my little book.

Reading that little book led to an interesting episode recently in my life. Hersheimer mentions how he helped start the "Friends of Chamber Music," a group that has been emulated in most major cities in the United States. We have such a society in Stockton, but attendance at these concerts has been poor for several years lately. While attending one of their concerts in May 2000, I was told that it was going to be their last concert ever, because they had run out of funds. I said to the few doctors I saw in the audience that I would match whatever amount they were willing to contribute to keep these concerts alive. Nothing became of that. But two days later, the society's president called the newspaper and told the music columnist about the chamber society's problem and my willingness to help out. The reporter called me at the office the next day for an interview, wanting more information. I talked with him on the phone about how uncultured our society has become; how the greatest examples of what's best in musical literature were composed for chamber orchestra; and, confidentially, how the non-supporting citizens in Stockton don't even deserve to have a chamber music series. By gosh, the reporter wrote most of what I had said in the next day's edition. I was mortified. But the publicity helped the Chamber Music group raise over one hundred thousand dollars, enough to keep the concerts going for another ten years. Stockton's chamber music lovers owe all this to Heinsheimer's book which inspired me (at that exact time) to proselytize for the cause of music in our community.

I recall one concert back in 1952, when I was still at Assumption College in Windsor. The long defunct Detroit Symphony was revived, and financed by Edsel Ford and family. They had enticed Paul Paray, a famous French conductor, to lead the orchestra. Ford auditorium was built across the river from Windsor. Edmond and I would take the tunnel bus and be right there, since the Music Hall was next to the Detroit side of the tunnel. I recall particularly Bruno Walter, pupil and friend of Gustav Mahler, conducting the Mahler Fourth Symphony. The program started with Mozart's Symphony No. 40 in G minor, and Richard Strauss's *Don Juan*. Sitting next to me was a properly dressed elderly gentleman with grey hair. He asked me in derision to wake him up when the Mahler one-hour-long symphony was over. In those days, Mahler was still thought of as avant-garde just like Messiaen or Schoenberg. When Mahler's Symphony was over, the elderly man was up clapping and shouting bravos. That was my introduction (and his) to Mahler at age eighteen.

Symphonic music is abstract in nature, so it did not lose any of its vitality when broadcast on the radio. Some of the legendary virtuosi that I had listened to live on radio broadcasts and annotated in my booklet were violinists Fritz Kreisler, Yasha Heifetz, Misha Elman, Yehudi Menuhin, Isaac Stern (the last two were San Franciscans), Nathan Milstein, Zino Francescatti, Joseph Szigetti, and Erica Morini; pianists Dame Myra Hess, Arthur Rubinstein, Rudolf Serkin, Vladimir Horowitz, Clifford Curzon, Robert and Jean Casadesus, Guiomar Novaes, Gina Bachauer, and Claudio Arrau; cellists Pablo Casals, Gregor Piatigorsky. M. Rostropovich, and Janòs Starker; singers Kirsten Flagstad, Renata Tebaldi, Maria Callas, Lauritz Melchior, Ezio Pinza, Jan Pierce and many others.

The number of Russian Jewish violinists was astounding. According to Russian Yiddish lore, there were many more Jewish violinists than pianists and conductors, because during a pogrom the violinist could put the violin under his arm and run away; whereas a pianist could hardly carry the piano on his back; and a conductor would have to leave his orchestra behind! When visiting Lebanon, I still listen to the Israeli radio stations broadcasting classical music or to the live concerts of the Israel Philharmonic, a great orchestra.

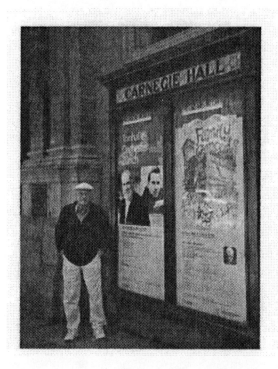

In 2004, I revisited the remodeled Carnegie Hall; I remember it as the former home of the New York Philharmonic during its golden age, under Mahler, Toscanini, and Mitropoulos.

I also recall the many great conductors I have seen in person make music in my lifetime: Eugene Ormandy, George Szell, Fritz Reiner, Guido Cantelli, Bruno Walter, Leonard Bernstein, Paul Paray, Pierre Monteux, George Szell, Stokowsky, Stravinsky, and many others. I learned much about music in those days. I was less familiar with opera than I am now, except for *Carmen, The Barber of Seville, Don Giovanni, La Traviata*, and a few others. It was much later that I began to idolize the operas of Mozart and Richard Strauss, but particularly, the epic grandeur of Richard Wagner's works. Lately, in conjunction with Maestro Kyung Soo Won and his son Justin, I find myself maturing in Wagnerian lore: the grandeur of the Ring Cycle and the mysticism of Tannhäuser, Lohengrin and above all Parsifal.

LEBANESE LEISURE

One summer, Renee and Paulette, Uncle Paul's daughters, came to Windsor from Venezuela to attend St. Mary's Academy, a then renowned Catholic girls' high school. Their parents wanted them to learn English in a Canadian school. We renewed our former friendship and passed some good times together. Along with them came the four daughters of the Matar family, a prominent Lebanese family in Venezuela.

We all went to Detroit's Metropolitan Beach one day, and took with us the old grandfather of the Matar girls—he had just come fresh from the old country, Lebanon. Sporting a huge handlebar mustache and sizing up all the bikini-clad girls at the beach, he turned to Dad, saying, "Ya Allah! Ya Youssef! *Meat* is very cheap in this country." (He meant to say *flesh*.) We all cracked up because we knew he was a *montagnard* from the Middle East, accustomed to seeing women covered in black from head to toe, and here in America he saw all these fashionably shaped women with their flesh exposed. Those were the early days of the "bikini" revolution. What also surprised the old man from Lebanon was the care these young American women took of their figures so the scant bikinis and the stylish beach clothes looked very good on them. I would hate to think of how Grandma Marzuka or Great Aunt Teresa would have looked in one of those bikinis; yet in my heart they remain more beautiful than all the idolized female models and movie stars in the world.

We passed our summer weekends at Mike's cottage. Every Saturday and Sunday was a feast. The dining table would be set up all day with *kibbi, tabbuli,* hummus, shish-kebab, and all sorts of Lebanese entrées that took hours to prepare and cook. By that time Irene had gotten a first-class Italian lady to help. Emilia is still with them, fifty years later at the ripe old age of 85. Emilia learned how to cook Lebanese food from Irene and Irene's mother, Mary Courey, and from my mother, Badwyeh. Emilia had consummate teachers. She already knew how to prepare all sorts of Italian foods and added to them her Lebanese entrées.

In those days Edmond and I discovered the perfect combination for happiness. We decided in one of those rare moments of poetic inspiration, that life would be unbearable if it was devoid of eating kibbe, drinking beer, listening to classical music on the radio, and watching our beloved Detroit Tigers on TV on Saturday and Sunday afternoons. I wouldn't say we were simple in our taste, but I will say that we were down to earth and firm believers in the primacy of leisure. We had pretty much little else to do all summer.

I've always enjoyed my times of leisure, and by that I mean time off from the constant rush to make a buck—yet not time off from physical exercise, or from intellectual, artistic and spiritual pursuits. However, to live the life of the leisurely wise, one has to have prepared oneself in the art of leisurely pursuit, by having spent a whole lifetime cultivating one's interest in matters intellectual, artistic and spiritual. There is no "free lunch," and "we sleep where we make our bed." Appropriate proverbs and sayings are wonderful reminders of the truth. I have always found it sad to see people over sixty-five, even in their eighties, still working to make more money when they have enough to last them several lifetimes. I have always felt that, instead, we ought to be spending our golden years in a sort of active leisure, engaged in intellectual and spiritual growth and perhaps in charitable giving helping the less fortunate (without passing judgment on them). Joseph Pieper, the German philosopher, had it right in his book *Leisure, the Basis of Culture.* "Leisure is an attitude of contemplative celebration," he wrote, "which draws its vitality from our approval of the world as it is." He suggested this ought to be the goal of any civilized or cultured person during retirement, the result being personal growth leading to self-actualization, and, if we're blessed, even peak experiences.

CHAPTER 11

PEAK EXPERIENCES

After that restful summer of leisure, I entered medical school. The theoretical and practical learning about the wonders of the human body immediately began in earnest, and after the first session of anatomy class, my interest in medicine rose to a high pitch from which it has never retreated. That enjoyment of concrete learning continued through physiology, pathology, and most of all neuroanatomy. Our anatomy professor, Dr. Alan B. Skinner, was a man of culture—right after my own heart. He was president of the Canadian Ballet Company and would explain to us the human skeletal muscles in terms of ballet. He was tall and portly with gray hair combed all the way back, a la Michael Caine in the movie *Dirty Rotten Scoundrels*. In short, he looked debonair.

His assistant, a surgical resident, was his opposite—a jerk of the first order. He scared us half to death on the first anatomy lab we ever had. He talked for two hours about how many students would flunk his tests, how much work we would be expected to do, and how stingy he was in grading tests. He was stingy, alright. After the first test, he took me aside in anatomy lab (before he posted the results on the board) to tell me that I had gotten "only a 67" (out of a 100). To me, a 67 was like being gassed. I was disappointed for two days until he posted the results of the exam on the bulletin board. He had the students' names listed from the highest to the lowest grades. I had 67 alright, but my name was on top of the list. I was relieved, but still felt an aversion for the man.

When anatomy dissection started in earnest, we were off to the races! Our group of six students had the "Corporal," the muscular corpse of an Afro-American who must have been a boxer or weight lifter. He was lean and muscular with little or no adipose tissue—a perfect specimen for anatomy dissection.

There was lots of studying in medical school, but that stressful routine was soothed somewhat by listening to music. The first year in London, when I was still in premed, I found a classical music station on the radio. It was the *New York Times* station (WQXR) and it came in very clearly. I would listen to non-vocal symphonic or chamber music while studying and I found the music conducive to learning. I remember one evening I was studying biochemistry and the Brahms third symphony was on the waves. When the music reached the extremely lyrical second movement, I looked at the formulas in my book and they began to appear like hieroglyphic symbols, a script of dry, technical formulations. I recall closing the book, leaning back in my chair and savoring every single note of the music. I knew the symphony well, and started thinking to myself, "What am I doing in a technical field when my greatest joys are music, aesthetics and the humanities? And besides, when am I going to get really serious about my spiritual growth?"

I had been reading (on and off) some of St. John of the Cross's poetry. The poems of this mystic that I learned in Spanish when in Venezuela are more lyrical in the original than in any translation. I still kept a book that had them all in Spanish. After closing the biochemistry book, I picked up St. John, opened a page at random and started reading the stanzas of his Spiritual Canticle (which is his rendition of Solomon's Song of Songs). In the following passage the soul is pining in search of her spouse Christ. The bride (the soul) asks the creatures in the meadow,

> *You forests, thickets, deserts,*
> *Which my beloved set in close array;*
> *You meadow-land so green,*
> *Spangled with blossoms gay,*
> *Tell me, oh, tell me has he passed your way?*

And the creatures reply:

> *Rare gifts he scattered*
> *As through these woods he passed apace,*
> *Glancing at us, as on he sped,*
> *He beautifully clothed every place*
> *With the loveliest reflection of his face.*

In another poem, the verses that express the longing to see God soar with expressions of love, particularly in the original Spanish,

> Vivo sin vivir en mi,
> Y de tan manera espero,
> Que muero porque no muero . . .
> Y sin Dios vivir no puedo.
> (*I live, yet no true life I know,*
> *And living thus only in hope,*
> *I die because I do not die . . .*
> *And without God, there is no life at all.*)

I fell in love with God through St. John of the Cross. And this was not simply an isolated perception. St. John's poetry gave more meaning to the abstract music I loved, to Bach, Beethoven, and Brahms. It was an experience of wholeness, of totality, a gestalt. The love of Beauty has led me to search for the transcendental love of Being, Truth, Goodness, and Oneness.

THE "ONE THING" NECESSARY

It was in periods like these that I started thinking about visiting during my next summer vacation, a Benedictine or Trappist monastery to see if I had a religious vocation. A puzzling thing to me has always been the indecisive nature of our willpower when it comes to proceeding with resolve to grow spiritually. I had read enough and meditated enough on the spiritual life to know that if I did my best and let God do the rest, I could become holy and happy, perhaps even a saint.

"There is *one thing* necessary," said Jesus to Martha, "and Mary has chosen the better part." Martha was the well-intentioned busy sister of Mary and Lazarus, exemplifying a busy, active life, always fretting about this or that, and not taking the time to practice "the better part" by which is meant contemplation. She was always occupied, like most of us, minding intricate details, doing various chores, and never stopping to take inventory of her spiritual response to God's call to holiness. Her sister Mary did. She chose "the better part," sitting at the feet of Jesus in loving contemplation.

At various stages of my life, I have stopped what I was doing and wondered about my commitment to reaching a higher stage of the spiritual life. I knew that has to start with purgation of my inclination to satisfy all my desires, while waiting for God to purify my self-love and my pride and greed, and hoping to reach, one day, the transformative union with the All in All. Call it nirvana! Call it self-actualization! Call it becoming a person of great moral strength! Call it by any name—it would still be a lofty and sacred goal.

The world has bit by bit lost the sense of the sacred. There is a tendency in democracies to bring down to a common level whatever is noble and elevated. Even God is now brought down to the level of friend and brother in exclusion of his awe-inspiring fatherhood as the mighty Creator of everything. Joseph Pieper has written a book on the new Church architecture in which he describes how shallow and sterile it has become compared to the Gothic and Renaissance temples of worship. He thought that modern church construction has lost the sense of the sacred. Just look at the tattered or immodest way people dress for Church on Sunday. There is an atrophied sense of respect left for the holy or the sacred.

Now that I am much older, I wonder how years have gone by without my earnestly following through on my recurrent resolve to grow spiritually. I would get inspired to meditate for a while listening to Bach's *Magnificat* or Beethoven's last quartets or when reading St. John of the Cross, Aquinas, or Dante. I would go to confession, receive Christ in the Eucharist and meditate with devotion. But I would do all these things without consistency, not following through on a regular plan of action. How could I have allowed all these years to pass me by, living with inconsistent progress, never getting past the first stages of the initiate? And whatever I have done in my life I could have done it all with conscious consistency as an offering *for the love of God*, and many times I didn't do that. To become a saint one needs to believe and work with resolve for the love of God.

St. Paul and later St. Augustine both said, "O Lord! How often have I known what to do and didn't do it, and what not to do and did it." Again, I quote the Homer I used to read to Penelope in class:

> *Perverse mankind! Whose wills, created free,*
> *Change all their woes on absolute decree;*
> *All, to the dooming Gods their guilt translate,*
> *And follies are miscall'd the crimes of fate.*
> —Homer, *the Odyssey* (Translation by Alexander Pope)

After having been given so many opportunities in my life to do "the one thing necessary," to put my hands to the plow and not look back, I ought to be careful not to run out of time in my spiritual pursuit of the God who is my all. I think that was why, when I was young, I would often close whatever book I happened to be studying and allow myself to be transported higher and higher by the slow movements of Brahms' second and third symphonies—or by the *alla danza tedesca* of Beethoven's Op. 130 Quartet, or by his third cello sonata, or by Bach's *Musical Offering* or his *Art of the Fugue*, or by Mozart's *Requiem* or his last string quintets—works of supreme beauty by artists at the peak of divine inspiration, nearing the end of their creative life and looking back at it all, with inspired wisdom and devotion. And still all that beautiful music pales when compared with kneeling in adoration in front of the exposed Blessed Sacrament. As St. John of the Cross, in one of his mystical moments puts it:

> To win love's chase, I took my way,
> And, full of hope, began to fly.
> I soar'd aloft and soar'd so high
> That in the end I reach'd my prey.
> —St. John of the Cross, *Dark Night of the Soul*
> (Translation by Allison Peers)

My travels have generated many inspired moments of spiritual highs, such as the one I felt upon entering the Arena Chapel in Padua (the *Scrovegni Chapel*) and looking at the sixty Giotto panels depicting the life of Christ, especially the panel I love the most, "The Deposition of Christ," which shows the angels' hands pressing down upon the clouds for solace and their childlike faces grimacing in pain at man's injustice to his own Creator. Meditating on that one panel, I knelt and wept while my soul soared higher and higher (*mas alto, mas alto*) in love with Giotto, in love with Italy, proud of my Catholic heritage, and grateful to God for his overwhelming love of me. In the poem just cited, St. John of the Cross goes on to say:

> "Quando más alto subia,
> Deslumbroseme la vista, . . .
> Por una extraña manera
> Mil vuelos pasé de un vuelo,
> Porque esperanza del cielo,
> Tanto alcanza cuanto espera,
> Y fui tan alto, tan alto,
> Que le di a la caza alcance.

(The dreadful force of dazzling light
Blinded me as aloft I flew,
In ways no mortal can explain
I made a thousand flights in one,
For he that hopes to reach the sun
His heart's desire shall surely gain . . .
I flew aloft so high, so high
That in the end I reached my prey.)

BRAINY THOUGHTS

In medical school, neuroanatomy soon became my favorite subject. It was taught by Dr. Murray L. Barr, already famous for his discovery of the *Barr body* (i.e. the sex chromosome seen next to the nucleolus inside the cell). Neuroanatomy was my kind of subject, complicated and difficult, and an example of the marvelous complexity of the human brain and the innumerable tracts of the spinal cord. The interconnections and maze of organized informational systems make the most complicated computer look like child's play. After all, computers were first designed in simple imitation of the human brain. Later on came more advanced computers, but still much simpler in engineering compared to the human brain—simpler because the computer is made up of dead matter, whereas the brain has all the advantages and superiority of living matter (instant adaptability, the flexibility of homeostasis, and the inner creative élan vital), that enables this living marvel to internally initiate appropriate action.

I studied my neuroanatomy by drawing the brain's tracts and association areas; by tracing the thousands of neural tracts in the spinal cord; and memorizing the hundreds of functional areas in the cerebrum, cerebellum, and basal ganglia. I was slowly getting the gist of this unbelievably complicated system. But it was not until the last night before the final exam that I fully understood it all in a flood of intuitive light. It was two o'clock in the morning; I had been studying for eight hours, and I had to get some sleep before the 8:00 A.M. final exam, when all of a sudden I saw the human brain in front of me, luminous and shining, surrounded by an aura of diffuse yellowish light-rays.

The whole vision had the sense of instant discovery, of a sudden flash of light. I thought I was looking at a strong lamp emitting bright rays which were illuminating my understanding. In fact, the human brain itself was aglow in front of my eyes and everything was suddenly understood with shining clarity! This vision of the human brain with all its distinct areas and connective tracts brilliantly illuminated, lasted for what seemed like several minutes. I was seeing everything I had studied for the past six months about the brain in three dimensions, both spatially in front of me and cognitively within me; I felt a sort of mystical vision of oneness with the brain as it is in itself; as it truly exists. I was beholding it both in all its details and in its abstract essence. When the "vision" left me, I was excited but exhausted and I immediately fell into a deep sleep.

The next day I aced the exam. For three hours I wrote, drew, and described the three-dimensional visual image that I beheld in front of me early that very morning. I got 97 points out of a possible 100. The next highest grades were 72, 68, and 63. Because of the 97, Dr. Barr could not use a statistical curve to adjust the grades higher. He told me that he was so impressed with the understanding I showed in my answers, that he didn't want to use a curve, even if he could have. I described to him the vision I saw in my room before the exam and he did not question it, because, he said, that's what happened to him when he discovered the chromosomal body next to the nucleolus of a brain cell—*the Barr body.* "It was instant recognition and oneness with the discovered object—Eureka! It was a peak experience," he said to me.

Eventually, I was awarded the neuroanatomy prize: a complete set of ophthalmoscopes and otoscopes, inside a velvety maroon case. I used these prize instruments in my clinical years. After graduation, I bought other instruments for use in my office and I put the originals back in the maroon box as a souvenir of my experience. I still have that precious reminder on the third shelf in my library at home. It rests there next to a bony skull, reminding me of both knowledge and dissolution—just as in representations of Saint Jerome, the Vulgate Bible is on one side of him, and on the other side, his lion and a skull.

What was the nature of that vision? It was a sudden illumination! But was it proof of long, hard work and final understanding? Was it imagination of learned detailed facts? The illuminated vision was immeasurably superior to any flat drawing or picture in any anatomy book I had ever seen. It was beyond doubt a peak experience for me. Abraham Maslov, the famous psychologist, described the stages of enlightenment: self-knowledge, self-actualization, and peak experiences. In self-actualization, knowledge of one's self becomes realized and acted upon (this becomes evident when one's internal and external performance show a high level of correspondence—are in sync—without contradiction between internal beliefs and external action). At its highest point it can lead to peak experiences, the summit of the mountain of self-knowledge that rises above our routine life and strips us of our inner fears. It is akin to St. John of the Cross's: "I flew aloft so high, so high, that in the end I reached my prey."

A TOUCH OF SWEETNESS

Another peak experience occurred to me at the Church of Santa Croce twelve years later, during a visit to Florence. The unexpected sight of the tombs and monuments of Michelangelo, Machiavelli, Galileo, Dante, Alfieri, Rossini, Cherubini, and many of the greats of Western civilization, coupled with the rainbow colors on the pews as the sun shone through the stained glass windows, produced a sublime moment in my life. The sudden appearance of processions, choirs, cardinals' red hats, and bishops celebrating Holy Mass accompanied by a choir singing Gregorian chant, all combined to lift me up ("*más alto, más alto*") to where I experienced a full appreciation of Western Civilization, actualized in front of me, in one location.

These experiences were perhaps in preparation for another moment of ecstasy I had about ten years later during contemplation while visiting a monastery chapel. I had gone alone to the Camaldolese (Benedictine) Monastery in Big Sur, south of Carmel, California. The monastery sits high on the coastal mountains overlooking the Pacific Ocean. I always thought I could see as far as Japan from up there! It was a silent retreat, interspersed with spiritual talks by an elderly nun. She lived as an anchoress (a hermit) in the mountains nearby. I remember she talked a lot about Juliana of Norwich and Hildegard von Bingen. Near the end of the retreat, she led us to the chapel to meditate for one hour in front of the Blessed Sacrament. I sat in a pew, closed my eyes, rested my hands on my knees, and allowed myself to enter into a quiet space avoiding any thoughts. In a dreamlike state, I entered into my existential self.

After about an hour (as I realized later), I felt a touch of sweetness as I've never experienced before. I must have remained in this state of oneness with God for some time. I was completely absorbed in the presence of God, swooned in his soothing love, until I slowly became aware of my surroundings. When I opened my eyes there was nobody left in the chapel. I remained in silence and the aura of sanctity filled my entire being and spilled over into my surroundings. I had never experienced such tranquility and peace. I've had feelings of closeness to God many times before, but never like this. I received a glimpse of "the peace that surpasses all understanding" (St Paul). In that Big Sur chapel, I knew full well that I was being touched by a Being, "of whom nothing greater can be thought" (St. Anselm).

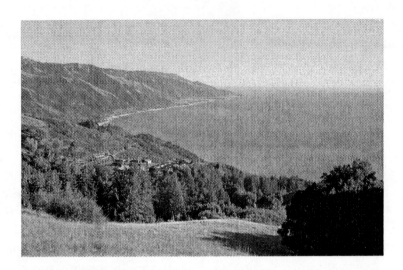

View of the Pacific from the Camaldolese Monastery, south of Big Sur, a spectacular meeting of land and sea. The monastery compound is atop the hill in the foreground.

With all these experiences under my belt, why have I vacillated in following the call to holiness? We are all called to be saints. Jesus says, "Be perfect therefore, as your Father in heaven is perfect." And he said further, "*There is only one thing necessary.*" The "one thing necessary" is contemplation of the ultimate joy, the loving of God with all our "mind, body, soul, and strength," and loving our neighbor as ourselves. In the metaphysical sense, the term *necessary* is pivotal. God is the only Being whose existence is necessary. Everything else is contingent (not possessing an intrinsic necessity to be, i.e. may or may not exist) and is dependent for its existence on the One Necessary Being, and existing only by participation with that Being's existence. When asked by Moses, "Whom should I tell them sent me?" God replied, "Tell them I AM WHO AM."

One reason we vacillate in desiring holiness is because we live where perfection is mixed with imperfection, and where the presence of good is imperiled at any moment by the possibility of its loss (i.e., evil, or the obstruction of grace by sin). In the absence of grace, all talk of Utopias is illusionary. In the ultimate analysis we know that we are still living on earth, a place of change and contradiction, so we resolve and yet vacillate—we decide and only partially execute, and it is only through God's grace that we can persevere to ultimately find perfection in Him Who is perfect. "We are pilgrims on the way," *siamo en via,* as the saints used to say. On earth we are still in school, slowly and tediously learning to do what we ought to do and avoid what we ought not to do. To strive for perfection, one needs a lifetime of patience; never giving up the goal "until the end of the race," as St. Paul aptly put it. That is why it is rare to come by advanced mystics like St. John of the Cross, St. Teresa of Avila, Henry Suso, Meister Eikhardt, Richard Rolle, the two Victorines, Juliana of Norwich, Hildegard von Bingen, the *Sufis* (Al Hallaj, Al Ghazali, Al Tusi)—and the few illuminated moderns like Saint Thérèse of Lisieux, Mother Teresa, Thomas Merton, or Pope John Paul II. After twenty centuries, they still count as a rare minority.

These great mystics have had to struggle and suffer throughout their lives on their way to perfection. Was not St. Anthony of the Desert constantly tempted by devils and monsters, even at his old age of one hundred years? Was he not in fear of God's Justice, which as the Holy Book says is "the height of wisdom?" In fact, the greatest of them all, Saul of Tarsus (St. Paul), who actually saw the ultimate vision on his way to Damascus and was blinded by the force of that vision, kept begging God to take away "the thorn in the flesh" that recurrently plagued him. And he was told by God that this affliction was necessary so that he would stay humble and grow stronger through God's grace. He wrote that his "strength is made perfect in weakness." Lord, help us through our hesitant vacillations! Lead us to your Father's love so that His grace can sanctify us.

AN UNFORGETTABLE JOURNEY

The school year passed by rapidly, for I was hard at work with no further peak experiences to speak of. Summer came and quickly filled my time with many activities and concerns, leading me far away from the peace and tranquility of the "one thing necessary," except for the one week I spent at Oka Monastery, near Montreal. My trip to the monastery took place, in 1954, when Mike and Tony and their families went along with Dad to Italy and Lebanon for an extended visit of several months. The trip provided Dad with material for a new book, *Travels in Italy and Lebanon,* in which he compares the two Mediterranean countries and describes some of the contrasts between East and West.

Mom, Edmond, and I stayed home in Windsor, for Mom didn't like to travel—she was happiest at home. I had always wanted to visit a Benedictine monastery and the opportunity came in mid-August. I didn't want to drive there alone nor did I have the money to do it, so I asked a friend if he knew of someone going up to the vicinity of the monastery. I was informed that a distant relative would soon be driving up to see his daughter in Montreal.

After making arrangements, the old gentleman drove his car from Detroit to pick me up in Windsor, which was on his way up to Montreal anyway. When I approached the car with my carry-on bag, I saw four people in it: the driver who was a seventy-five-year-old man, Tony, my friend, sitting in the front passenger seat, and two others I had not met before. I took the right side of the back seat, next to the window. Dad always said it was the safest seat in case of an accident.

It was a Saturday morning when we drove off on a "picaresque" journey that I will never forget. The old man behind the wheel was a terrible driver and all of us alternated begging him to let one of us drive for a while ("to relieve him of the driving chore"). And every time he would answer saying, "I can't allow any of you to drive, because I've assumed the responsibility of your personal safety. Besides you're all in *my* car, and I will not have anyone of you put us at risk." Wow! What a *pagliaccio* he was!

All the while the old man was crossing over the continuous double lines to pass cars, even around curves. I was constantly sitting at the edge of my seat during the whole ordeal from Windsor to Montreal. As we approached Montreal, the passenger sitting next to me belatedly saw fit to inform me that this joker driving us had killed his wife a year earlier running a red light in front of a bus coming from his right. The wife died instantly. He was cited and almost sent to jail, but instead he was severely reprimanded by the judge, and the rest of his family forbade him to drive anymore. Yet this maniac had driven us already a distance of over one thousand miles and it was only by the grace of God that we made it safely to Montreal. I couldn't wait to get out of the car and leave this whole group of truant elders. The entire episode reminded me of a picaresque novel in 16th-century Spain—the *Lazarillo de Tormes* himself could not have been a greater buffoon than this foolish clown who drove us for two days.

SALVE REGINA

From Montreal, I took a bus to Oka, a small enclave which sat on the banks of the Ottawa River, where the Trappist monastery of "Our Lady of the Lake" was located. Thomas Merton mentions in his *Seven Story Mountain* this Oka monastery as the first one he considered visiting to discern a possible vocation to the contemplative life. Unfortunately, he never visited Oka, but instead ended up visiting and taking vows at "Our Lady of Gethsemane" in Kentucky, which became famous because of his writings.

Our Lady of the Lake Monastery at Oka was a large compound of buildings, barns and silos, built around a most elegant church, its white steeple rising prominently above the surrounding countryside. I arrived late in the afternoon, and was ushered by the guest master into a room facing the front of the church. I could hear the bell every time it rang, drowning the crowing of the roosters and the bleating of the sheep in the countryside. There were monks going hither and thither, doing their farming chores at all hours of day, except the times of communal prayer. I was asked to be in the refectory for supper at five o'clock, and I used the time in between to unpack; and then began reading a Thomas Merton book.

The silence and the peace of the monastery were evident by the minute. I could observe through the window the monks ending their daily chores and moving toward the dining hall. There were over sixty monks dressed in their white habits and as we ate nobody talked; all were listening to one monk standing up, reading a passage from Holy Scripture. When we finished eating I went walking outside, at which point the novice master approached me wishing me a good stay, but never once asking me if I was just visiting or considering joining. Shortly later, the bell began to ring again, summoning everyone to Vespers. It was still light outside.

By the third ring, the guests were all seated on the balcony in the back of the church, overlooking the sanctuary below, where the monks, seated in individual stalls, started to sing the evening office. The plain chant was beautiful and inspiring. After the evening prayers ended, the lights were turned off and in semidarkness all the monks assembled in front of Our Lady's altar to sing the *Salve Regina*. It was unforgettable to see and hear them bidding good night to their Lady Queen before retiring for the night. I often think back to the atmosphere of that moment—it was so reverent. It had a touch of medieval chivalry—the bidding goodnight to the lady the knights had dedicated themselves to honor and defend.

> Salve, Regina, Mater misericordiae;
> Vita, dulcedo et spes nostra, salve.
> Ad te clamamus, exules filii Evae.
> Ad te suspiramus, gementes et flentes
> In hac lacrimarum valle.
> Eia ergo advocata nostra, illos tuos
> Misericordes oculos ad nos converte.
> Et Jesum, benedictum fructum ventris tui,
> Nobis, post hoc exsilium, ostende.
> O clemens. O pia, o dulcis Virgo Maria.

(Hail, Holy Queen, mother of mercy;
Our life, our sweetness and our hope.
To thee do we cry, poor banished children of Eve.
To thee do we send up our sighs, mourning
And weeping in this vale of tears.
Turn then, most gracious advocate,
Thine eyes of mercy towards us,
And after this exile
Show unto us the blessed fruit of thy womb, Jesus.
O clement, O loving, O sweet Virgin Mary.)

After a few nights, I started chanting along with them from the balcony, but very softly. That hour of the evening was the most tender moment of each day and has remained in my memory as one of the times in my life I was happiest and most at peace. I've seen this scene repeated at the Camaldolese monastery in Big Sur, but it could never have the charism of the first time I saw it and heard it. Ever since, I've prayed the *Salve Regina* every night before going to bed; it is *my* bidding goodnight to the woman who is the most holy, pure, and immaculate in creation.

I was at Our Lady of the Lake monastery for over a week reading, meditating, and praying. I learned the three steps of *Lectio Divina* (Divine Lesson), the steps that all monks and mystics in all parts of the world and throughout the ages have practiced in their daily reading of Holy Scripture. This method consists of first reading the text, second meditating on it, and third entering a tranquil space of contemplation so that the soul can be purified by the grace of God, the Holy of Holies.

On the seventh day I packed my bag, said good-bye to a few of the monks in the kitchen (where I visited often because I could talk there and eat better) and left for Montreal, going back to the world. I guess I was still young and full of expectations of worldly success in my chosen profession. My twenty years had not taught me patience and tranquility yet. Deep down, *I never really left that monastery*, or for that matter, that world of devotion, contemplation and peace. I have come back to that tranquil state intermittently and often during my whole life. Yes, I have sinned many times. Yes, I have done what I was not supposed to do, but I would run back to grace-giving confession and communion every time, for I could never stand to be separated from my Savior for any extended period of time. It is a supernatural thirst for grace and peace that I have, and I thank my Lord for that precious gift.

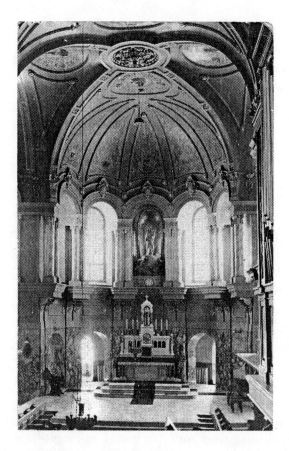

The Chapel of Oka Monastery: there the monks sang the Salve Regina every night, at sunset. Note their choir stalls at the bottom of the picture.

IRENIC DAYS

I returned to Windsor and spent the rest of the summer with Mom and Edmond. In midsummer, my brother Johnny came from Venezuela to marry Irene Farah. I had dated her with the express purpose of keeping her for my other brother, Philip, who had visited and met her the year before. As it turned out, Philip ended up marrying Lydia, the Italian-Venezuelan contessa with whom he was in love, prior to meeting Irene. But he encouraged Johnny to look up Irene, and finally he sent him to marry her, (in a way, maybe to assuage his own conscience for having left her). Now, I have known Irene since childhood when we were children in Serhel. Her family lived one door from us and we used to play with her sisters and brothers in the fields behind our homes. (By then my siblings were too old to play children's games with me.)

She was and still is *elegant-winter* in color scheme, with black hair, dark eyes, and a beautiful beauty mark on her cheek, where the movie stars used to paste them to look attractive. She always had an effervescent personality, so I was quite happy to entertain her for the rest of the summer, until my brother Johnny came to Windsor and married her. I knew then that their marriage would last a lifetime, and so far it has lasted forty-five years. They were able to have a child, Antoinette, who has grown into a cultured, beautiful woman with two children of her own and a wonderfully supportive husband, Dave. They live in Amhersburg, close to Windsor, and as of late, my brother Johnny and Irene have moved there from Quebec so they can be near their daughter's family.

When I think of Irene, I recall the story of her great-uncle Hanna (John) Farah, who lived in Serhel on the outskirts of town. Apparently, one cold winter day Hanna went down to Tripoli to buy meats and groceries for the family. Upon returning that same evening, he was dropped off at Karm Sadde, the closest place to Serhel that cars could get to in the middle of the snowy season. The ground was lightly dusted with fresh snow and, as Hanna was coming home, he heard one, two, and then three howls behind him. He looked back and saw a wolf, then two, then three, following him at a distance. He started walking faster, but soon the pack, having swollen to five wolves, appeared to be closing in on him. He had to think fast of a way out of this desperate situation and an idea popped into his head, even though he was scared half to death. He began to take food out of the bags he was carrying and throw it to the wolves. First, he tossed one steak, then two, then three. They would stop and fight over the meat and tear it away from each other. They were obviously very hungry. In the meantime, he upped his pace to almost running while he continued tossing groceries right and left over his shoulders to the wolves: ham, eggs and sausage, whatever he had bought.

As he approached his home in the village, he was left with only oranges to toss out, and toss them he did. But the oranges started rolling behind him on the down-sloping road to the village. He said he mistook the racket caused by the rolling oranges for the wolves and started running even faster until he was finally at his own doorstep, huffing and puffing, exhausted from the ordeal. When he looked behind him, all he could see were the oranges rolling down towards him. The wolves were gone. That was the story he told us when we were still children in Serhel. He swore that it was true in every detail. It has always been one of my favorite stories and I've been telling it to our children and grandchildren for years. And now every time I read a Jack London wolf story, I think of Irene's great-uncle and the five wolves at his heels.

Back in Windsor, and before the summer of 1955 was over, I fought a severe bout of hay fever. I stayed in my room on Reginald Street, with my eyes itching for days at a time. I passed the time listening to the radio with my eyes shut tight which relieved the itch. I started getting interested in major league baseball because I was listening daily to the radio broadcasts since I couldn't open my eyes. My eventual hero, Al Kaline, had just signed with the Detroit Tigers to play right field. He was drafted straight out of high school and never spent a day in the minor leagues. When I could open my eyes to watch TV, I remember seeing him catch a fly ball in deep right field and throw it the whole length of the field right into the catcher's mitt—the longest strike in baseball. "Out!" would shout the umpire, should any player dare to come home from third base on a fly ball to Al Kaline. He was a great batter, too, and very humble at that. I fell in love with his awesome talent. And the fact that he was born the same year I was born gave my ego a boost! We were both twenty-one years old in 1955, and I identified with him. I suppose everytime I witnessed him hit a long homerun I experienced a "tiny" peak experience!

CHAPTER 12

A GOOD DOSE OF MEDICINE

At the end of that wonderful summer, I went back to London, Ontario, for my second year of medical school. Since Tom Poisson, my former roommate at Mrs. Aziz's home, began earning free room and board by working a few hours at night at the mental hospital in St. Thomas nearby, I decided to do the same. I started the school year living at the hospital but didn't stay any longer than I did at the Oka monastery. Within one week of my arrival, a paranoid schizophrenic stabbed a hospital employee on the ward I was servicing. It occurred to me that I would never become a doctor if I died at that hospital, so I decided to leave before some maniac killed me!

I went straight to see Mrs. Aziz, but she had already rented the room I occupied the year before. My schoolmate Don Murphy solved my dilemma by introducing me to his landlady, who gladly rented me her last available room.

My new landlords, the Boyces, belonged to the United Church of Canada, an amalgam of once disparate Protestant sects, believing in instant salvation by "accepting Christ as their personal savior." Good works were desirable to them, but not necessary since "all who acknowledge Jesus are saved." They believed that their faith by itself guaranteed their salvation, so they saw little need for spiritual advancement, nor was this desirable to them. At the time I thought such a belief bordered on religious presumption, which is a form of pride. The Boyces practiced a sort of democratic religion, in which all believers would be equally saved, as if Christ had never said, "In my Father's house there are many rooms," or that "the first shall be last, and the last shall be first." We had a few heated discussions at first, but the Boyces were well-meaning devout Christians just the same, and after a few days I quit talking religion and enjoyed my one-year stay in polemical silence. They were nice to me and I decided to keep quiet and enjoy the peace.

This was the year we studied the pathology, bacteriology, and physiology of the human body, and were just beginning our clinical instruction. In the second semester we were finally allowed on the hospital wards in the afternoons, and we followed the surgeons and internists as they made their rounds on their patients. That was 1956, the year when the Cold War between the Western Capitalists and the Russian Communists got into full swing. Each side kept building and testing bigger and more destructive atomic and hydrogen bombs. I saw Mrs. Aziz's son, Mitch, in a restaurant after the New Year; and something he was reading in the newspaper (about the United States and the Soviet Union threatening each other with the use of hydrogen bombs) enticed me to tell him an old story from the time Antoine Yamuni and I were still living in Lebanon. "One day in 1945," I told Mitch, "we were led to believe that the end of the world could possibly come the very next day."

This was back in August 1945, when the big war with Japan had just ended. The United States had just dropped an atomic bomb on Hiroshima and two days later another one on Nagasaki. Shortly afterwards, the U.S. military announced that there was soon going to be an atomic test on Bikini Island, in the middle of the Pacific Ocean. I had heard all this on the radio and with my limited knowledge of elementary physics at age eleven, I told Antoine Yamouni to prepare for the end of the world. As I understood it, atomic fission was going to spread from one atom to another until the whole world got engulfed in the conflagration, and we were all going to die in the cataclysm. Antoine, who lives in Stockton now, reminded me not long ago, that when we heard this, we both went to confession and took with us his younger brother, Michel, whom we had convinced of the necessity of being in the state of grace in case we were all to die shortly.

Two days later, the Bikini natives were taken off the island they had inhabited for thousands of years and the bomb was dropped amid great pomp and a spectacular show of naked power. The event was broadcast all over the world by the news media and touted by them as a pageant not seen since the days of Nero in ancient Rome. Of course, following the atomic blast nothing happened, other than for a huge crater on Bikini in the Mid-Pacific, and the incineration of all the island's flora and fauna. Since we didn't die, I was taught a valuable lesson in natural philosophy on the errors of scientific extrapolation based on insufficient experimental evidence.

Mitch listened to my story and cracked up laughing, telling me that he and his brother Victor were old enough in 1945 to have undergone a similar experience about the explosion on Bikini Island. However they did not go to confession because as he told me, "That sacrament is no longer in common use among the Greek Orthodox in this country, and you know that's what we are. But do you remember," he went on, "that right after that atomic test the Bikini bathing suit became popular, supposedly because that's how the aborigines on Bikini Island dressed—scantily."

A LOVE AFFAIR WITH BASEBALL

The Boyces' boarding house was only four blocks away from the medical school and two blocks from the university's Victoria Hospital. In second year we acquired a considerable amount of basic medical knowledge. Dr. John Fisher taught pathology, the principal course during the second year. It was a protean course lasting the whole year, because the study of the myriad diseases and anomalies and their effects on tissues is probably the most important course in medicine. Dr. Fisher was the hospital's chief pathologist and a great teacher, but he was also an avid fan of the Cleveland Indians, who played baseball across Lake Erie, a stone's throw from London, Ontario. He got me interested in listening to their radio broadcasts, which I enjoyed that fall and again in the spring of that school year. I still sing to my grandchildren their advertising sponsor's jingle. Between innings, a girl's alto voice would come over the radio waves singing:

> *There goes that call again,*
> *That friendly, cheerful call again:*
> *Mabel, Black Label!*
> *Mabel, Black Label!*
> *Carling-g-g's Black Label beer!*

I have no idea why that jingle has stayed in my mind all these years. I recall another jingle, one about tooth-paste that was aired on the Detroit Tiger broadcasts:

> *You'll wonder where the yellow went,*
> *When you brush your teeth, with Pepsodent! Pepsodent!*

I've sung those silly jingles for years to our grandchildren as bedtime lullabies. I also remember many plays and incidents from those baseball broadcasts, including one night game, when the Cleveland Indians had used every single pitcher on the roster in relief (over a long fifteen-inning game) and the visiting team had the bases loaded, with nobody out at the top of the ninth inning. Suddenly, the Indians' manager surprised everybody by calling in Rocky Colavito from the outfield to pitch. Now, Rocky was their regular right fielder and home run hitter who was known to have a strong throwing arm. He would throw runners out at home plate with a single toss of the ball from right field straight into the catcher's mitt, just as Al Kaline used to do for the Tigers. So Rocky came to the pitcher's mound that night, threw a few practice tosses, and then proceeded to strike out the next three batters, leaving all three runners stranded on the bases. It was awesome! A delight and a surprise to every fan!

It was during that same season that Cleveland's great strikeout pitcher, Herb Score, was struck in the face by a line drive off the bat of Gil MacDougall of the Yankees. I was listening to the game! They took Score to the Cleveland Clinic Hospital, but he never recovered full binocular vision after that. The stricken eye ended up with less than 20/50 visual acuity. At that time, young Herb Score had a great future and was the Indian management's hope for many years to come. It was a tragedy for all baseball lovers in those days.

Another Yankee, Bobby Richardson, robbed me of much joy when, in the 1962 World Series, he robbed Willie McCovey of a line drive to center field with an outstanding leaping catch at second base. The San Francisco Giants were one run behind and had two men on base in the ninth inning when that catch was made. It was our first year in Stockton and it demolished all hope for a San Francisco Giants World Series championship. That is one incident that has remained clear in my memory, because I was teaching a Stanford eye resident in the surgery room at San Joaquin General Hospital, at the very moment when we heard the announcer say: " . . . And there goes a hard-hit line drive to centerfield . . . Oh! What a catch . . . Bobby Richardson just leaped and snagged the ball! The game is over! The Yankees win the Series!!!" At that very instant the Stanford resident, who was also an avid Giants fan, almost dropped the cataract he was extracting from the eye. I remember cajoling him, "Frank! Please, let's not have two tragedies in one day!"

I listened religiously to the Cleveland Indians broadcasts in the spring and fall, when I was at school in London. But when in Windsor during the summer, I was the Detroit Tigers' greatest fan and I would listen to them on radio or watch them on TV. About a year ago, I went to a Stockton Ports ball game, because octogenarian Bob Feller was going to throw the first pitch and Zeiter Eye was sponsoring the game. Feller was Score's predecessor as strikeout king for the Cleveland Indians. When he was signing autographs, I went up behind him and sang the "Carlings Black Label" jargon. He turned around and patted me on the back, nostalgically saying to me, "You must be from Cleveland, I haven't heard this jingle for forty years!"

"WHAT ELSE GOES UP, BRUCE?"

In bacteriology we had to memorize the Latin names of the genus and species of bacteria and other microbes. I recall that *Pasteurella pestis* was the Latin name for the plague bacillus. *Bacillus anthracis*, the anthrax germ that used to infest cattle, was identified by the great Louis Pasteur, who developed a vaccine to save France's cattle industry. There were *Clostridium botulinum, Clostridium tetani, Pseudomonas aeruginosa,* and many others. Now the botulism poison is used for injections to beautify women by masking the aging lines on their faces, whereas in those days we thought of it only as the deadliest poison on earth. We had to remember all those names, at least for the exams. I was good at it because I knew Latin and its derivatives. I would pronounce every syllable slowly and distinctly on purpose. It sounded like Italian opera. In Latin and its derivative languages, one pronounces all vowels audibly so that they don't come out as garbled, guttural pronouncements. The vowels a, e, i, o, u, are always pronounced the same no matter where they occur in a word—in any word!

All of the subjects we took in medical school were interesting and attested to the wonderful organization found in that phenomenon called man. I had to pass both written and oral exams for the finals. I was always the last student to be called in for orals since my name started with a Z. I thought it unfair, though, to have the students whose names were at the end of the alphabet always be last. By that time the professors ran out of fundamental questions and started asking about obscure subjects or esoteric minutiae.

This happened one year to Bruce Squires, a classmate who underwent a very embarrassing yet hilarious episode during his orals. His examiners were Drs. Stevenson and Stavraky, physiology, Dr. Burton, physical chemistry, and Dr. Rossiter, biochemistry; all sitting together for the oral exam. Bruce was six or seven students in line ahead of me. As his turn came up he entered the room and the door closed behind him. I guess by the time the professors got to the letter S (Squires) they had run out of the usual basket of questions. So they asked Bruce to describe the physiology of intercourse (coitus). Along with the function of the muscles of the back, coitus was hardly ever mentioned in our lectures. Bruce hesitated, and then said: "Well, sirs, in coitus the blood pressure and the heart rate go up."

"Very good! What else goes up, Bruce?" asked Dr. Burton, who was always a maverick.

"Well, sir, the respiratory rate, I guess," answered Bruce.

"That's good! And what else?" continued Dr. Stavraky.

"Well sir, the blood-sugar level skyrockets." Bruce was now sweating.

"And what else goes up, Bruce?" rejoined Stevenson of physiology.

Bruce was starting to get mad at their insistence. He said to himself, he told me later, "What do they want me to say?" And then instinctively he blurted out, "Well, the organ in question gets engorged with blood and goes up like a warning flag asking for satisfaction, sir!"

"No! No!" said Dr. Burton, "the adrenalin level goes up, young man, and that's what causes your . . . well, I won't say the word . . . to get engorged with blood. That'll be all, Mr. Squires, good day, sir!"

Bruce came out of the door pale and trembling all over. He thought they had flunked him. When my turn came up, and I went into the examining room, the professors were simply out of questions. Dr. Burton looked at me and said: "Zeiter! We're going to ask you only one question: 'What did Mr. Squires look like when he came out of here?'"

"Well sir, his face was as white as a sheet, and he thought that he had flunked. I know it's none of my business sir, but what happened? Bruce looked very depressed." They all roared with laughter. Stevenson actually described to me what happened, savoring every word, and the other examiners were still laughing. "Go out and tell him we gave him an A minus for effort." It was obviously a set-up and Bruce fell for it. Bruce was gentle and artistic and went on to specialize in gynecological endocrinology and years later became the dean of the medical school.

BIOLOGICAL GRANDEUR

I found medicine interesting and awe inspiring because the human body and its functions are of incredibly intricate complexity. It is a grandeur all its own, unequalled among God's great creation. In fact, it is mind-boggling that the human body (made up as it is of an organized hodge-podge of protoplasm consisting of 95% water) works at all. The old question of "the presence of evil in the world" is often summarized by another question, "How could there be a just God when a five-year-old dies of leukemia?" The answer to that question begs for medical knowledge. That is why priests and philosophers, with little, if any, medical knowledge, find the question puzzling and have always had difficulty giving it an adequate answer in their sermons or writings.

The fact is that the human body is so complex and is composed of so many organs, systems, cells, enzymes, hormones, and millions of biochemical reactions occurring simultaneously, that it is a wonder that not all children die before the age of five from any of the many malfunctions that may occur at any time to such a complex system. That the overwhelming majority of children do not die of leukemia or other diseases and live to a ripe old age is the greatest proof that there is a God who designed a system (with or without the help of evolution) that works well and predictably when it follows *His* chemical, physical, and other laws of nature. Even more unfathomable is to think that the *natural laws* themselves, which govern such intricate order and precision, developed by blind evolution or just came into being by pure chance. I find such a notion preposterous.

Strict evolutionists approach nature from the point of view of the genesis and development of life, rarely from the perspective of how does one explain the natural laws themselves which govern the process. It is one thing to gloss over the complexities of biological systems and try to explain this enigma through mutations and selection of the fittest. But it is an entirely different matter to try to explain away the perfect, immutable laws of chemistry, physics and mathematics as part of evolution. Did Nature—which, incidentally, is a word used to avoid saying God—try several methods of addition, subtraction, multiplication and division, before settling on an immutable rule of how these calculations ought to work? Did Nature, before it settled on its immutable laws, try several contradictory formulas for calculus or make various trials at the laws of gravitational pull, electromagnetism, and hydraulics? Did it try different spectral colors, various wave lengths for light and sound, and several variants and mutants of the laws of thermodynamics, friction, and critical temperatures prior to selecting the final model? As Einstein said a few years back, "God does not play dice with the universe!" The theories of evolution—I said theories, not laws—are totally inadequate when used as the only explanation of how the bulk of the natural laws themselves came into being. To advocate strictly material postulates to explain why we have the natural laws we do (to summarily rule out any form of intelligent design) amounts to reductionism in its most virulent form.

In fact, that may explain a puzzling phenomenon. Why is it that the preponderance of those dealing with the very inexact biological, sociological, and psychological sciences, tend towards agnosticism or atheism; whereas the majority of the scientists dealing with the hard facts of physics, chemistry, and mathematics, are less sanguine about explaining away the link between God and His universe? Maybe that is why good old Father Dwyer, instructed us in our first philosophy class, to go about for a whole weekend touching every object we came across, confirming to ourselves in loud words that, "It is! It exists! It has being!" That it was not an ideal figment of our own making!

A house may have one or two thermostats. The human body has thousands, maybe millions of counterbalancing controls that keep it from totally breaking down through entropy into the billions of simple atoms which otherwise function so marvelously together. It is these controls that allow the physiology of the human body to always tend towards homeostasis, towards equilibrium, as Claude Bernard noted. All living matter (let alone man) is a masterpiece, a perfectly functioning organized society of member organs and cells, working much more smoothly than the social and political institutions which man has created artificially. Under normal circumstances the body works to perfection, controlled by an internal autocratic governance of a myriad of automatic reflexes and responses. Aberrations and malfunctions are the exception to the rules and laws that govern the system.

Other things that I found interesting about the study of medicine are the legends surrounding medical discoveries. Many of these are serendipitous. Alexander Fleming discovered penicillin by accident—and yet not by pure accident. The discovery could only have been made by a mind prepared to notice the unusual. One morning, Sir Alexander was inspecting the cultures in the agar plates that he had placed on a windowsill in his laboratory a few nights before. One of the cultures attracted his attention because it looked different from the others. A colony of a strain of staphylococci exhibited an area in the center of the plate where there was a concentric circle of no-growth about two centimeters in diameter. He also noticed that in the middle of the no-growth zone was a filamentous, fungal-looking clump of extraneous matter. A janitor cleaning the laboratory would have completely missed the significance of the finding and might have washed the agar plate clean. Dr. Fleming's mind was trained to notice oddities on culture plates and to seek a reason for them, so the discovery of penicillin was not purely an accident.

Dr. Fleming examined the foreign invader and found it to be Penicillium, a common mold. He figured it must have accidentally fallen into the staphylococci culture from the breeze blowing through the open window and must have secreted the substance that inhibited the growth of the bacteria in the center of the agar plate. After more research, he made the world-shaking discovery that these Penicillium secretions do indeed inhibit the growth not only of that particular strain of bacteria but of several others as well. Eureka! He discovered penicillin, the secretion from the fungus Penicillium. Thus began the whole antibiotic industry that led to the treatment and cure of bacteriological diseases. The pharmaceutical companies now grow these bacteriocides in barrels and vats and help save millions of lives all over the world every day.

More discoveries were made eventually. After penicillin, other antibiotics began to be manufactured, streptomycin (which was used to control my sister Mary's tuberculosis), erythromycin, the tetracyclines, ampicillin, amoxycillin, augmentin and numerous others. At present we have effective antibiotics which, taken once a day over five days, will root out infections that used to kill millions of people barely a decade ago. Can philosophy, religion, economics, politics, or art, and particularly can the practice of law, of legal enforcement and judicial proceedings, claim such tremendous advances in their centuries-old methods? They cannot! That is why I have so much respect for my profession, and for the helping hand it has given humanity and still gives it every day. Tragically, the blood of willful abortion and euthanasia is spilled by the very same profession that paradoxically works so hard at saving life, even a single life.

Another story that fascinated me was the discovery of the benzene ring by Dr. Kekule. Up until then, most known organic compounds were thought to be chains of carbon atoms linked together in a straight line. Kekule found that certain compounds did not behave as straight hydrocarbon chains and was at a loss to come up with the reason for the difference. One night he dreamt of a snake curled on itself in a circle, biting its own tail. When he woke up, he had intuited the circular chain of the benzene ring, that hexagon-shaped chemical structure present in many organic compounds from simple benzene to the most complicated hormones and enzymes without which life would be impossible. That discovery opened the door for the mass production of steroids, prostaglandins and hormones, such as cortisone, androgens, progesterone, and estrogens. Presently, the pharmaceutical industry is one of the largest components of the gross national product. It is obviously an industry that is fundamentally necessary for our well-being, immeasurably more important than other industries such as entertainment, sports, or the consumerism of the Christmas shopping season!

We learned the history of medicine from Dr. Taylor who wrote the thick (over a thousand pages) book that we used in that course. In biochemistry, every now and then, Dr. Best, co-discoverer of insulin with Dr. Banting, would come down from Toronto to London to lecture to us and tell us the story of their discovery.

My interest and love of the scientific history of medicine induced me to join the Osler Historical Society and increased my enthusiasm to become a medical doctor. After all, history had always fascinated me. It had always explained to me what was happening presently in our world. I firmly agree with George Santayana's dictum that "He who does not study history is bound to repeat its mistakes." I was surprised to find medical science as fascinating as the humanities that I loved. It was a glorious feeling to know that I was supplementing my knowledge of the humanities with a deeper knowledge of natural science and medicine, and I was participating in the awesome responsibility of doing God's work by diagnosing, treating and curing the sick, and helping the lame. I never had so much passion for life and learning as during my years in medical school.

PSYCHOTIC ART

I was eligible to enter Alpha Omega Alpha, the honor medical society, when I was in my third year of medicine. To enter, I wrote a thesis, "Psychotic Art," using the concepts of "*catharsis* and *cathexis*" from Aristotle's *Poetics*, his treatise on art. To discuss deviant art I had to start with the concept of what is beautiful and what type of art meets, or fails to meet, this concept. First I considered Plato's theory of what constitutes beauty as found in the *Symposium*. I continued with Thomas Aquinas's definition "*pulchra sunt quae visa placent*" (beautiful are those things the sight of which pleases), found in his *Summa Theologiae* I, Q 5, Art. 4; and I continued with his subdivision of the elements that constitute beauty: wholeness or completeness, the harmony of the parts, and clarity or brightness of expression (*integritas, consonancia et claritas.*).

I then followed with a discussion of the modern investigations of Benedetto Croce, Suzanne Langer, and Ernst Kris. I planned to use pseudo-psychotic art illustrations from Hieronymus Bosch's paintings, Caravaggio's violent scenes, Hogarth, and especially Goya's "*Capricios*" and "*Proverbios*," some of which he sketched on the walls of his mental asylum. But I still needed fresh contemporary material drawn by actual neurotics or psychotics in a clinical setting. So I went down to Detroit where the Lafayette Psychiatric Clinic was encouraging the use of art as therapy for its inmates. I had made an appointment to investigate this with the clinic's director, Dr. Luby, since he was the force behind this trend. I went straight to the receptionist and asked her if I could see "Dr. Loony." She started laughing at my Freudian slip: "It's Dr. LUBY not Dr. LOONY!" she corrected me.

In spite of the faux pas, his staff was accommodating and happily gave me loads of material. I took back to London several original watercolors done by inmates and worked for two months on my subject.

The presentation of the thesis was successful. The very title aroused interest, especially since earlier in the year we heard talks on such unexciting subjects as "The Effects of Hypertension during the Third Term of Pregnancy" and "Vaccination, an Early Preventive Approach to Kala Azar." One paper's title was actually "The Isolation of the Alpha-Allantoic Enzyme in the Chick Embryo." So what would have been anywhere else a loony subject, *Psychotic Art*, hit the members of Alpha Omega Alpha like a breath of fresh air. In short, it was well received and long discussed.

Eventually my thesis found its way into *LIFE* magazine's Science Library Editions, in the volume entitled *The Mind*. In that publication, (the chapter called "Strange Landscapes from the Realm of Mental Illness," pages 136-51,) several of my paragraphs and reproductions were used—the ones I obtained from Dr. Luby at Lafayette Clinic. I was sent four copies of the *LIFE* publication and given a mention in the "acknowledgements" at the end of the book. That was the extent of the commercial benefit I derived from my work!

During my long medical career I have always been amazed by the great attention given to minute details by many of my medical colleagues, and particularly by those involved in research. Of course, the cure for many diseases has been discovered by dint of labor and minute research. But the Medical Honor Society prided itself on its interest in the general and philosophical aspects of medicine. *Psychotic Art* brought out many psychological, artistic, historical, and socio-philosophical questions. After I had finished my presentation, the discussion was intense.

My psychiatric mentor was Dr. Robert Harris; we became close friends following our association during the writing of my paper. He was also interested in the humanities, a bent not uncommon among psychiatrists. At Western Ontario Medical School we had to take one semester of psychiatry every single year, from the first to the fourth. This intense focus on psychiatric teaching was, and still is, unusual in a medical school program. I think it occurred due to the fact that the dean, Dr. Hobbs, was a psychiatrist. That kind of knowledge and experience, however, proved useful in my medical practice, because of the intense psychological overlay in many malfunctions, both physical and mental.

DAYS OF LEISURE

When third year came, we began to spend many clinical hours in the hospital during most of which we were on our own. So, I came home for long weekends and enjoyed talking to Dad and chatting with Mom, who was very solicitous about my comfort and health, especially when I was away at medical school. She understood that I had to be away to pursue higher learning. She would never ask me to come home if it meant skimping on my training for the future. This was evident several years later during her dying days when I was an intern in Detroit, across the river.

"Don't worry about me, *ya habibi* (my love). Go back to the intern quarters and get a good night's rest. You probably have a lot of work to get through tomorrow."

Dad was always interested in medicine. After all, he was once slated to go to medical school. He would listen to my stories with total attention, as if he was going to school himself.

During the summers, I kept on working at Mike's office each weekday morning. I would schedule patients for him, call the hospitals to schedule his surgeries, and talk with his nurse Dorothy when I had nothing else to do. He also paid my annual medical tuition, which in those days was $625 Canadian for the whole year. Now it's in the tens of thousands! Dad took care of my room and board expenses. The extra money I made working in Mike's office was pocket money.

In the summer afternoons I would spend the time reading, going to ball games, or just visiting my friends. Bob Kennedy, who was now a supervising engineer at Chrysler-Canada in Windsor, seemed to have plenty of free time on his hands. We would get together often and critique the politics of the moment or meet friends at Pilette Park, which became our gathering place. The park was on the Detroit River and had a beautiful view of that city's skyline across the water.

At presidential convention time in 1952 and 1956, we followed each day's deliberations of both the Democratic and Republican conventions. I was for either Robert Taft or Eisenhower on the Republican side, while Bob preferred

Adlai Stevenson. I learned about dirty politics early when the so-called "moderate wing" of the Republican Party brought back General Eisenhower from Europe and chose him over Robert Taft (who was *Mister* Republican for years) to be their candidate for the presidency. I felt sick for Taft and apparently he felt sick for himself because within six months of his defeat he developed cancer and died. Ike won the election in 1952 and again in 1956.

My interest in the Detroit Tigers never abated. I would pass sleepless nights wondering what would have happened if Al Kaline had caught Mickey Mantle's line drive that just made it over the right field fence. It was a feat Kaline actually accomplished quite often. He consistently robbed batters of home runs by leaping high against the fence and grabbing the ball. One of my fondest memories was seeing the televised game when the Yankee's Don Larsen pitched the only perfect game in World Series history. I rarely followed other sports. It was much later that I became interested in American football and basketball. Most of my summers between medical school years were the same. They were days of leisure that I recall with nostalgia. I would work at my brother's office in the morning and then spend the afternoon reading, listening to serious music and chatting with friends.

CHAPTER 13

THE CITY BY THE BAY

Around November, 1957, I had a crisis of acute anxiety that lasted several weeks. It was my final year of medical school and I had to decide on a hospital for internship. The final choice was between going to the University of California at San Francisco, a difficult hospital to get into in an exciting but distant city, or Harper Hospital in Detroit, which was close to home but not as adventurous. There were pros and cons to both choices. All this indecision came about because I had fallen in love with San Francisco the previous summer where I spent two months doing an externship. Following my visit to that beautiful city, I constantly daydreamed about living there.

I had driven there from Detroit with Dr. Phil Courey, a dentist and relative engaged to marry my cousin Sue Barkett in Stockton. He was to take the written part of the dentistry licensing exam to practice in California. I was chosen to spend two months of externship at the U.C. San Francisco Medical Center. It was July 1957. We had a great trip across the United States, being both eastern Canadians traveling to the western United States for the first time. Three years before, Dad and I drove from Detroit to Omaha, Nebraska, to attend the graduation of Dr. Joseph Barkett at Creighton University in 1954, but that was as far west as I ever went. Phil and I brought with us Phil's great-aunt, Mary Courey, seventy-five years old then. Phil and I were twenty-two, and we enjoyed listening to her life stories during the whole trip.

We got to Colorado Springs and wanted to take the bus ride up to Pike's Peak, over 14,000 feet in altitude, but Mary refused to go up the winding road to the top of the mountain. We made a big mistake in insisting that she go up with us, because the whole way up she was scared to death looking at the abyss below her. We went up and up and she started to panic and shake.

But when we finally got to the top and saw the majestic scene of the surrounding snow-capped mountains, she was happy and thanked us. We continued on to California, and entered that forested state by way of the Nevada desert at Reno on Highway 40 (now Highway 80). It reminded me of crossing the Syrian Desert and entering green, mountainous Lebanon to the west, before reaching the Mediterranean coast.

I remember when I first experienced the view of Lake Tahoe driving on old Highway 40. The lake was the deepest blue I had ever seen. I thought then that it was the most beautiful lake in the world. I distinctly recall the drive from Brockway Springs to Tahoe City on the north shore of the lake, a most beautiful view of limpid deep blue waters and snow-capped mountain crests seen filtered between tall pines and cedars. Little did I know then that I would come to spend many future summers in that scenic area.

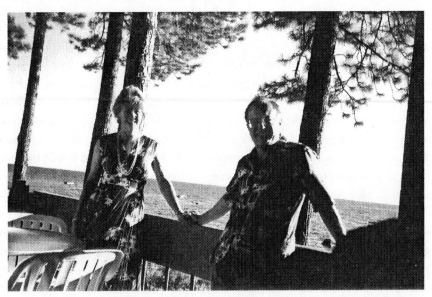

The view from the veranda of our Brockway Springs condo at
Lake Tahoe, just before sunset

We left Lake Tahoe and descended into Stockton where all the relatives lived. I was immediately impressed by Stockton's wide streets and easy living. I stayed at Uncle Tannous' house for the weekend before going to San Francisco with his son Joe. My cousin Joe had come from the Bay Area to take me back with him to the big city. He had been living in San Francisco for several years and had studied law at Hastings Law School, before suddenly quitting two months before graduation. To most people, walking away from a three-year investment in a profession would be unthinkable.

Walking away from a career, allowing a marriage to crumble through divorce, or letting a real estate investment go back to the bank would never be a consideration of mine. One ought to fight like a lion to see all these things come to a successful, or at least face-saving, completion. There is a commonly used Lebanese proverb which says, *wislet al likmeh littim,* ("when the morsel of food is one inch from the mouth, don't throw it away! Eat it!")

VIEW FROM THE BATHROOM

Six months before I first met my cousin Joe, he underwent a tragedy that changed his life and made him a disgruntled old man at an early age. It may have been the cause of his loss of interest in completing his career. His wife whom he adored died in childbirth. He had always held her in the highest esteem, respecting and loving her faithfully, "and then she dies just like that," he told me. He didn't even conceive of her as a regular human being. "She was full of honey," he once told me, "and when she spoke, I would hear sweet music accompanying her voice." The child, who survived (Douglas), was given to Joe's parents to bring up, (Uncle Tannous and his wife Frasiah). Joe rarely saw him because when he did he was reminded of his wife's death, so he normally avoided coming to Stockton altogether.

My visit to San Francisco helped him come out of his shell. He had undegone six months of solitary seclusion. We became the closest of friends, confiding everything in each other. We solved many problems together, starting with finding me a place to live, since he lived in a tiny one-bedroom flat above someone else's garage and I couldn't stay with him. I rented a room in the pharmacy students' fraternity across the street from Herbert C. Moffitt Hospital, the UC Medical Center where I was to be working the next day. That house, full of many memories, has been demolished since then in order to build an addition to the medical center.

That room was my heavenly abode for two months. It had a panoramic view all the way to the Pacific Ocean. It was on the second floor in the northwest corner of the fraternity house. Built at the top edge of a big drop in one of San Francisco's hills, it had a view of the Golden Gate Park below, the Arboretum and the little-league baseball diamonds to the right, and old Kezar stadium to the left. It looked beyond San Francisco, onto the Pacific Ocean. I could see the Golden Gate Bridge in its resplendent rusty red and Marin County beyond. To me, it was like looking at Rome, the Bois de Boulogne in Paris, the French Riviera and the Kadisha Valley all at the same time.

My work kept me in the hospital from 7:00 a.m. to 1:00 p.m. and Joe worked the midnight shift at the Youth Authority Center from 11:00 p.m. to 7:00 a.m.; so I worked while he slept, and he went to work when I was ready for bed. We had between 1:00 p.m. to 11:00 p.m. each day during two months to explore every nook of one of the prettiest areas in the world. We saw not only San Francisco, but the whole Bay Area including the east bay cities of Berkeley and Oakland, Marin County to the north, and the magnificent Pacific Coast from Santa Cruz to Monterey, Carmel-by-the-Sea, and Big Sur. I fell in love with this incredible expression of God's beauty, enjoying His creation— mountains, forests, and sea—and loving Him all the more for it.

I recall the entire two months as if it was yesterday. It was one of the happiest, most pleasant periods of my life. I was learning practical medicine in the morning, hiking the Golden Gate Park in the early afternoon, and cruising around San Francisco Bay each afternoon and evening with Cousin Joe in his red Nash Metropolitan. He had lived in "the City" for several years, but it took my presence to prod him to explore areas he'd never seen before.

The first weekend we explored the Cliff House area at the west side of the Golden Gate, where the Bay opens into the Pacific Ocean. The Cliff House is a restaurant that hangs on a cliff overlooking the ocean, and in those days there was a series of smaller snack bars on the cliff to the northeast. (They've been torn down since.) They sold hamburgers, hot dogs and sandwiches; so we stopped to eat at one of them, since neither Joe nor I could afford to eat at the Cliff House Restaurant nearby.

In any case, while we were eating our hamburgers, I paused to go to the bathroom. I squeezed into this tiny room that I could barely move in, but it had a small window with a view of the Pacific Ocean to the left and the Golden Gate Bridge to the right, with a fantastic panorama all the way to the massive mountains of Marin County across the water. I recall thinking to myself that the view from this small john in this insignificant little snack bar has got to be the most beautiful view in the world. I came out of the tiny enclosure and sat down next to Joe, finishing off my hamburger and chips; then Joe got up and went to the bathroom. He came out with a smile on his face: "Henry, I bet I know what you were thinking when you were in the bathroom."

"What was I thinking?" I asked him.

"You know, we're very much alike and we know each other well now," he said, "so I bet you thought what I thought when I was there. I looked at the view and thought it was the most beautiful view in the world." And as time went on I became obsessed with the Bay, and I decided then and there that I would come back someday and live in San Francisco.

JUST CRUISING

For two months while exploring the area, I was externing at the UCSF Medical Center. I took histories, attended conferences, examined patients and ordered treatment under the supervision of Dr. Paul Sanazaro, Peter Forsheim, and others. The latter impressed upon me the rule that diabetics must follow.

"If you are a diabetic," he would say, "you may have two of the following vices, but never all three: Obesity, the love of sweets, or smoking. But it is better not to have any, or you'll go blind from the disease." It is amazing to me how people crave their poisons: People with hypertension crave salt; diabetics love sweets; and asthmatics gobble up chocolate and love to have flowers around the house!

During internships (and more so in externships) there is usually a lot of scud work to do, but this externship did not include menial labor. It was designed to teach the basic principles of medicine, without taking advantage of the students. By the time I went back to Canada, I had learned plenty and was ready to enter fourth-year medical school.

In the meantime, my cousin and I were exploring the Bay Area to the hilt: Foreign movies, concerts, plays, parks, museums, and nightclubs with live Jazz bands. I recall one evening in particular. As we started driving over the Golden Gate Bridge on our way to Marin County, we turned on the car radio and Beethoven's Ninth Symphony had just started. We drove over the Golden Gate Bridge to Sausalito, then over the Vallejo Bridge to Berkeley, then to Oakland and the Ninth was still playing. We continued south and crossed over the San Mateo Bridge to the west bay and back up on Highway 101 to San Francisco and the symphony was just ending; which tells us either how little traffic there was in those days, or how long Beethoven's Ninth Symphony is—about an hour and seven minutes.

I recall visiting the De Young Memorial Museum and seeing for the first time, El Greco's *Saint Francis in Ecstasy*. "How appropriate for that painting to be in San Francisco," I told my cousin Joe. We then drove up to the Palace of the Legion of Honor Museum, which was a gift from France to the United States following World War I. One Sunday afternoon we went to hear the Budapest String Quartet that was scheduled to perform one of the mystical last quartets of Beethoven, the Opus 130 in B-flat major and my favorite. We got to the Civic Center and saw a long line of people slowly moving to the entrance to buy tickets, so we joined the line.

After about half an hour in line I told Joe, "There is no way all these people are lined up here to hear the Budapest String Quartet. I am moving up the line to see what's going on and I'll be right back." I inquired from a person half a block ahead, what are we in line for? This huge line of people was apparently waiting to hear Harry Bellafonte at the Opera House (the larger auditorium), close to where the Budapest String Quartet was to perform (at the smaller hall in the Art Institute next door). So we walked half a block, saw no line, bought tickets and went in. There was a small-sized chamber music audience of about 300 people. "That's more like it," I told Joe.

My favorite place in San Francisco was Golden Gate Park and all the many beautiful spots within it. I explored all of them for days on end, usually alone. Then the time came for me to go back to Canada and agonize over where to have my internship.

A SPRINKLING OF GOOD AND BAD

I was in my fourth-year medical school; I was unable to pull it off and go to San Francisco for my internship. I was accepted at UC Medical Center, a choice place to get into. But to go there I would have had to leave Mike, Edmond, Mom and Dad, and my friends, and probably never come back to Canada. I started rationalizing that I could always go there later after internship or residency (which eventually I did), but I couldn't make up my mind between Detroit and San Francisco and time was running out.

My psychiatrist mentor and friend, Dr. Bob Harris, came to my rescue when I told him about my indecision. He counseled me on how to make a final choice by telling me that the objects of a choice always consist of a sprinkling of both good and bad. The choice would involve having to give up the lesser good perceived in the thing one rejects, for the greater good present in the thing chosen. That made a lot of sense to me. He told me that making a choice is usually difficult because of our inability to sacrifice (give up) the good present in the thing one does not choose, for the greater good that we find in the thing chosen.

So, I chose to give up on San Francisco, in spite of its beautiful weather and scenery, for the greater good of closeness to home, a surer chance of residency at Harper Hospital, and peace of mind for the moment. And it all turned out for the best. Had I gone to California, I would have never met my wife, Carol; I wouldn't have been close to my mother at the hour of her death; I would have missed out on the good advice I continued to receive from both Dad and my brother Mike, and I wouldn't have trained at a great eye residency at Harper hospital under Dr. Ruedemann, who was then president of the American Academy of Ophthalmology.

Besides, Detroit had occupied a prominent place in our family history, ever since my parents lived there for ten years in the 1920s. I remember that when I was a child in Lebanon Dad told me that Detroit was French Territory at one time. That was before we learned at our French school that the whole Mississippi Basin, all the way south to New Orleans, belonged to the French until Napoleon sold it to the young American republic in 1803 when he needed funds for his military campaigns. We were also taught in French school that Napoleon was France's greatest hero and that he was unjustly maligned by the English, "that nation of shopkeepers," as Napoleon called them. So I was surprised when I came to Canada and took up history in that dominion of the British Empire. The perception and the teaching there was that Napoleon was an evil dictator who was set on conquering "the peace-loving Britons" and the rest of the world. Unfortunately, quite often in history, the victor's interpretation of what took place prevails, and the loser's version rarely survives.

I made the decision to intern in Detroit on December 6, 1957, on my father's birthday and five months before my graduation as an M.D. The minute I made up my mind about where to intern, I was at peace with myself. So I decided to enjoy my last year by concentrating on the clinical aspects of medicine and ignoring studying for the grades. Anyway, the final year was more practical than theoretical—we spent much more time in the wards than in the classroom (where we received grades). I was finally experiencing what it was like to be a practicing medical doctor, and I enjoyed every minute of it.

LEON WOLFE, A RENAISSANCE MAN

I recall the close friendship I developed that year with Leon Wolfe, a classmate whom I really respected. (He died in 2002.) He was one of the older students, having been a Rhodes Scholar at Oxford where he obtained a doctorate in entomology. He was in his thirties and I was twenty-three. I recall thinking that he was very old. The only older student in the class was Al Breuder, a former pharmacist, who also passed away in 2003.

Leon was brilliant and scholarly, a true Renaissance man. He was a mountain climber, a skier, a poet, an actor, an accomplished musician, and was respected by all, even the professors. I used to study with him before exams. One afternoon he took time out from study for three hours to explain to me all the techniques of mountain climbing. I never realized that mountain climbing was such a complicated sport, an art and a science all to itself. On another afternoon after class, close to the end of the year, we were studying for the finals, when he said: "Henry, let's rest from studying for a few minutes. I'll play Beethoven for you."

That took me by surprise; I didn't know that he played the piano. We moved to the family room and he asked me what Beethoven piano work I would like to hear. I told him in jest, play me something from Beethoven's last sonatas. He sat down at the piano and started playing the allegro first movement from the Sonata in B-flat major Op. 109. It was one of the mature and mystical late works of Beethoven, very difficult to interpret with the feeling it was intended to convey. I was mesmerized and couldn't believe my ears. He played the piece flawlessly. He continued with the Scherzo and then suddenly stopped and said to me: "Let's go back to studying, we're running out of time." I learned later that playing the piano was Leon's way to take a break from study. Tom Poisson and I would go to the ice cream parlor for a break, but Leon Wolfe played Beethoven's last sonatas for relaxation. I was saddened by the poverty of my own musical talents.

Here's a man who was a Rhodes scholar at Oxford, who climbed mountains, who had a Ph.D., and was now studying to be an M.D., who played the piano like a master, and who had many other talents, too numerous to mention. And yet two years earlier, during our second-year of medical school, he went home at noon one day and found his wife in the arms of the wife of his best friend. He was shocked and informed his friend, Dr. O'Brien, another Rhodes Scholar who studied with him at Oxford. They both left their wives. Apparently the lesbian affair had gone on for some time. Leon would have been a perfect catch as a husband, yet his wife preferred another woman.

Leon eventually went on for postgraduate training in neurophysiology at McGill University and became a Wilder Penfield fellow in neurophysiological research at Montreal General Hospital for forty years, with several discoveries to his name. I often saw him at our class reunions. He was still healthy, handsome, polished in conversation and wiser than he was at the previous reunion. He is dead now.

ANOTHER PHYSICIAN-MUSICIAN

While still in fourth-year medicine, I had another chance to meet a polished physician-musician while on my obstetrics rotation. I had moved to the intern's quarters at St. Joseph Hospital in London for two months, for we had to be on call to deliver babies. I was lying down in bed studying gynecology with my room door open when I heard the strains of Mozart's *Don Giovanni* overture coming from the hallway. This kept on for about four minutes when I decided to go see who was playing my favorite music.

I walked out into the hall and tapped twice on the door the sound was coming from. There was no answer, but the door was ajar. I quietly pushed it open, and to my great surprise a tall fellow, with his surgical greens still on and a baton in his right hand, was standing in front of a thick musical score conducting music that was coming out of his stereo record player. He stopped waving his arms, embarrassed, and introduced himself to me. He was much older than me, about forty.

We started a conversation through which I learned that he was a Hungarian surgeon repeating an internship in Canada in an effort to get his medical license. He had recently been the permanent physician-surgeon of the Budapest Opera Company when the whole troupe asked for political asylum while on a tour in Canada. At the very same time the Russian Army was cruelly crushing the 1956 Hungarian uprising. So the whole Opera Company, with its *corps de ballet*, its singers, and its accompanying orchestra members and their surgeon, opted to stay in Canada as political refugees. It was a great gain for the Canadian world of music and a boost to its cultural life. The make-believe conductor and I became good friends and started attending together the London Symphony concerts for several months, until I left medical school, though I don't recall his name now.

TAKING THE OATH

The study regimen was so concentrated that there was simply no time left for anything else, including normal eating habits. I wasn't always that way.

When I entered medical school, I was the only student who still enjoyed his food and ate it slowly. The other students would gulp down their food and rush to the afternoon anatomy lab, telling me to hurry up, so I wouldn't be late for class. I used to tell them we're all training to make a living and eat well, so why should I shorten the *end* that I was slaving so hard to achieve? Finally by the close of second year I was stripped of my Middle Eastern ease, even in my eating habits. Slowly and inexorably, I was becoming older, busier, and more utilitarian, but less imaginative and tranquil. Childhood was finally dying in me. I killed my artistic imagination for three years while I was embroiled in the process of becoming an efficient scientist and a precise technocrat.

I was evolving from a carefree child into an adult preparing himself for a demanding career. Instead of composing music in my head, I wishfully imagined myself becoming the world's greatest researcher. One day I would find the cure for cancer, or at least become the physician who would stamp out contagious disease from the face of the earth.

First and second year medical school captivated me because I was learning so much and finding the human body and mind so intricate and challenging. When third and fourth year came along, I was doing more serious thinking about a future medical practice and specialty. A plethora of medical careers kept me interested: the "Sherlock Holmes" investigative nature of the internal medicine diagnostician; the philosophical-cultural aspects of psychiatry; the structural design of the eye in ophthalmology; the pictorial-visual aspects of dermatology, but most of all, the caring, curative, and charismatic components of the whole medical profession.

I became convinced that no matter what one likes or dislikes; no matter what talents and abilities one had; no matter whether one delighted—horrible dictu—in blood or had an acutely sensitive nature, there was a medical specialty he could go into. If one hated blood, for instance, one could go into radiology or psychiatry. If one liked precision, one could go into ophthalmology or neurosurgery. Similarly, if one disliked people, he could go into pathology or research, and so on. Even such diverse interests as aviation, oceanography, or history can be satisfied by specializing in aviation medicine, marine medicine, or the history of medicine as a teaching career. Medicine, I thought, was the most protean field in human endeavors. After fifty years in the field, I know that this is true and probably more so now, because of the proliferation of medical specialization. I was for choosing medicine as a profession, because my interests were equally protean.

So in my final year of medical school I considered psychiatry, dermatology, internal medicine, otolaryngology, and ophthalmology—in that order. I even considered joining the Foreign Service as a medical examiner of those applying for entry into Canada or the U.S. I was told that it was a great choice because physicians are rotated and sent every six months to a different European or Asiatic capital. The person who told me that, Dr. Poulin, had done it for three years and enjoyed it immensely. However, when the time came to choose a branch of medicine, specializing in ophthalmology gave me the satisfaction of mastering one circumscribed field, leaving me time to pursue interests in the arts, humanities, and sports—but best of all to live a satisfactory family life.

Medicine has taught me to respect nature and its Creator. It has strengthened my faith in God because I acquired (first-hand) the awe-inspiring knowledge of the complexity of the human body and mind. And because of the nature of medicine, I have been given the chance to practice Christ's injunctions to cure the sick, help the poor, visit the shut-ins, and counsel the perplexed—in short, to make the world a better place to live in, both physically and spiritually. I thank God, as well as my father and my brother Mike, for inspiring me to become a physician.

Before we graduated, we had to take and sign the Hippocratic Oath. I still have it with my signature, framed and hanging behind my desk.

> *I will abstain from whatever is deleterious and mischievous.*
> *I will give no deadly medicine to anyone if asked, nor suggest any such counsel;*
> *And in like manner I will not give to a woman a pessary to produce abortion.*
> *With purity and with holiness, I will pass my life and practice my Art.*
> *Into whatever houses I enter, I will go into them for the benefit of the sick;*
> *And will abstain from every voluntary act of mischief and corruption; and*
> *Further, from the seduction of females or males.*

What noble notions and precepts these are. They are to be developed as a habit in our life as physicians, by our constant following of what we have sworn to uphold. This oath was taken by the Greek and Roman pagan physicians. We are living in a post-Christian society that refuses to honor the Hippocratic Oath. We have not so much become "pagan," considering that the oath itself was formulated during pagan times. Rather, we have sunk lower than they, practicing, as we do, the culture of death as no other culture in history has practiced it. Today many medical schools do not require their graduating students to take the Hippocratic Oath, and most of those who do, have a revised, watered down oath. Our civilization is surely headed in the wrong direction.

CHAPTER 14

INTERNSHIP AND RESIDENCY

I was fortunate to be ready to start my internship one month earlier than the usual first of July. I began the first of June because I had graduated two weeks earlier, on May 15th, and this made it possible for me to take July off without disrupting the internship rotation. I had planned to take the second part of the National Board of Medical Examiners in San Francisco in July, which, if I passed it, would allow me to get a license to practice medicine in California or for that matter, anywhere in the U.S., following my internship. On May 31, 1958, I crossed the river from Windsor to Detroit and was assigned a room in the intern's quarters across the street from Harper Hospital. I was informed that my salary would be $200 per month. Internship commanded slave wages in those days; and so did nursing. That was one of the reasons why the cost of medical care started to skyrocket when interns, nurses, and hospital personnel started to insist on living wages.

I was to start in the surgical service of Dr. Eugene Osius, the chief of staff at Harper Hospital. He was a big, burly man of German descent. Harper was a thousand-bed hospital in Detroit, and starting internship on the service of Dr. Osius was providential in my life. It turned out to be of major help in my obtaining a first-rate residency appointment.

In the meantime, I spent the last two weeks of May at home on Reginald Street with Mom and Dad, until I moved to Detroit. They were both pleased and relieved that I was not going to be far away from Windsor, Ontario—only across the river, in the city where they had lived for ten years during the roaring twenties. I passed my time at home listening to music, conversing with my parents, watching my beloved Detroit Tigers on TV, and visiting my brother Mike. He had promised me that once internship was over and I had my license, he would let me make his house calls in the evenings I had free from hospital duty. This way I could make some extra money to supplement the puny $200 a month that I would be making at Harper Hospital. So I passed my time pleasantly until I moved to Detroit, which was half an hour away from Mom, Dad, and Mike, should I want to visit.

I was scheduled to work in the emergency room for two weeks before going on to Dr. Osius' surgical service. In the Emergency Room my schedule was to be 24 hours on and 24 hours off. I would start at 7:00 a.m. with the morning nurses' shift. Then they would leave when the 3:00 p.m. shift started; and eight hours later, the 11:00 p.m. shift would take over until 7:00 a.m.; and all this time I would be still on call in the ER checking patients, only now half asleep. It was grueling working in the ER for twenty-four hours straight while witnessing three shifts come and go. And yet it had its good side, because at 7:00 a.m. I would go to my room and sleep until noon; then I would wake up and have the whole day to myself till the next morning. I would visit my parents in Windsor or go to the Detroit Art Institute or to a baseball game. The two weeks I spent in the Emergency Room passed by quickly.

One thing I remember was the incredible number of women who came to the ER with PID (pelvic inflammatory disease from gonorrhea). The nurses would set them up in stirrups to be examined by us. The stench was awful. We learned fast, to grade the severity of the PID as +, ++, +++, or ++++ according to how far we had to stand from the patient to smell the stench. Smelled at twenty feet away it was ++++; at only five feet away it was only one +. I decided then and there never to go into obstetrics or gynecology.

After two weeks, I was glad to be on Dr. Osius' surgical service. He specialized in stripping varicose veins, mornings and afternoons. He was famous all over Michigan for that. I would work on his side on the right leg while the chief surgical resident and the first-year resident would be stripping veins on the left leg, on their side of the surgical table. After two weeks of that routine I was bored to tears. I began to wonder whether it was better to work hard in the ER and be tired, or to do little in surgery and be bored! This state of boredom was the perfect time for me to go to California at the end of June, which I gladly did, though I still had two more weeks to complete the full month rotation with Dr. Osius when I returned.

THE YOSEMITE/KADISHA RESEMBLANCE

I drove to California with Phil Courey, just as we had done the year before. Cousin Phil was now getting married to my cousin Sue Barkett in Stockton, and it was convenient for me to travel with him to California. He drove all the way, and I hated driving. While traveling he asked me if I needed any dental work, and without realizing what I was getting into, I told him, "Yes, I do need work on a cavity I have in one of my left upper molars." He immediately signed me up to be his guinea pig for the second part of his practical exam (for his California license in dentistry). I sheepishly accepted. What could I do? He was driving me all the way West! It all turned out to be a breeze for both of us, for he got his license and I had a cavity filled gratis. In time, Dr. Courey became a very good dentist; he eventually was my father's, mother's, and my Brother Mike's dentist until he moved with Sue back to California twenty years later when he became my dentist.

I traveled all over California that month, after first having visited my uncles and relatives in Stockton and attended Phil and Sue's wedding. I wanted to explore places other than the Bay Area this time around. Cousins Henry Barkett and Raymond Rishwain took me to visit Yosemite National Park the first weekend I was in Stockton. Henry was the only member of his family to be born in America after the Barketts left Lebanon in 1938. The event of the Barketts' emigration from Lebanon is one of my earliest memories from childhood. Henry's mother, who was also my godmother, later told me that she named him after me, because she liked my American name.

Beholding Yosemite was visually and spiritually moving. The natural beauty hit me the minute we entered the park. There is a great resemblance between Yosemite Park and the Kadisha Valley in North Lebanon where I was born. But on that first visit to Yosemite, I was not aware of the reason for my passionate reaction of awe and wonder. Only when I returned to Lebanon in 1968, ten years later, did I realize why I swooned over Yosemite. My reaction on seeing Yosemite for the first time is exactly what is meant by the term *déjà vu*: an experience of intense familiarity with a place seemingly never encountered before.

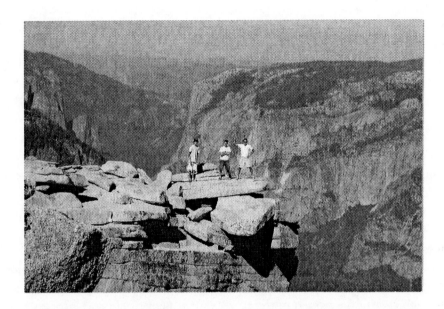

Standing on top of Half-Dome in Yosemite National Park, California

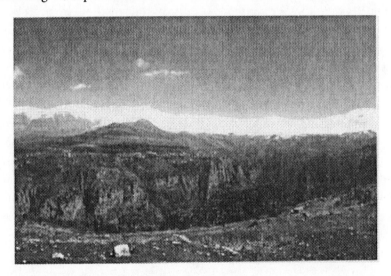

An impressive view of the deep gorge of the Kadisha Canyon, beneath the snow-laden crests of the Mount Lebanon range; it was that range that Uncle Paul and brother-in-law Michel Braiz had to cross to reach the Bekaa plain on the other side, where they sold their farm produce. In this photo Serhel is just to the left of the scene. The village in the center at the very edge of the gorge is Hadchit, from the French *haute chute*, meaning high drop—into cliffs.

The image of the Kadisha Valley stored in my memory and imagination was conjured up by the panorama of Yosemite Valley, a place I had never seen before. Re-cognition consists in *remembering* at the very moment of perceiving an object, that one has either seen it before, or has undergone a similar prior experience. That is what happened when I saw Yosemite.

It was the view from Glacier Point on top of Yosemite Valley that impressed me the most. A hundred snow-covered mountain crests are seen from up there; and at the same time, from the same spot one looks down and sees the impressive drop into the valley below, a sheer drop of four thousand feet, making the giant pine trees below look like toothpicks!

On the way back from Yosemite we took the southern route toward the Wawona grove of giant sequoias (*Sequoia gigantea*). A number of these huge trees are two thousand years old, still thriving from the time of Christ. I was flabbergasted by the immense size of the trunks on those trees. The "tunnel tree" was still alive and standing when we visited in 1958. Cars used to pass through the tunnel carved in the trunk of this giant sequoia. Unfortunately, this majestic tree eventually died and fell because of an ill-conceived human attack on its trunk. We counted several hundred of these huge trees. They grow in groupings called *groves*, like a family of three to five members bunched together. The thick and furry bark of these trees has enabled them to withstand forest fires over the centuries.

At the end of a pleasant day, we took the road to Fresno and came up the valley toward Stockton. It was a supremely hot July day in the San Joaquin Valley. The temperature was over 110 degrees. When we saw a watermelon stand on the side of the road, we were attracted to it like bees to honey. We stopped to eat watermelon to cool off. Henry Barkett went to the back of the car and opened the trunk to get his large army knife, and a few minutes later Raymond, noticing the trunk still open, went back and closed it. We ate tons of watermelons in the shade and when we were ready to continue toward Stockton, Henry searched for the car keys and couldn't find them in his pocket. He realized then that he had left the keys on top of a suitcase in the trunk that Raymond had inadvertently closed. We called AAA and, while waiting for what seemed an eternity, ate more watermelons until we were sick. We eventually got back to Stockton late at night when the valley had cooled off to 70 degrees.

It was on that day that I learned how hot the valley could get in the summer, but also how, as evening approaches, the temperature drops to 60 degrees or lower. It was a phenomenon I had never experienced in the Midwest, where the humidity and the heat normally persist day and night. I learned that on a hot summer afternoon in the Central California Valley, the heat causes the atmospheric air to gradually expand and rise up (as it becomes lighter), so that by evening a vacuum is formed at ground level. And since nature abhors a vacuum, the cool air from the Pacific Ocean is sucked into the valley's lower atmosphere to fill the vacuum. This current of cold air first cools the Bay Area, bringing with it the notorious San Francisco fog, and then proceeds on its way to our central valley to fill the vacuum created there. The current passes through the wide opening in the coastal range of mountains (the Carquinez Strait) where the San Joaquin and Sacramento Rivers form a delta before finally emptying into the Bay.

This physical phenomenon does not occur up north in Redding or down south in Fresno, because there is no major break in the coastal chain of mountains through which any major river flows. It gets hot between 1:00 p.m. and 6:00 p.m. when people are still at work in their air-conditioned offices, but around Stockton it always cools off at night to make for pleasant evenings and sound sleeping at night. The coolness persists in the morning till noon, even on the hottest summer days, so that playing golf or tennis starting at 7:00 or 8:00 a.m. is quite pleasant. I play tennis every other day, winter or summer, always at 7:30 in the morning. It is cool at that time in the summer, and in the winter we wear heavier outfits. Having a regular foursome to play is a real blessing.

Following my visit to Northern California in July 1958, I went south exploring the Los Angeles and San Diego areas. I was impressed by the vast spread of the Los Angeles area and its varied cities, each different from the other in scenery and climate. One night I attended a concert at the Hollywood Bowl when Janos Starker was soloist in Dvořák's Cello Concerto. Starker is still the best living interpreter of that greatest of all cello concertos. Attending that concert was to prove epochal in my life. I went back to my internship at the end of July, inspired by my trip and now more than ever in love with California. I returned to Dr. Osius' surgical service and to stripping varicose veins.

HOSPITAL POKER

Originally, when I came to Harper Hospital for an internship, I influenced some other medical students to intern in Detroit. Several of them were Windsor residents like Hal Wagenberg, Tom Klein, and David Schwartz. A few of us at Western went down to Detroit Receiving Hospital several months before internship started, to check it out. We returned to London with many exaggerated stories. We invented them in order to tease the medical students who were staying in Canada for internship (at Victoria and St. Joseph's Hospitals in London or at Toronto hospitals). We told them that pathology was so abundant in Detroit that at Receiving Hospital there was one ward for patients with *lupus erythematosus cum lupe* (with a reddened face) and another ward for *lupus sine lupe* (without the reddened face). That was an immense exaggeration to josh them, even though we were actually impressed with the three or four cases we saw in Detroit. *Lupus* is a rare disease which we had studied, but we had never seen a single case while in medical school. Of course, Detroit drew interesting cases from the entire state of Michigan and parts of Ontario, Ohio, and Indiana.

During both internship and residency I belonged to a poker group that met every night at the interns' quarters; at times we played past midnight. We used to rationalize that with the pitiful stipend they were paying us, and with food and lodging free, all we could use the stipend money for was to play quarter-ante poker. I don't know how we were able to get up in the morning with so little sleep and then work a full day on the wards or in the operating room.

A group of Filipino doctors at Harper sat with us at the poker table nightly. I remember particularly Sam Hernandez and Benito Liu. Sam would play the game until he was ahead by twenty dollars or so, and then would leave the table, giving us some lame excuse or another. Poker etiquette dictates that one doesn't leave the game *early* while ahead, because it is only fair to give the other players a chance to recover some of their losses. I asked Sam one evening if he was ever ashamed of taking advantage of the other players.

In reply, he took me to his room, opened his closet doors, and showed me about twenty brown suits, twenty brown sweaters, twenty brown shirts, twenty brown ties, and twenty brown shoes neatly grouped inside the closet.

"Here are my poker winnings!" he told me; "When I get back to Manila I am going to be known as Doctor Brown!!"

Sam could be very funny. Four years later, when both of us had completed our last day of residency, he and I were leaving the hospital through the front entrance. At that very spot there was a ramp leading to an information booth around which patients and relatives always gathered to ask for directions. As we approached that booth, Sam increased his pace, jumped high up in the air in front of the booth, and coming down let out the grossest fart I've ever heard. "Good Bye Harper Hospital," he shouted on his descent.

One poker evening, Dr. Wally Romano, the radiology resident, got called to X-ray a broken arm at Children's Hospital. He got off the poker table and asked me if I would go along with him, as Children's Hospital was in a dangerous part of town. We arrived at the emergency room, and sure enough a five-year-old boy was holding up a swollen forearm that was probably broken. Sitting next to him was his hefty mother. I couldn't help but notice the boy's name on the front of the chart while Wally was taking the X-rays in the other room. Strangely enough, the boy had the name of a famous baseball player. I asked the mother if she knew that there was a baseball player by that name—a great homerun hitter, who played as catcher for the Baltimore Orioles. She said, "Ya, that's his daddy." I concluded that on a certain hot summer evening when the Baltimore Orioles came to town to play the Detroit Tigers, some wild oats were sown!

One evening, while he was still in training, Alfred Ruedemann, Jr., my old chief's son, brought home from the butcher shop a whole jar of pigs' eyes so he could practice corneal transplantation on them. He placed the jar on the top refrigerator shelf, but inadvertently left the lid loose. The next morning when Ruby, their old maid, opened the fridge door, the uncovered jar fell from the shelf, and fifty eyeballs rolled over the kitchen floor all around her feet. The maid went berserk, screaming: "Lordy, Lord! Lordy, Lord! Have mercy on me!" And she ran out of the house never to be seen again.

MEDICINE AND MUSIC

I was eventually accepted into the ophthalmology residency at Harper thanks to Dr. Osius. Here my love of music turned out to be a great advantage. After I returned from the California trip, Dr. Osius asked me, while we were in surgery one morning, what I liked the most about California. I don't know what possessed me to tell him that it was a concert at the Hollywood Bowl where I heard Janos Starker in a performance of the Dvořák Cello Concerto. He looked surprised and asked me if I liked cello music. I promptly told him I did. "Then come to my house on Wednesday afternoon at two o'clock," he said and gave me his home address.

When I got to his house on Wednesday I was a few minutes late. His butler ushered me into a large living room overlooking the Detroit River. To my surprise Dr. Osius and three other doctors from our hospital were sitting in a circle playing a Schubert string quartet. Osius towered over a glistening cello, playing with expressive gusto. He was going through his cello part marvelously. I realized then why he looked so pleased when I told him I liked cello music.

A few days after, he asked me if I liked seafood. How could I say no to the chief of staff! He invited me to eat at Joe Muir's, Detroit's finest fish restaurant, and taught me how to eat lobster in-the-shell, a delicacy I had never been able to afford. Two weeks later, I took my Filipino friends to the same restaurant. As I was showing them how to dissect their lobster, I heard a booming voice behind me saying: "Yesterday, a pupil, and today a master, eh, Henry." I turned around and Dr. Eugene Osius was hovering above me. The next morning in surgery, he asked me if I had applied for a residency program at his hospital and I informed him that I had applied to Dr. Ruedemann's eye residency (there were 72 applications for two spots in that residency). He smiled approvingly and asked me about my grades in medical school. I told him they were very good. Then he said to me, "Henry, don't you worry about getting in! Ruedemann and I were classmates from first grade in Detroit to the end of medical school at the University of Michigan." I saw right away that this new connection with Dr. Osius would put the frosting on the cake as far as getting a residency. And so it was! Within days I received my letter of acceptance to the Eye Residency at Harper Hospital and its affiliated Kresge Eye Institute.

THE KRESGE EYE INSTITUTE

This institute came into being as a gift from Stanley S. Kresge, the department store mogul who happened to have been operated on by Dr. Ruedemann for retinal detachment. Retinal detachment surgery was not advanced in those days and the success rate compared to cataract surgery was notoriously poor. S.S. Kresge was admitted to Harper Hospital after a sudden loss of vision in his right eye. Dr. Ruedmann diagnosed the cause as a retinal detachment and operated on him the next day. Retinal detachments were not one of our chief's fortes, but he was a so-called "cutter" (i.e. happy with the knife), and would operate on a sick eye without hesitation. He undertook the surgery; in spite of the poor success rate for detachments in those days the result was a success. Sight was fully restored, and S.S. Kresge was very grateful. Ruedemann didn't charge him the usual fee and asked the hospital to waive theirs as well. Several months later, on one of his follow-up visits, S.S. Kresge asked his surgeon how come he hadn't been billed yet for the surgery and for the hospital stay. My future chief wisely said to him, "Because you are a prominent philanthropist and have donated money to several hospitals in the area in the past. Harper is grateful to you."

Actually, he had never donated to Harper Hospital and Ruedemann knew it. "What can I do for you?" asked Mr. Kresge.

"Sir, I have many young upcoming eye doctors training under me; I am teaching them how to restore vision to blind people just as I have done for you. If we only had a specialty institute to teach them the basics, I could double the number of doctors I am training to help people see."

Thus began the Kresge Eye Institute with a two-million-dollar grant from the Kresge Charitable Foundation. The donation was used to buy the building on Mullett Street, in downtown Detroit, and to furnish it with the latest in equipment and with the best basic science professors. In time the eye residents from Henry Ford, Sinai, and Grace Hospitals, as well as Harper and Detroit Receiving, all began to send their first-year residents to the Kresge Eye program. That's where both I (1959-62) and thirty years later our son, John Henry (1989-92), took our residency training in ophthalmology.

As time went on, Dr Ruedeman and Mr Kresge developed a very close friendship. One winter, they were vacationing with their wives in Palm Beach, Florida. S.S. Kresge woke up in the morning and couldn't see to read the newspaper; alarmed, he told ADR he couldn't see to read. Ruedemann asked him,

"Where did you leave your reading glasses?"

"In Detroit," was the answer.

"Well, for cat's sake, that's the problem," said Ruedemann. "Let's go to one of your stores and pick up some reading glasses for you."

At the store, the booth where the reading glasses were located was unattended. So Dr Ruedemann, the President of the America Academy of Ophthalmology, started trying various spectacles on S.S. Kresge, the owner of that store and many others. Within minutes the grey-haired lady attendant of the booth ran over and began castigating them for messing up her display of reading glasses.

"What do you think you're doing?" she quizzed the Doctor.

"I am fitting him with glasses," he replied politely.

"What do you know about fitting glasses, you old codger?" She said raising her voice.

At this point both of them had an urge to laugh, but decided to go along with her. She found a pair of glasses that allowed Mr. Kresge to read clearly. But before they left she gave them a severe warning,

"Next time I see you messing up my table, I'll call security and have you thrown out of the store! Do you hear?"

They paid her and walked out. Dr. Ruedemann told us later that the minute they passed the front door, they cracked up laughing. They told their wives the story and all four would start laughing every time they thought of the incident. That went on for the whole two weeks they were in Palm Beach.

All first-year residents had to spend each morning at the Kresge Eye Institute on Mullett Street, learning the basic sciences of the eye—the principles of optics, the anatomy, histology, and physiology of the eye with its bacteriology, pathology, and neuroophthalmology. Since I was the neuroanatomy whiz from medical school days, I was asked to assist Dr. Maurice Croll teach that subject. He was professor at both Kresge Eye and Wayne State University. For optics we had Dr. Emil Ludwig, "the man with the wooden leg." He was a superb physicist who knew both physical and physiological optics backwards and forwards. Early in the course, he put a stop to the gossip about his leg by telling us the real story of how he lost it. Apparently, while on a fishing trip in the Amazon basin in Brazil, he fell accidentally from the canoe into the river. "That river was infested with piranhas," he told us, and stopped his story right there. He didn't want to talk about what happened next.

Dr. Everett Kinsey taught us ocular physiology and Dr. Ralph Pino taught us the principles of refraction and the prescribing of eyeglasses. He also taught a short course on the practical aspects of managing an ophthalmology practice. Why is it, I have often asked myself, that the practical aspects of managing one's professional practice are given only a passing mention, if at all, in the years of training? Whether the field is law, dentistry, medicine, architecture or accounting, the know-how of running the practice is given short-shrift. This shortfall in our educational system is universal, affecting all the professions. What a shame! The graduate leaves academia without any knowledge of how to manage his or her practice, or even his own household budget. I have met several accountants and attorneys who are experts at tax shelters and at balancing books, but who don't know how to buy or sell a piece of property or how to run the finances of their own practices?

I learned a lot from the tall, bespectacled, always trim and slim, octogenarian Ralph Pino. Within a year of having established my own practice in Stockton, California, I hired an optometrist to do the refractions and fit glasses. Dr. Pino had warned us about the unnecessary jealousy and rivalry that exists between optometrists (O.D.s) and ophthalmologists (M.D.s).

OPTOMETRISTS V. OPHTHALMOLOGISTS

"The optometrists are trained to check and fit the patient with glasses," Dr. Pino would tell us, "and yet they want to do medical ophthalmology as well. On the other hand, ophthalmologists don't want to accept the fact that they are not as good at refraction for glasses as are optometrists." It is similar to the rivalry between orthopedists (M.D.s) and chiropractors (D.C.s). "Why don't ophthalmologists hire one or two optometrists in their practice to do their refractions and fit their patients with glasses?" he preached, "and free themselves for the task of medical treatment and surgery?" Then he would add with a wink, "This way we can keep them off the streets and under supervision, so they wouldn't do any harm practicing outside an ophthalmic office!"

In those days one rarely saw ophthalmologists and optometrists working together. Now it is common practice. I started that trend by hiring optometrists shortly after opening my practice in 1962. I had Barry Wooledge, O.D., working with me for many years. Now, the busy practice (Zeiter Eye) that I left under the care of my progeny, Joe and John Henry, consists of seven offices strategically located around San Joaquin county, employing five optometrists to work with us. Besides, we are often invited to other optometrists' offices to give them instructions in post-surgical care and to confirm or deny a surgical necessity. This way, the trust the patients have in their optometrists is automatically transferred to the surgeon and vice versa; and the patient's anxiety about undergoing surgery is much allayed. It is a win-win situation all around. Since then, this policy has been adopted by most ophthalmologists. Gregarious Dr. Rob Paterson, O.D., has been with us for over twenty years. Dr. Gerry Burke is our contact lens fitter, and Dr. Linda Hsu has her own practice but comes a few days a week to work in our various offices.

But the marvel of them all is Dr. Howard Abrams, who still comes and puts in one day a week at age ninety. Howard started referring patients to me forty years ago when I first came to Stockton. He told me that he observed when I first started that I "cared for optometrists and was humble enough to think and behave towards them as colleagues of equal worth." Dr Craig Hisaka, professor at U. C. Optometry School, has said the same thing to me. When Dr. Abrams closed his own practice twelve years ago to retire, he couldn't stand the boredom of staying at home, so he sheepishly asked Dr. Joe and me if he could work in our office. We were delighted. I told Joe at the time that if we don't take him in after all his years of loyalty to our practice, God will punish us! Howard still skis in the High Sierras in the winter and is active in the Lions internationally, helping in eye missions overseas. We are personal friends and on the best professional terms with all of our optometrists and ophthalmic technicians. The whole office staff is like a family working together with the same objective: helping people.

"Even if you don't have optometrists working for you," said Dr. Ralph Pino, "respect them and befriend them because they are your best source of surgical referrals, and besides they know a cataract from macular degeneration when they refer the patient to you."

Thanks to Dr. Pino's advice, I befriended the optometrists, from day one, as equal professionals in the practice of helping people to see. They've always known that my feelings were genuine, and they have helped me build my practice by sending me all their referrals. I will always remember Dr. Pino for his practical philosophy.

MY CHIEF, DR. ALBERT D. RUEDEMANN

At Harper Hospital, the eye service ward was on two-west, or the western wing of the second floor. One evening I had a curious experience there. Tennessee Williams, the celebrated playwright, was mistakenly admitted to the eye ward, because it had the only hospital bed available that night. He was literally picked off the street by the police and dragged into the hospital. He was drunk, belligerent, and arrogant. The worst part of his behavior was his condescension towards the nursing staff. I was chief resident on call that evening and I had to do a physical exam on him, which was impossible because of his condition. Before the morning sun came up, he signed himself out of the hospital, and that was the last I saw of him. Dr. Ruedemann would have had a fit had he remained on his wing of the hospital. When I informed him the next morning of what took place the previous night, he said to me, "I could never stand that filthy, liberal, decadent worm, nor did I ever like any of his plays."

Dr. Albert D. Ruedemann was conservative politically. He would listen to Paul Harvey (the Rush Limbaugh of his day) on the way to the hospital in the morning, and then he would repeat to us his guru's opinions as he was operating, emphasizing to us everything Harvey had said on the radio.

I remember the time A.D.Ruedemann Jr., came back from Essen, Germany, having acquired a photocoagulation machine from the German ophthalmologist-inventor, Gerald Meyer-Swickerath. It was the first to be brought into the United States. The machine was huge. It occupied half the surgical room. By contrast, now we have small lasers which the surgeon holds in one hand that accomplish the same task a hundred times more efficiently than did the original two-ton machine—just as computers have become much smaller. The progress in medicine in the recent past, and particularly in the technical field of ophthalmic surgery, has been monumental.

MY MOTHER'S GLORY

While in eye residency, I underwent a trial of lost love and it's after effects. It was not a loss of romantic love, but the loss of my mother. She was operated on for gall bladder inflammation the year before. For a whole year she was nauseated, uncomfortable, and sickly—the symptoms of the so-called post-cholecystectomy syndrome, common after gallbladder removal. What my brother Mike and I, the two doctors in the family at the time, failed to realize is that these symptoms merged into those of her colon cancer. Mike and I were thinking all along that it was a post-gallbladder problem.

She was finally admitted to Hotel Dieu Hospital in Windsor and a diagnosis of cancer of the caecum was made. Her abdomen was opened, but the cancer was found to be inoperable; it had spread throughout the abdomen and the wound was closed. Prior to the surgery, when we saw the x-rays we were encouraged because cancer of the caecum, as contrasted with cancer of the descending colon and sigmoid, is not a penetrating or metastasizing disease and is usually caught in time. But not in her case; she had a deadly penetrating form of cancer on the wrong side of the colon, where it was not expected to occur. Her cancer was of the worst kind.

For three months she had palliative treatment in and out of the hospital. It was during her final days in the hospital that she would send me away nightly so I would not see her suffering. She would tell me that I had to get up early the next morning for hospital rounds and I needed my sleep. I did not let her know that I was in no state of mind to think of rounds and hospitals. Finally, early on the morning of November 16, 1959, my brother Mike called me to tell me that she had passed away at two in the morning. I had been at her bedside until midnight, but she had sent me back to the interns' quarters, telling me as usual that I needed my rest. Mike said to me that he did not want to wake me up earlier because there was nothing I could do. My oldest brother has always been gentle and considerate. When I finished talking to him, I hung up the phone and played Mozart's *Requiem* on my hi-fi set. I cried while listening to the Latin words of the *Dies Irae* and the *Pie Jesu*.

Then I left the interns' quarters and drove to Windsor to make the funeral preparations. When I arrived at the hospital, my mother's body was en route between the morgue and the funeral home. I spent all morning with the preparations, but the task of choosing a casket was the worst. I felt I was speeding up her time of burial. When the body was finally exposed in the funeral parlor, I cried every time I saw it. Freud once said that upon seeing someone dead, the first thought is, "I'm glad it's him/her and not me lying in there." I didn't feel that way when I saw my mother in the casket. Far from it—it really hurt—but then I was still alive!

Three days passed in grief, then came the funeral. The people at the funeral parlor took her golden wedding ring off her finger and gave it to me. I kept it until my wedding day. On the inside of it there was an inscription in Arabic that said,

"Married to Yousef Zeiter, 1932"

I kept it on my ring finger for 30 years until John Henry, my eldest son, got married. At his wedding, he forgot to bring the ring to the Church, the one his wife had picked out for him. That's children for you! Panic ensued. He ran to me and asked me if he could borrow my wedding ring "just for now." I lent him the ring for the ceremony, but have never been able to retrieve it from him. His wife, Lynette, a romantic (in fact a landscape painter), was adamant that it was *the ring* used in their ceremony, and therefore, the true ring that John must wear forever. Such is life! Fortunately, my worldly prudence came through again. I started using Dad's ring. At his death in 1986 I was given *his* wedding ring when he passed away, 27 years after my mother's death and three years before my son's wedding. It had inscribed in Arabic on the inside: "Married to Badwyeh [Antoinette] Zeiter, 1932"

Now I wear that ring. As life would have it, providentially, I wear the ring that has mother's name inscribed inside of it. What a tribute to my love of her! I did not intend it that way, but God made it so!

The cross that was on the casket at the time of burial was also given to me before my mother was lowered into the grave. I recall hugging the crucifix to my chest and keeping it there while crying all the way home from the cemetery. That crucifix now hangs in our house.

CHAPTER 15

CAROL

I never dated very frequently. Up to this point, if I knew a girl, it was as a friend. Within three months of mother's death I began to date a few of the nurses and trainees at the hospital. They were for the most part a few years younger than I. After several months of getting nowhere, I met Carol, the girl of my dreams. I took her to a concert on our first date, and right away I knew that I was going to marry her. The character traits I hoped for in a wife Carol filled to perfection. In fact, I fell in love with her on our first date.

While at a medical conference at Ann Arbor the week before, I had seen a poster advertising a concert on May 8, 1960, Mother's Day that year. The Philadelphia Orchestra under the baton of the celebrated Eugene Ormandy was to perform the Verdi Requiem, with three university choruses massed together. I had always been a requiem buff (for years I used to collect requiem recordings), so I bought two tickets, figuring I would invite one of the nurses or my brother Edmond to go with me.

On a Thursday morning, three days before the concert, I entered the hospital cafeteria to have breakfast, and my eyes immediately settled on a group of seven or eight nurses just off their night shift, drinking coffee. I had seen most of them around before, so I walked over to that table, informed the group that I had two tickets to a concert on Sunday, and casually asked if any one would like to go with me. The nurse at the center of the table (by far the prettiest one) put her hand up and asked me, "What are they playing at the concert?"

I had seen this girl around, because my co-resident's wife, Mary Stief, who worked with her on the pediatric ward, had pointed her out to me and told me that we would make a great pair. I learned later that she was saying the same thing to Carol.

When this cute nurse asked me what they were playing I was surprised at the question, since most of the nurses I had ever taken out before didn't care to know what kind of music they were listening to with me in the car. More often than not, they would change the station from my beloved Mozart to some station playing popular music. I told her that it was the Philadelphia Orchestra playing the Verdi Requiem. Her face immediately lit up, and she told me that she would love to go with me.

"Besides," she said, "my dad is taking my mother to the same concert and I planned to be with them for the whole Mother's Day weekend. So if you can get a ride there I'd love to attend the concert with you, and we can return to the hospital in my car if you wish."

We made arrangements to meet in Ann Arbor. Three days later on Sunday afternoon, I met her at the concert hall. She introduced me to her parents and we sat one row behind them. Now I was puzzled, because I had already bought the tickets one week before. How could her parents be one row ahead of us? Did she plan for them to meet me? I didn't know then; but I doubt it, since now I know Carol is very straight and not a bit devious. I learned from her later that I was the hundredth date of her young life. Her mother, who was a slightly handicapped Polish immigrant, wanted her in the worst way to be popular, so she allowed her to date starting at age thirteen.

The Requiem started with the *Requiem dona eis Domine* and then the *Kyrie Eleison* as usual, and I turned to whisper in her ear how beautiful the music was, when she said to me: "Wait until you hear the *Dies Irae*, you're going to be blasted out of your seat." She had no idea at the time that I was a fan of serious music, or that I had heard the Requiem before.

I thought to myself, "What is going on here? This girl seems to know and like my kind of music more than I do! I had better keep quiet and see what happens!"

The *Dies Irae* came and it was stupendous. When she noticed that I was getting excited again, she whispered in my ear, "Wait 'till they get to the *Tuba Mirum*, they'll probably bring the trumpets and the trombones to the back of the hall for a greater effect in that *Last Judgment* segment."

I said to myself, "Holy mackerel! I can't believe this is happening to me! This girl is one in a million. She really knows and loves great music."

When the concert ended, we exchanged pleasantries with her parents, and immediately took off in her car back to Detroit, with Carol behind the wheel of an old turquoise-green Pontiac. As we drove back, she told me that she was working on her master's degree in pediatric nursing at Wayne State University.

She mentioned taking an elective course at the University of Detroit to get some extra credits. I asked her if she knew that the University of Detroit was Catholic and Jesuit-run, and she said yes. Then I asked her, "What are you taking at U.D.?"

"I thought I'll take a course in philosophy; I know so little about the subject," she said. I asked her what kind of philosophy and she replied, "Metaphysics."

Now metaphysics, the study of being, was, and still is, the love of my life. So I was flabbergasted. My questions then flew in succession:

"Do you have a favorite philosopher?"

"St. Thomas Aquinas," she replied.

"Are you Catholic?" I asked.

"What does that matter?" she remarked.

"It matters to me," I said.

"Yes, I was born Catholic. As a child I wanted to become a nun."

The completeness and congruity of my assessment whirled in my head for the duration of only ten seconds: a blue-eyed, beautiful blonde, in a medical field; a connoisseur of great music, my kind of music; a Catholic who is taking metaphysics of all things; and an admirer of the Angelic Doctor's philosophy. What more could I ask for! Of all the things on God's earth, aren't these the things that I love the most? I was in ecstasy as I turned my head toward her and said with the most assertive and yet tender voice I could muster:

"Carol! You know something? I am going to marry you!"

That was on our first date! I had just befriended the girl that very same day! I was impulsive for sure, and a romantic to boot. But it was a well-judged, well-considered sort of impulsiveness. It was not exactly love at first sight, but more like a precious discovery. Well, I don't know about that not being love at first sight, either! I thought that I had just found in this barren world "the pearl of great price" and I wanted to sell everything I owned and to buy it, as Jesus said in the parable referring to God's Kingdom. Yes, it was love at first sight. It was the sort of educated first impression that had all the ingredients of a stable and lasting love rather than a whim of a moment. It was akin to a peak experience that comes very rarely in life; or more accurately, it was the point at which I wanted to shout to the whole world: "Eureka!"

She looked at me and said, "You are crazy! You don't even know me. Don't get carried away on a first date!"

She was practical and had dated much more than I had. I was an impulsive, romantic, academic sort of a fellow. Little did she know that after fifteen

·

minutes of conversation, following her reactions at the concert, I knew enough about her to allow both my mind and my heart to be captured by her. She was all that I had dreamt of for a long time. It was rather like Sir Alexander Fleming recognizing the importance of his serendipitous find—a lifetime of preparation enabled him to understand the importance of his accidental discovery of penicillin.

We got back to Detroit and Carol was dropping me off at the residents' quarters before she went home. I started to get out of the car, when she asked me, "Aren't you going to kiss me goodnight?"

Like a fool, I said to her,

"I don't normally kiss girls on the first date."

She grabbed my arm and said, "You're going to kiss this girl goodnight."

So we kissed, and the habit of kissing her has not worn off after forty-five years.

My heart said to me, what a wonderful, passionate woman she is! I loved her then, I love her now, and I will always love her. Over the years, we have grown culturally and spiritually at different paces and at different times, but, just the same, we have grown closer in love, in appreciation one of the other, and in caring for each other's well-being.

Having experienced her love of music first-hand, I invited her a week later to a New York Metropolitan Opera production (in Detroit) of Giordano's *Andrea Chenier*. The opera was a first for both of us. A few months later, she told me that she was upset with me that night because, after telling me she had just finished reading Ayn Rand's *Atlas Shrugged*, I said, "I don't read cheap novels." She was right to be upset because I had spoken out of turn and out of ignorance, for I had never heard of Ayn Rand. Yet Carol might have spoken to me of Ayn Rand's philosophy and I might have informed her of my distaste for so-called philosophers who sneak their personal philosophy seductively into their novels.

As to the matter of Carol's musical expertise which impressed me during the Verdi Requiem, she confessed to me a few months later that her knowledge of that Requiem was the result of her taking a music appreciation course at the University of Michigan while an undergraduate. The course included the analysis of five musical works: Bach's *Magnificat*, Puccini's *La Bohème* (which to this day is our favorite opera), Handel's *Messiah,* Bach's St. *Matthew Passion* and, of all things, the Verdi *Requiem.* Her musical knowledge did not extend much further than those five works. However, Carol did take piano lessons for ten years as a child and, through frequent practice, she has become a fine pianist, with me her biggest fan. Quite often I try to listen to her playing, unseen in order not to disturb her.

NURSING A RELATIONSHIP

For our third date she invited me to supper at her home, having sent her parents away to the movies. She surprised me with delicious stuffed grape leaves, *hummus*, *tabbuli*, and of all things, *kibbe,* my favorite dish. She knew from Mary Stief, her fellow nurse, that I was Lebanese. I was surprised when I saw Lebanese food on the table, and further stupefied that she knew my likes and dislikes already.

We kept on dating, but for a long time she wouldn't tell me that she was in love with me. That was disappointing, but I was patient and in love with her. She would often tell me that she liked me, but that she did not love me yet. Of course, in philosophy loving and liking are interchangeable. They both lead to the desire of the loved object, just as hate leads to aversion from the hated object. So what was this "I like you, but I don't love you" all about? I wasn't well versed in that lingo. I learned later that it was common for people to act as if there is a partition or a divide between loving and liking. People put more emphasis on one or the other at various times of their relationships.

Finally, one night, three months later, she confessed to me that finally she had "fallen" in love with me. It was the night of her sister Judy's wedding. Two weeks before, I had gone up to Mackinaw Island as a cruise ship doctor and brought back with me a small jewelry box made of cedar wood and mother-of-pearl inlays. She really liked it and appreciated the thought behind it. We were fast becoming close friends.

That particular night when she told me she loved me seemed to be a starry night for both of us. I was actually at another wedding, that of Angelo Camburis, the chief surgical resident. I had taken Dr. Nancy Caputo, an internist on the staff, as my date to that wedding. Carol knew I was at the Detroit Yacht Club for that wedding, so she phoned me there about 10:00 p.m. to coax me into coming to her sister's. I excused myself, awkwardly, from the first wedding party and drove my date to her home, then reversed course and went to Carol's sister's reception. Actually, I was exhilarated by Carol's confession, and wanted to tell her face-to-face that I loved her too. That proved to be a long night, encompassing two wedding parties. I think I drank too much wine at Carol's sister's reception; I recall I was trying to keep up with Rod (the groom), who actually outdrank me. I didn't return to my quarters until 2:00 a.m. I was finally satisfied that the girl I was in love with, was also in love with me.

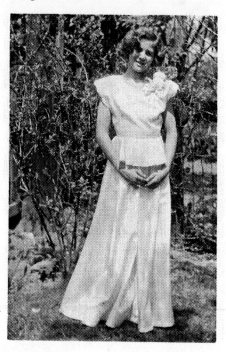

Carol Schooff, 13, getting ready to go to a dance

Carol was the third child in a family of four. She was born to a Polish mother and a German-Dutch father. Her maternal grandfather was a Polish patriot who edited the Detroit Polish newspaper in Hamtramck, the Polish quarter in Detroit. Her paternal grandfather Gerhardt was a police captain, apparently a Germanic disciplinarian. Carol also encountered discipline at school. When Carol was in kindergarten, the teacher had her and several classmates sit in the corner and "talk to the wall," because they were talking. Carol was scared and started moving her lips in prayer while the others kept still. The teacher who told them "talk to the wall" thought that Carol was obeying her command and sent her back to her desk, but kept the others facing the wall. Little Carol was happy that God had granted her request, so she thought she would thank him by wanting to become a nun.

At seven, she received her first communion. She was dressed in white and was fixing her hair in front of a mirror when she suddenly said to her sister, "I look darling today, don't I?" The older sister, Camille, went and told her mother that Carol was proud and vain. But Harriett told Camille, "Today is Carol's day. She can say whatever she wants and, besides, she is right! She does look darling!"

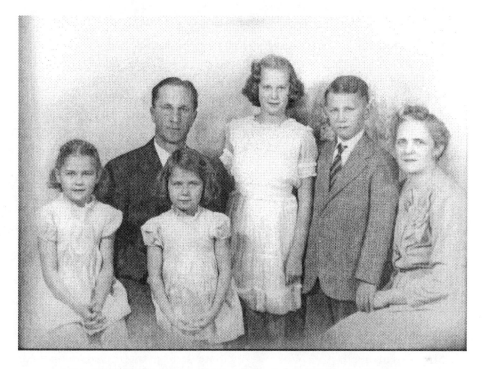

The Schooff Family in 1944—From left to right Carol, 8 years old, George Schooff, 40, Judith, 6, Camille, 10, Kenneth, 9, and Harriett, 39. Both parents were high school teachers in Detroit, Michigan. George was a high school football, swimming, and golf coach, and Harriet taught English Literature.

As she grew up, Carol loved to play tackle football at school and in the backyard. That pleased her dad, who was so interested in athlethics. She tells me she was the fastest runner in school and she recalls the day when she entered a 50-yard dash and won, beating even the eighth-grade boys. However, she was not allowed to continue playing football as an adolescent. Her parents had never mentioned anything to her about the facts of life before she found herself starting puberty. That was when she stopped being a tomboy, and decided to be fully a girl.

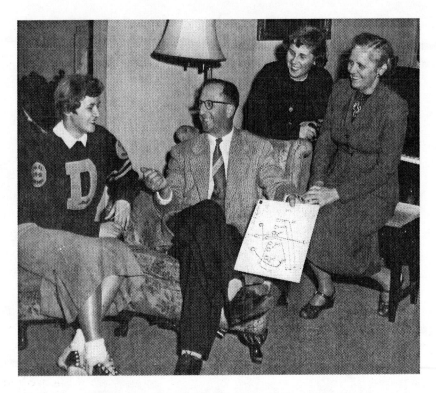

Carol's father seen explaining his football strategy for the
game which gave his team the State championship that year.

She was in her last year of intermediate school when that happened. Seventh, eighth, and ninth grades were rowdy and undisciplined, but not for her, she told me. She thought often of becoming a nun like St. Thérèse of Lisieux. She finished high school and enrolled in the University of Michigan's Bachelor of Science program in nursing. When I first met her, she had graduated and had just come back from a three-month tour of Europe. On her return she was hired as a nurse at Children's Hospital. She later transferred to Harper Hospital, and that's where I met her.

In the meantime my learning went on as usual in the residency program. In my first year of basic science, Dr. Ruiz, (who is now a retinal surgeon and head of the department at the University of Texas in Houston,) was kind enough to let me do part of a cataract extraction and several pterygium excisions. Years later when I saw him in Houston (when John Henry, our oldest son, was at Baylor Medical School), I thanked him for his kindnesses to me during our residency program.

In second-year residency we started performing surgery, but the learning was still mostly in eye diseases and medical ophthalmology. That year was not the most exciting time of residency, except for our wedding, which took place on January 21, 1961.

LA VITA NUOVA

The wedding was originally planned for June of that year. Carol's mother started pushing for an earlier date while my father was all for the later June date, as he thought we were hurrying things too much. I can understand Carol's mother's feelings, since in those days long courtships were frowned upon. Now, we encounter couples living with each other for up to ten years or more before deciding to officially get married, if at all. Why should they marry earlier when they are having the privileges of marriage without its responsibilities? That was thought of as strictly immoral in my day—a travesty of married life. Harriet thought an early marriage would be safer and more honorable, God rest her soul.

I drew up a list of pros and cons to an early marriage as opposed to a later one. It was a long list with pros on one side and cons on the other. There was no clear winner, as happens with most of such lists. I threw the list away and agreed to a January marriage. We chose my brother Mike to be best man and Carol's sister Camille to be matron of honor. We included in the wedding party Carol's youger sister Judy, and their brother Ken.

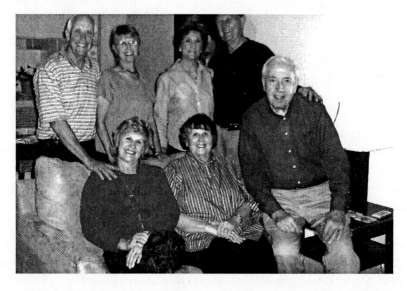

Carol's siblings and their spouses in 2004; from the left: seated are Carol, Camille and Bob, her husband; standing are Rod and Judy, and on the right Betsy and Ken

Our wedding day was a cold Saturday in January. The previous day, a snowy January 20, 1961, was the inauguration day for the "Sir Lancelot" president, John Kennedy. I hardly slept the night before and we had to wait in the vestibule of St. Matthew's Church in Detroit, for the end of a funeral service that was scheduled before our wedding. We passed a full hour of anxious waiting time, a kind of macabre prelude to our wedding. I was hoping that the coincidental juxtaposition of the funeral with our marriage ceremony was not an omen of things to come.

"Good Lord, we don't need this dark beginning for our marriage, following the end of someone else's life," I thought to myself. "Here I am marrying into a culture different than mine, when all my siblings married a second or a third cousin. They weren't willing to undergo the risk of marrying a blue-eyed Nordic blonde, like I am doing now. Am I taking a big chance entering into a marriage between two cultures? But I *do* belong to two different cultures—may be even three, considering my (Hispanic) high school education in Venezuela. I have lived in America for over ten years already," I continued thinking, "and I have acquired quite a bit of its habits and ways of life; so much so, that I feel I have two layers of skin, one Middle-eastern, the other Western; and I am still barely twenty-six years old."

Presently (2005), at my age of seventy-one, I can recall the many times when I faced difficult situations where I used the ways of one culture or another—and more often than not, a blend of both—to solve my problems. What a great advantage this has proven to be in my life; just as over the years being multilingual has added an exciting rainbow of colors to my interest in the history, geography, and literature of different countries.

However, on our wedding day, I could barely be expected to have the hindsight that I have now. So on that cold day forty four years ago, I went on ruminating, "When will my *vita nuova* begin? How will I function in a novel, unpredictable, and different state of life? Will I succeed, or will I fail in marriage like so many others have?" Yet even then, I knew that rain or shine, whatever is going to happen in the future must have been experienced by many others before me. I knew that there is precious little that's new under the sun. I would be neither the first nor the last to take the plunge into marriage.

The funeral went on and on as I continued with my thoughts, since I was still alone in the sacristy and protocol would not allow me to be anywhere near Carol before the ceremony. I kept thinking that there is no happiness without trial, vexation, and suffering. I thought that the whole notion of the disposability of a partner is immature, because it denies the married couple the chance to progress in the same union to the eventual fulfillment reached in lasting marriages.

On my wedding day I was still untested and did not have the lifetime experiences that mellow a person. I had not yet gone through the "dark night" that cauterizes and heals, as St. John of the Cross would have put it. The periods of trials and vexations came later, but before the wedding I knew none of that.

Well, it was still snowing when the funeral ended and that put a stop to my philosophizing for the moment. Now the guests were able to vacate the vestibule after a long wait and enter the church proper for a high nuptial Mass. My brother Mike was our best man. He was considerate enough—he is the greatest guy in the world—to have paid for our rehearsal dinner the night before, for he knew that we were both penniless at the time. Camille, Carol's older sister, was our matron of honor. We were married by Father Rattenkeller, a Passionist priest who had given us marriage instruction for three months. He was the one who told us that taking one another for granted would eventually ruin a marriage. "If you don't grow in love daily, you'll slowly fall out of love," he said to us a few weeks before the wedding.

I look back every now and then at our wedding pictures: Carol was stunningly beautiful with her well-groomed hair and beautiful, spotless face. She had both physical and inner beauty. The physical beauty has amazingly remained over the years, but, oh, how the spiritual beauty has flowered—way beyond my expectations at the wedding, and definitely more than I allowed myself to hope for during the midlife years of turmoil and trial that we went through. To reach this serene bliss, I would go through the rough times again if I had to, for there is no other way for personal and spiritual growth and a satisfying life. The oldest organization in the world, the Catholic Church, has always known and taught that the way to redemption (and thus perfect happiness) is the cross. At times, marriage can be the way of the cross.

The wedding Mass was over in one hour and all of us went to the reception hall. Unfortunately, the caterers had put the food out too early, and it was almost gone by the time the wedding party arrived, since many guests had skipped the wedding ceremony and arrived at the reception hall early.

After the reception at the hall, the family retired to the house of my in-laws, where the partying continued till midnight. I remember Aunt Mildred (who was Wayne University's purser and my father-in-law's eldest sister) warning me not to buckle under the rule of Harriet, my mother-in-law. According to her, Harriet had dominated her husband and her two sons-in-law ever since their weddings. As I learned later, this was only partially true, but Aunt Mildred's cynical remarks stayed in the back of my mind for the first several years of marriage. In a way, this made my relationship with my mother-in-law fair at best, rather than more giving and loving. Mildred's injunction turned out to be (in its own small way) akin to Iago's whisper in Othello's ear about his wife Desdemona's supposed infidelity—what Mildred said poisoned my ear and soured my taste for a while, until I got to know Harriet better.

There was also widowed Aunt Florence, who was always glued to her sister Mildred. Florence always talked about her daughter, a nurse who was doing missionary work in Africa. My father-in-law, George, and his two sisters were devout Catholics. Harriet had been Lutheran, quite rare for a Pole, but she converted to Catholicism upon marrying George. I am convinced that Harriet was an extremely intelligent and practical woman who saw the necessity of fitting into her new Catholic family as a dictate of practical wisdom. Carol inherited that virtue from her. I have noticed throughout our marriage that whenever Carol finds herself at the edge of a cliff through impishness or foolishness she always wisely and promptly backs off, never allowing herself to fall into the precipice. When the chips are down, she has invariably exhibited a keen intuition for practical wisdom and common sense.

We newlyweds left our family's home that same night exhausted from the festivities. We stayed overnight in a Detroit hotel, before proceeding to a honeymoon in Florida. The next day we drove all the way to Tennessee, where we consummated our love for the first time.

We drove further the following day until we reached Fort Lauderdale, Florida, with a one-night stop in Georgia. We drove carefully through the South because we were told that the police in these small towns give traffic tickets at the drop of a hat, since ticketing was the town's main source of revenue! When we arrived in Florida, we checked into the Kimberly Inn, right on the ocean.

The honeymoon in Florida was an exciting and happy time. We spent our time on the beach or at the swimming pool during the day and indulged ourselves in yet more pleasant activities at night. The weather was perfect as compared to Detroit in January, and we were grateful for that.

We had our first argument during our honeymoon. Carol still owed her parents money for the car she had bought from them and planned to continue making the payments on it. In Mediterranean culture, this is inconceivable, since parents are expected to be generous with their children without expectation of a payback, other than in love and respect. I was still not completely aware of

Western ways, so we argued over the car loan, but ended up paying her parents back for the car in instalments after we returned home.

The first week back in Detroit was a time to shop for furniture for our small one bedroom apartment in the married residents' quarter. With our meager income, we visited used furniture stores on Michigan Avenue and ended up furnishing the bedroom, dining room, living room, and the small waiting room for a total of $300. When we vacated the premises eighteen months later to come to California, we sold the same furniture for $500! In those days, Carol and I used to jokingly remind each other that if we were paid any less at the hospital, we would have had to live on sardines, liver, and kidneys, which were plentiful and very inexpensive in those days.

THE "SWEETER THAN HONEY" YEARS

During that wonderful first year of marriage Carol was getting her master's degree in nursing, finishing up her thesis while working at Harper Hospital's pediatric wing. I continued learning the intricacies of ophthalmology, and was allowed now to do some surgical procedures in preparation for the final year, which normally was predominately surgical. Kerwin Stief was my co-resident at Harper, but I was mingling more and more with fellow residents at the Detroit Receiving Hospital, since they were part of the same Kresge Eye residency program.

Around April, Carol went to a conference in Cincinnati that was part of her master's program. I missed her, even though I was busy enough at the hospital and making house calls for my brother Mike besides. I would come back to the quarters every night exhausted and would crash into bed and fall asleep. I realized how romantic Carol was when I received the first letter she ever wrote me. I had just gotten home from work, tired and missing her terribly, when I read it and it lifted up my spirits. I have saved all her letters over the years.

Love and affection were openly and frequently expressed and not taken for granted early on in marriage; it is unfortunate that couples don't know enough at that stage to keep that initial spark of love growing. In those early years everything looks sweet and wonderful. These are the honey-sweet years. So, less than a few months into the marriage, my spouse wrote to me several letters from her hotel in Ohio. This letter is particularly precious because it was the very first:

It's Morning, 11:00 a.m.

Hello Dearest,

Darling, before I go on, let me stop and tell you how much—how very much—I love you. I adore you. I love you so much—the greatest part of it too, is that I feel a new and different aspect of it; i.e. that it is eternal. I know, darling, I'll not only always, always, always love you, but I Always have loved you. I hope this letter doesn't sound too mushy. And if it does, that's too bad 'cuz I love you—so there! Oh well, guess you must know by now how much I miss you. Last night I dreamt of our marriage and of our love. When I woke up, I just laid in bed for about an hour thinking of you and of how much I love you and how wonderful you are. What a perfect adorable, wonderful husband and father you'll be . . .

Two more letters followed in two days, full of the same expressions of love and affection, overflowing with adulation and veneration. How beautiful and hopeful were those first several years of marriage. A woman leaves her father and mother, giving herself entirely and with full trust to a husband who, she hopes, will reciprocate her faith in him and will love her, protect her, and look after her needs. It would be a great tragedy if the man did not respond in kind or betrayed that trust. I have seen bitter disappointment in many marriages when that hope is crushed. Carol's sentiments increased my love for her and made me aware of her trusting and generous heart.

Feelings do change with time, vacillating as the years go by. It's the usual course of events, and so it was with us. Love is romantic at first; but then the ups and downs of midlife arrive unannounced to complicate matters. Finally, with patience, acceptance and forgiveness, the years of sublime intimacy follow, which I hope will keep growing until the end of life. When two souls are so entwined, they anticipate each other's thoughts. That is the fruit of perseverance, where the word "divorce" is unknown by one's parents, by one's church, and by one's precepts. God can be very helpful if we let Him do His work.

Before we had any children, Carol obtained her master's at Wayne State University. As a student, she would get us tickets to the Detroit Symphony concerts for only $3.00 each. What a bargain that was! We went every Thursday evening throughout the whole concert season. Once, we had seats right in front, close to where E. Power Biggs played the organ in Saint-Saens' Third Symphony, the *Organ Symphony*. Carol never forgot the power and majesty of that work by Saint-Saens. She always reminds me of the great experience she had upon hearing the organ thundering near us on the stage. Another exciting moment during those years was a performance of Mozart's *Don Giovanni* by the music department of Wayne State University. In the final scene of that opera, when the basso voice of the invited statue thunders the line, *Don Giovanni!!! m'invitasti a cena, i son venuto* (You have invited me to supper, and I have come), we had goose pimples; and at the end of that scene when Don Giovanni is dragged down to hell for his misdeeds on earth, the whole stage, draperies and all, was on fire during that production's ending. I don't know how it was done, but it was spectacular.

On weekends, we planned outings or picnics with friends and it would inevitably rain. The weather in the Midwest is unpredictable, both summer and winter. I suffered through many allergies in that area of the world, and used to go to see Dr. Levin, the allergist, for help. It was a shame, though, not to be able to enjoy one's outings without the rain falling. And it was exasperating having to cancel one's plans so often. We really couldn't wait to get out of Detroit—the hot and humid climate in the summer and extreme coldness in the winter—and come to California where the weather is more predictable.

I used to go to a dentist, Dr. Kennedy, on Woodward Avenue, who over time extracted three of my wisdom teeth. I remember that he always mentioned the fact that he played clarinet for Guy Lombardo and his Royal Canadians band. He had left the band to go to dental school. Years later, when I met him, he was positive he would have made a fortune had he stayed with Guy Lombardo, whose band reached fame and glory after the doctor left. Dr. Kennedy never charged me for his services, saying to me every time that I was a fellow Canadian and, besides, an intern with no money.

Another person who never charged me for his services was my barber at Harper Hospital. The second week I was an intern I walked into the hospital's barbershop in the lobby of the hospital and sat in the chair. The barber saw my name tag, and asked me if I was the son of Joe (Yousef) Zeiter of Windsor. When I said yes, he hugged and kissed me, telling me that I was his long lost cousin. (I traced this relationship in the Family Tree that I included in this book.) It turned out that he was a descendant of the Abi-Samra branch of our original Mukari family. His name was Joe Summers, a derivative of (Abi-) *Samra*, another example of the Americanization of an immigrant's family name; probably by an immigration officer's spelling error—or by the original members of the family wanting to have an Anglicized name. We became the best of friends and always called each other "cousin," just as in Stockton I greet and am greeted by all the relatives as "cousin." Joe the Barber stood at our wedding and he was one of the truest friends I ever had.

Joe's son (Joe Jr.) was a salesman for Capitol Records, whose subsidiary was Angel Records, the classical music recording company. Through him I obtained all the music records of my favorite soloists. Joe Jr. used to bring me lots of these recordings at one dollar each. I started learning about every piece of music and the artists by reading back covers; that became my encyclopedia of music.

A beautiful interlude took place in the spring of 1961 when Carol's brother Ken (who was in psychiatry residency at Chapel Hill, North Carolina) invited us and his parents to visit and attend the baptism of their newborn son, George, for whom Carol was asked to be godmother. Carol alternated the driving with Harriet, my mother-in-law, while George and I alternated in the front passenger and back seats. When we arrived in Knoxville, Tennessee, we started ascending into the Smoky Mountains. Next, we passed through Gatlinburg, Tennessee, which guards the western entrance of the national park. Spring had arrived all of a sudden, while in Detroit winter was still raging. We stopped for lunch, and Harriet chose a restaurant that looked good but ritzy. George fought her all the way, because he wanted to eat in a place less expensive. She ordered him to get into the restaurant and stop complaining. I was shocked by her assertiveness. When she saw a look of surprise on my face, she took me aside and told me, "Henry, don't worry about George. He doesn't know what's good for him!"

It took me a few years and several vacations with my in-laws to realize how true that statement was. George was a bit tentative and she would have none of it. She wanted him to "let his yes be a yes! And his no be a no!" I began to appreciate Harriet, whom I recognized as the driving force in that family. I learned from them that every family needs at least one assertive member, or the family gets nowhere.

We continued on to Ken and Betsy's apartment in the vicinity of the University of North Carolina. There were white and pink flowers on trees everywhere—It was springtime, and I fell in love with the area. Entering North Carolina from Detroit was like emerging from a place of doom and gloom into a place of hope and beauty. I got to know Ken better during that trip. He was a bon vivant who liked good wine and good food and we had many other similar interests.

A SON IS BORN

Our first son was born on December 21, 1961. Carol looked beautiful following delivery, and the baby boy looked just like his father—at least everybody said so! Dr. Morgan, a staff physician, was the obstetrician. I wanted to name the baby Henry, but Carol's vote outweighed mine; we compromised on John Henry, after the great Catholic convert, John Henry Cardinal Newman (not after the hammer man whom I had never heard of at that time), and after my brother Johnny. The Henry was shortly chopped out of the John Henry by both Carol and her family members, and dropped by John Henry as well as he grew up. I guess the word john, by itself, sounded better to everybody!

We spent Christmas at the in-laws, eating turkey with all the trimmings while Carol was convalescing. Three weeks later we all attended Carol's graduation. The rest of the final year of residency passed uneventfully. I was chief resident in 1962. Dr. Windsor Davies, the professor of ophthalmic pathology, who also had the busiest practice in Detroit, wanted me to join him in both teaching and practice. I declined, graciously. I wanted to move to California and start my own practice there, away from academia, and Carol agreed.

On Memorial Day, we went with other resident couples to a picnic at Kensington Lake on the outskirts of Detroit. Carol and I lay on the beach by the lake and reminisced about our courtship. Every Sunday, my brother Mike and Carol's parents would call us in the morning to invite us over for brunch. We enjoyed our visits with each of them, but we wanted to reserve at least one Sunday a month to be alone or with our Harper Hospital friends. So we agreed to alternate Sunday brunch between Carol's parents and Mike and Irene's. The third Sunday we decided to keep to ourselves, and everyone was happy with this plan. On the Sundays we went to Irene and Mike's, we always planned to get there early, right after Mass, so Carol could learn from Irene or her mother how to prepare Lebanese food.

LEBANESE COOKING

Since then, Carol has become a wonderful chef, and cooks all the varieties of Lebanese food: *kibbe*, both raw or cooked, stuffed grape leaves, stuffed cabbage leaves, *koosa mahshi* (skewered squash stuffed with rice and meat), *batinjane* (eggplant stuffed with the same), *mjaddra* (lentils and browned rice), *lubieh* (green beans cooked in olive oil with tomatoes and spices), and all the forms of hors d'oeuvres: *hummus*, sometimes used as a dip, *tabbuli* (a special kind of Lebanese salad), and many others. The other things she learned but rarely prepares now are the dozens of Lebanese pastries such as *baklava*, *knafeh* (delicious two-layered custard pie), *burma*, *ma'mul*, and others. They are too labor-intensive, requiring hours for preparing the ingredients, let alone putting them together, mostly in layers upon layers of filo. My sisters-in-law, Madelyn and Yvonne, living close to us in Stockton, have obviated the necessity for Carol to slave over preparing these sweets. They are always making these sweets for their families and occasionally send some of them over to us, especially at Christmas time. I've had a sweet tooth, since childhood, and I still do.

Sunday lunch at Mike and Irene's has always been a culinary feast, and still is to this day. Whenever we visit the Midwest, we always look forward to going to their house to visit and eat, and we bring back with us many dozens of Francis Bakery's thin *pita* bread. We haven't found anything as delicious anywhere outside of Lebanon, because his loaves of pita are thin and their two layers separate easily. The use of Lebanese bread is very versatile. Small pieces are torn by the fingers and used variously as a scooping spoon (especially with yogurt which is a normal part of the diet); as a dull knife to separate portions of food; or as a wiper of lips and fingers in place of napkins; and all this over and above pita's simple use as a necessary food staple.

Over time, Carol learned how to prepare and cook most of these dishes. A few years ago *Readers Digest* claimed Lebanese food to be the healthiest food in the world. And after attending a conference on nutrition several years ago, Carol returned home all excited. "The director of the meeting was a neurosurgeon, who was well informed in matters of nutrition" she told me. "He told us that *hummus* and *mjaddrah* are the healthiest source of protein you can eat."

Part of Lebanese culture is the disappointment or hurt the host feels if the guest doesn't eat enough to "fill a camel's belly." The host will keep insisting, "Have some more!" "You didn't eat anything!" "You eat like a bird!" In the Eastern Mediterranean, mothers, sisters, wives or neighbors use food as a form of endearment, and, in a way, this is understandable since the food itself takes a lot of time to prepare and is delicious, besides. That is why they love to share it with both friends and strangers—it is part and parcel of Lebanese hospitality.

One evening we invited Dr. Frank Sennewald, my old friend from medical school, and his wife, Joyce, to a Lebanese supper cooked by Carol. We were still living in the residents' quarters. Frank was familiar with Lebanese food and loved it, but what surprised him most was Carol's yogurt, a home-made recipe she learned from Irene, her sister-in-law. Yogurt is made by boiling milk and then waiting till its temperature drops to a certain point before adding the starter (i.e. a tablespoonful of yogurt from a previous batch) and stirring it into the still warm milk. Now, Dr. Sennewald's German method was to add the yogurt when the milk's temperature dropped to 148 degrees as measured exactly by a thermometer; whereas Carol added the starter when she could withstand leaving her index finger in the hot milk and counting one to ten before she had to pull it out. That was the practical Lebanese way, learned from sister-in-law Irene. Frank wouldn't believe her until he went home and tried that same technique, and then called Carol to tell her that, in fact, her system works and her yogurt tasted better than his.

This was high praise, coming from a German scientist, as I later came to appreciate when I visited Dr. Sennewald's country in 1971 and saw, first-hand, how exacting and meticulous Germans are—at least to my eyes. I had taken my two boys to visit Germany. They were seven and eight at the time, and I couldn't help but notice how fussy and precise the Germans were in everything. At the Frankfurt Airport, the taxicab driver called me back from about a hundred yards away—and that after I had paid and tipped him—to show me how my boys had spilled two (yes, two) popcorn kernels on the backseat of his taxi. He wanted me to clean the mess of "two popcorns" left on his backseat. This was the textbook definition of obsessive-compulsive behavior—puritanical cleanliness in its most excessive form.

When we arrived in Lebanon shortly thereafter, we were delighted to see a few scraps of paper, orange peels and cigarette butts on the curbs next to the sidewalks. We felt liberated! People had a carefree "who cares" attitude. The children and I felt emancipated, free as birds, and in love with the Lebanese "*chacun à son gout*" attitude. For one thing, the Lebanese are mavericks and have always refused to live in a straight-jacket. Little John and Philip never thought they would witness such a relaxation from the rules of obsessive cleanliness. After all they were taught in America that cleanliness is next to godliness! The boys fell in love with Lebanon also for many other reasons, of course. I remember when they stood at the base of the six gigantic columns at Baalbeck and looked at them in wonder. John Henry said to me, "Dad, each of these columns is bigger and taller than the towers of Cologne Cathedral," which they had seen and appreciated a week earlier while in Germany.

So, Dr. Sennewald, good and true German that you are, I salute you for confirming the superior technique of yogurt-making to the Lebanese!

CHAPTER 16

FIRST YEARS IN STOCKTON

When the time came for us to leave Detroit, Carol and I bid everybody goodbye, packed the old Buick I had inherited from my brother Edmond, and happily set off for California. The eye residency was officially over now. I had just completed twenty-three straight years of schooling. Finally, I was anxious and ready to begin the private practice of medicine and ocular surgery. It was an exciting time for us.

In anticipation of settling there, I had flown to California in November 1961 to talk to a busy San Francisco ophthalmologist about joining his practice. Dr. Albert Serrail had graduated from Kresge Eye Institute ten years before me. Dr. Ruedemann remembered him as an outstanding resident. "He came to me from California and became my chief resident," the chief told me. "He was a hard worker like you and an aggressive surgeon." Serrail had opened a practice in San Francisco and Ruedemann had heard that he was looking for an associate. I flew to San Francisco, already picturing myself in practice on the fourteenth floor of the 450 Sutter Medical Building, the most prestigious medical address in San Francisco. I was disappointed when we began talking salary and the length of time it would take me to become a full partner.

I knew I was well trained at Kresge Eye and Harper Hospital, and that I was repeatedly asked by my clinical professors (Drs. Davies, Frey and Crossen) to join their private practices while I was still in Detroit. But I wanted to go to San Francisco, and here I was dealing with this penurious physician who was unwilling to offer me more than $1,000 a month? I decided to drive to Stockton where all my relatives resided. It was where Grandma Marzuka originally made her small fortune and the place she had often described to me as the land of milk and honey. The San Joaquin Valley of California was etched in my brain long before I had fallen in love with San Francisco.

Well, my cousin, Dr. Joseph Barkett, had just erected a medical building and needed to fill it with doctor-tenants, so the time was right. He welcomed me with open arms and generously offered me four months free rent, since I was his young cousin just starting out in practice, and had no financial resources as yet. He told me that both he and his partner Dr. Brunetta had a huge practice and would send me more eye patients than I could handle. It was a deal! I felt at home right away and all the relatives, including Dr. Joe, were happy when Carol and I told them we were coming to Stockton to stay.

My cousin Joe fulfilled every one of his promises. In anticipation of my first day in practice, July 23, 1962, he had filled my appointment book with twenty-three new patients. If ever there was a gesture of goodwill guaranteeing a new doctor unmitigated success, that was it. During the first few years in practice, Dr. Barkett, Dr. Brunetta, cousins Peter, Ed, George, Ben, Mike and Joe Rishwain, cousin Jeanette Michaels, the offspring of uncles Tannous and Ass'ad, and the rest of my relatives were referring to me their families, their friends and anybody they came across who had the slightest eye problem. I started with a busy practice right off the bat. As a matter of fact, one day a patient limped into my office with crutches because of a broken ankle. He was referred to me from Dr. Barkett's office. Both the front secretary and I started laughing. It turned out that my dear cousin intended to refer him to Dr. Serra—an orthopedist that I had brought to Stockton from Detroit, along with Drs. Primack and Brennan—but Dr. Joe just couldn't get his cousin Henry out of his mind that day. I called Joe to tell him that he sent the patient to the wrong doctor, but he just laughed and said to me, "Go ahead and check his eyes anyway, I'm sure he's due for an eye exam, and then send him on to Dr. Serra!" Hilarious! Drs. Joseph Serra and Marvin Primack eventually went on to become respected leaders in the medical community, very active in the Medical Society and to the present great friends and colleagues.

Carol had wanted to live in California all her life. Even before she met me she had applied to several hospitals in California, desiring to move to that state. She hated the Detroit winter because it gave her the Midwestern winter blues—a common condition when the sun is not seen over an extended period of time and the winters are full of snow, sleet, rain, and dark clouds.

In my case, I also wanted to leave the flatness of the land—no mountains or hills to be seen anywhere, in contrast to my memories of picturesque northern Lebanon or even Caracas, Venezuela. Carol and I thought California would be the high point of our dreams, full of mountains, sunshine, and an enchanting coastline. Ironically, we ended up in Stockton in the central valley, a flat area with the mountains as far as thirty miles away on either side of us. Still, we have the mountains nearby and plenty of sunshine with a weather that is pleasantly dry and pleasant during the long autumns and springs—mild in the winter, but with some hot summer days. That heat, nonetheless, comes only in the afternoon, leaving the evening, night and morning a cool 65°F.

During the spring prior to our final exodus, I had flown with Carol to California so she could see firsthand what to expect. She had never been out West before. The relatives welcomed her with open arms. She met Dr. Barkett, our cousin and sponsor, and his wife Marie. At the time of our trip, our cousin Jeanette Michaels was in real estate and helped us locate a house to rent. Carol also met many other relatives of mine and was amazed by their hospitality and sheer number. We returned to Detroit full of expectations for a new and wonderful life that would soon be ours in California.

WESTWARD BOUND

The last weekend of June, 1962, we left Detroit in our old Buick, packed to the gills, with barely enough vacant space for little John Henry's car seat in the back. Carol and I alternated driving all the way to California. We decided to take the northern route and make an adventure out of the trip, since we knew we would be passing through the scenic mountainous part of the United States and Canada.

We intended to explore everything there was on the way, starting with the wide prairie land of these United States. The sky was crystal-clear and we were full of life, love, and hope for a new venture in California, a *vita nuova*. The Buick that I acquired from my brother Edmond was old but serviceable. We took the freeway west through the vast plains of Michigan, Illinois, Iowa, skirting Nebraska to go into South Dakota by way of Sioux City and Sioux Falls. I had made that trip before, but Carol hadn't. She was amazed at the immensity of this country. We drove for three days through the plains, but were still far away from our goal. Every now and then we saw signs advertising caves to visit, snake charmers to see, petting zoos and all kinds of oddities reminding us of movies we had seen about the West, such as *Buffalo Bill* or *Annie Get Your Gun*, and the hundreds of movies with Randolph Scott, Gary Cooper and John Wayne.

We saw a live passion play in Lawrence County, which I recalled years later when I saw the famous passion play in Oberammergau, Bavaria. We visited Spearfish, Sturgis, Deadwood and Lead, four beautiful towns. They were a stone's throw from Mount Rushmore, where we admired the famous sculpted heads of Washington, Jefferson, Lincoln, and Roosevelt. We felt patriotic and the whole history of this nation swirled through our heads—the ideal realism of the forgers of our great Constitution and the founding of the government as a lasting Republic with "liberty and justice for all."

When we arrived at the foothills of the Rockies in Wyoming, we began a steep rise just past the town of Buffalo, an ascent which proved almost fatal to the faithful Buick. We started seeing smoke rise from the hood and it was getting worse the higher we ascended. At first, we thought it might be due to an empty radiator; so we added water but the car kept on smoking and we kept creeping up slowly to almost 6,000 feet. We made it with the car still half-alive. I remember passing through Billings, Bozeman, and Butte, the Montana three B's—no relation to Bach, Beethoven, and Brahms, the other famous three B's. At Butte, we made a ninety-degree turn and headed north through Great Falls for another ascent to Glacier National Park and into Banff and Lake Louise, where we stayed overnight. Oddly enough, the vehicle didn't fume this time. Exhausted, we checked into a hotel, fell on top of the bed, and went to sleep right away. It was not until the next day that we recalled the wondrous beauty of Glacier National Park which we had passed through the day before. But on opening our hotel room window, we witnessed an even more impressive sight: Banff and its surrounding lakes and mountains.

We continued the next day for a short distance beyond Banff to Lake Louise. Jasper Park further north was a sight to behold. The mountains were gigantic and the lake in the middle of the park was crystal clear. The next day we returned to Banff and continued on to Vancouver by the Queen's Highway in Canada, just north of the U.S. border. The whole way through the Canadian Rockies was overwhelming, its grandeur awe-inspiring. We saw lots of snow on the mountain tops, still in July. It was virgin country with tall evergreens reaching to the sky and the scent of the pine trees in the air.

We had decided to go to Vancouver first, and then drive down through the Washington, Oregon, and California coasts. We visited Victoria, the provincial capital on Vancouver Island, and its Bush Gardens, full of flowers and exotic plants. We hated to leave Victoria and its gem-like charm, but we continued down to Seattle where the World Exhibition (1962) with its remarkable Space Needle—still a landmark structure in Seattle—had just been completed.

For three days we drove down the Oregon and California coasts captivated by their marvelous vistas, the best meeting of land and sea God ever made. I recall the blowing of whales swimming off-shore, and the abundance of wild flowers on the sides of the road. Fortunately, we were given beautiful weather throughout the whole trip and we escaped the fog that usually hangs over that coast in the summer.

I recall, in particular, two events. One is seeing Coos Bay on the Oregon Coast with the whales offshore and the dramatic cliffs descending into the Pacific. The other is our drive down Highway One through hundreds of *Sequoia sempiverens*, the tall big trees of Humboldt Grove. What a sight! It was like driving through the gigantic colonnade of a Gothic cathedral, except that these trees were a *living* testimony to almost two thousand years of unimpeded growth. Their elegant posture was breathtaking, tall and straight up to hundreds of feet in height, with furry red-brown bark, thick and resilient enough to protect them from forest fires. The beauty and grandeur of these trees inspired in us respect and admiration for their Creator.

We continued down the coast, through the lush hills of the Napa Valley, sprinkled with vineyards and fruit trees, to San Francisco, the Baghdad of the West. In those days, you could count the seven hills since tall skyscrapers had not been built yet. San Francisco, in 1962, was still a quaint city with buildings of small elevation that were well kept and always freshly painted with the beautiful decorative colors and carved stones of the late nineteenth and early twentieth centuries. The buildings were entirely different from each other in architectural structure, in contrast to the impersonal, tall, plain cubic buildings that now dwarf these older structures. Fortunately the newer bland skyscrapers are limited to the downtown business area and do not extend into the small neighborhoods which have retained their charm, exhibiting the stamp of the various nationalities that have given color and excitement to this city by the Bay.

We stayed at the Shaw Hotel, a small, three-cornered, old building just behind Market Street, accessible to areas of interest and one we could afford. On my part, I explored San Francisco all over again, since both my cousin Joe Zeiter and I wanted to show Carol how beautiful a city it was. Joe and his second wife Peggy—his first wife had died in childbirth—and Carol and I drove around the City and the Bay Area the whole weekend. We particularly enjoyed a visit to the Larkin Theater where foreign movies were always being shown. We loved foreign movies—more imaginative and less gaudy than Hollywood's. For three days we ate at our favorite restaurants and explored the Golden Gate Park from one end to the other. We loved going to Sausalito, on the other side of the Golden Gate Bridge, and from there, looking back at San Francisco's white buildings glowing in the setting sun across the water.

FRESH START

On Monday morning we drove to Stockton and stayed at my Cousin Bernice's home for two days. Bernice was my first cousin, the daughter of my Dad's sister Ziara, and her husband, Tony, was my second cousin (great-aunt Teresa's son). Jeanette, their daughter, had found us a house to rent not far from her parents, but we had to wait two days to get in since it was being repainted. We couldn't afford to buy the house so we had to rent. The home on Inman was furnished, so we moved there immediately and found it to have a nice yard with fruit trees that occupied Dad with husbandry every time he came to visit.

I immediately set out to buy ophthalmic equipment for the two examining rooms that I had rented from my cousin, Dr. Barkett. I was scheduled to see my first patient on July 23 and it was already the sixteenth of the month, giving me seven days to furnish the office, find a secretary, and set up a procedure to deal with my initial patients. Fortunately, Dr. Barkett suggested a secretary to me, Laverne Bruno, a tall, beautiful twenty-year-old local Italian girl, just out of high school. She was presentable but utterly inexperienced in the management of a medical office. The truth is that I was no better than she was at that time in running a practice. We both learned about medical practice, in tandem. Laverne worked for me until she got married two years later. She became a very capable and efficient secretary as time went on and was of great help in my starting up the practice.

The first day in the office was encouraging because Dr. Barkett had scheduled twenty-three patients for me. Two of the patients I will never forget, since they both had mature bilateral cataracts and needed surgery. A week later I operated on the first surgical patient (Celeste Rizzi, deceased now), a seventy-five-year-old farm hand; and while he was still in the hospital, I operated on his other eye, which had a cataract as mature as the first one. The result was 20/20 vision in both eyes, but he had to wear the thick cataract glasses—this was ten years before we began to use intra-ocular lenses. The fact that I operated on both eyes during the same hospitalization—three days apart and until now never on the samer day—caused great consternation among some of the ophthalmologists in Stockton, who were trained never to operate on both eyes during the same hospitalization. Over the years I introduced many innovations which the other eye doctors resisted until they became state of the art procedures; they had to adopt them then.

The second cataract patient was a rich farmer from Tracy (Marco Marchini, deceased now). I successfully operated on him a few weeks later at Dameron Hospital, rather than at St. Joseph's, even though both patients were Catholic and would have preferred to go there. Dameron gave me hospital privileges immediately, asking very few questions, whereas St. Joseph's had to investigate every detail of my curriculum vitae, but gave me surgical privileges also, two months later.

My first cataract patient wanted to pay me five hundred dollars, as I recall, even though the fee was three hundred per cataract. He said there should be a discount for two as opposed to one surgery. If he hadn't offered, I wouldn't have asked him to pay anything, since he routinely came to the office in tattered clothes, and looked very poor. However, he pulled out of his pocket a thick wad of one hundred dollar bills—more than I had ever seen in my life. I guess he was an Italian farmer who had saved quite a bit of money. Several months later I took care of another farmer who knew him well; he told me that Mr. Rizzi had never married and had tons of money stashed away. I learned early in practice not to judge a patient by the clothes he wore!

Another surgical patient in my early Stockton practice was Dr. Barkett's grandfather, Sarkis Barkett, who was over ninety years of age when I first saw him. He was a member of the first group of immigrants who originally came from Serhel, Lebanon, to Stockton. That group included Paul Abdallah, John Nehme, Grandma Marzuka Zeiter and her sister Teresa, and Sarkis Barkett himself. One of his grandchildren brought him to my office bleeding copiously from his face. I observed a twig about 3/16th of an inch in diameter sticking out one inch from his face just below his right eye. I asked the grandchild to tell me what happened.

Apparently the old nonagenarian was reaching out to trim a rosebush in his front yard, when he lost his balance and fell on the just-trimmed rosebush in front of him. He must have landed on top of one of the newly cut twigs, which entered his face and snapped, leaving one inch of twig sticking out of his face. It looked at first as if the eyeball was gone, but it did not turn out that way.

We took old Sarkis to St. Joseph Hospital with the twig sticking out of his eye, and only God knew how deeply it had penetrated. I realized it had to be pulled out, but what if it had penetrated deeply enough to pierce the internal carotid artery or the circle of Willis in the lower part of the brain? Pulling it out would unplug these major arteries and would cause a fatal hemorrhage. My imagination started to go wild on me. After all, this old man was Dr. Barkett's own grandpa. I recovered from my imaginings and reminded myself of the old medical aphorism, "To be a good surgeon is to have courage while wielding knife and facing blood!"

I decided to pull the twig out, right then and there in the emergency room. I injected first a little local anesthetic and then pulled out the three-inch twig and nothing happened. It had penetrated the orbit below the eye and there was no resulting loss of vision. Old Sarkis was as hard as nails and lucky besides. He was not afraid of pain. I kept Sarkis in the hospital one day. His blood pressure was 120/80; his blood count perfect; his heart had no murmur; and his pulse was a regular, steady 72. I realized that there in front of me, was this perfect specimen of an old Lebanese *montagnard* (mountain farmer) from Serhel. His fifty-year sojourn in the U.S. had not softened him up.

Old Sarkis reminded me of Dad, who lived 94 years, of great aunt Teresa who lived 102 years, and of great uncle Abuna Boutros, the monk, who had to be martyred to die, at age ninety-six. Indeed, on one of Dad's first visits to see us in California, he still thought he was a young man in Lebanon: he placed a ladder against an apricot tree in the backyard and reaching for the outlying branches to prune them, slipped from the ladder and fell about ten feet to the ground, fracturing one ankle and badly spraining the other. Carol and I were out somewhere or we would never have allowed him to climb the ladder, knowing that he was over seventy years old. By the time we got home he had crept to the back door of the house and entered by dragging himself on all fours. He was fortunately quite healthy, and his ankles healed in less than two months.

MY COUSIN JOE BARKETT

These old Lebanese had their own traditional habits, well grounded in common sense and the hard knocks of life. They lived a long time without fretting about diet, jogging, or running on a treadmill. Maybe what lengthened their life was the *"not fretting"* about having to add a few years at the end of their lives by a planned regimen of frenetic physical exercise! An example of their matter-of-fact approach to life was the story, my cousin, Dr. Joe Barkett, related to me just a few years ago. It was a tale having to do with his father Anthony (in fact old Sarkis' son) about how to use one's wits.

One afternoon after school (1941), when Joe was twelve years old, he came to his father's grocery store to help him for a few hours. His father looked at him quizzically and pointing to a sack of beans on the floor asked him, "Joe, do you know how many beans there are in the sack over there?" He didn't know, and his dad did not persue the issue. A few days later, when a customer bought a half-pound, Joe decided to count the beans in the half-pound and then multiply that number by the number of half-pounds in the sack (after he had weighed it). He came to his father with the number and then in turn asked his father if he knew the answer. "Heck no," his father replied. "I just wanted to find out if you can think!"

Joe then told me that when his daughter Lisa was leaving the house to go interview for her first job he instructed her, "They'll probably ask you for a resumé; but you don't have one since you haven't worked yet. Just tell them that you know how to *think*." She was puzzled, but when asked for the resumé she looked the interviewer squarely in the eye and said to him, "I don't have a resumé, it's my first job out of college, sir, but I assure you I have learned *how to think*." She was hired immediately, and the interviewer told her, "I've never heard that line before."

Joe recounted another family story concerning his mother Sadi'a, my first cousin and godmother—God rest her soul. A few years after his father died in 1954, Joe found a house in a nice neighborhood for his mother to move into—I remember well the house, on 844 Elm St. It needed to be furnished, so Joe phoned Sid Stein, a patient of his who owned a furniture store downtown, and told him to take care of his mother. She went downtown and chose several pieces to be delivered to her the next day. When the furniture arrived, she inspected the pieces and immediately called Joe to tell him that they were not the *same* pieces she had chosen. Joe told her that it couldn't be so, that he knew Sid Stein to be as honest as the day is long. But knowing his mother's strong resolve, he told her that he would meet her at the furniture store after office hours so they could investigate the problem together. Down at the furniture store Mr. Stein assured Dr. Joe that he sent out the furniture his mother had ordered. It turned out eventually that it was the exact furniture style, model, and manufacturer, but not the *very same* pieces she had picked. Yet, my godmother, who never went to school and had never learned how to read or write, insisted that it was not the same furniture, and she was right. While in the store buying the furniture the day before, she had marked with a piece of white chalk the back of every single piece she had selected; and she knew for a fact that the pieces that were sent to her house the next day were not the same ones that she had picked!

The first few months of practice taught me several lessons about proper office management. I was fitting contact lenses and allowing the patients to charge them on credit, just like any other office visit, rather than asking them to pay for the contacts upon receipt. That was a big mistake. Regular visits incur no cost for materials provided; hence the patient is allowed to wait for the monthly statement to pay. Contact lenses and eye glasses, however, entail a substantial material cost above and beyond the physician's services. When the end of August came, I received a huge bill from the contact lens manufacturers, but I couldn't honor it on time, because the patients had not yet paid for their contacts and I had no money in reserve. Besides, as it turned out—and that is a major lesson for every businessman—the clients or patients or customers who have not paid upon receipt for the object bought are less satisfied with that object and tend to either return it or complain about it (possibly an unconscious wish not to pay what they still owed on it). In my practice, the contact lens patients who had paid in full for their lenses appreciated their worth and tried harder to wear them, eventually succeeding more than those who had not paid yet. The latter group often came back to me with complaints of all sorts. So, I started a policy of full payment for contact lenses and glasses upon receipt of same.

I found out after a few years in practice that the little that Dr. Ralph Pino, back at Kresge Eye training, taught us about the practice of ophthalmology was merely a rudimentary start for what I had to learn on my own. In a very short time, I learned much more from the actual experience of running an office. The business side of ophthalmic practice required dealing tactfully with patients, secretaries, nurses, hospitals, suppliers and other doctors—and this on top of having to deal with wife, children, parents, and relatives. It was a three-ring circus to be managed with efficiency and tact. When I became savvy and in control of my practice, I found myself at the end of a normal day asking, "Lord, why only five problems today? Why haven't you sent me the usual ten or fifteen?"

PHILIP, SUZIE, AND CAMILLE

In the meantime, Carol gave birth to our second son, whom we named Philip after my brother in Venezuela. We always chose Christian names. We named John Henry after Cardinal Newman as well as my brother Johnny, and Philip after my other brother and one of the apostles. We hoped for a girl and soon Suzanne was born. We named her after St. Suzanna and the other great Hebrew heroine by that name.

Yet all the saints' names were not able to save our last three children from a medical problem at birth, which stemmed from my being a Mediterranean Rh positive and Carol being a typical Nordic Rh negative. John Henry, as the first child, came out scot-free, although he sensitized his mother's blood for all future children. Her Rh antibodies—the original research was done on the *rhesus* monkey, thus the Rh nomenclature—affected Philip, who needed one blood exchange transfusion after birth, the treatment then for that blood condition. But poor Suzie needed three blood exchanges over several days. Finally, when Camille, the youngest, was born, she also needed an exchange. It was hard on Carol, even though the children came out of the ordeal healthy and strong.

THE CURSILLO

Philip was baptized at St. Bernadette's Church by the pastor, Father James De Groot. We belonged to St. Bernadette's parish for two years, before we started to earnestly look for a house to buy. We found Father De Groot friendly and pious. He had come from an immigrant Dutch family of sixteen children, five of whom had religious vocations, three sons becoming priests and two daughters, nuns. The parents were local San Joaquin Valley dairy farmers, a very religious and devout family. It would be an understatement to point out that religion and morals have deteriorated markedly in the Netherlands since that time!

When we came to Stockton in 1962, the Catholic faith and the other faiths were very much as they had been for centuries. That same year the Second Vatican Council convened. Except for a few exceptional and notorious modernists, the world still believed in the sacredness of the family; in heterosexual relationships; in keeping God in the schools; it disapproved of moral turpitude (in both private and public spheres); frowned on premarital sex and immodesty in dress; and in general tried to save a marriage from divorce, except for Hollywood. The public at large was still singing, "How Much is that Doggie in the Window?" and "Love and Marriage go together like a Horse and Carriage." Even though we had been through two world wars in the first half of the century, in 1962, the average citizen was still living in a stable world of centuries-old morals, behavior and culture. It was in this atmosphere of faith and devotion that I was invited to make a "Cursillo" retreat in October of 1962. In Spanish Cursillo means a short course of instruction. I participated in it and eventually became more involved in this movement of Catholic renewal of faith.

At first I was a pupil at a retreat, but later I became one of the instructors. The Franciscan Pastor of St Mary's downtown, Father Alan McCoy, was the rector. He was a very holy man and is still alive at age ninety-three. There were Cursillos for men and for women. There were Cursillos in Spanish and in English. The movement had started in Spain years before, like so many other Catholic movements. Those making the Cursillo gathered in the old Assumption School on San Joaquin Street, only one block from my first medical office. For three days we attended Mass in the morning, took instructions in the faith during the rest of the day, and slept army style in individual cots after 8:00 p.m. sharp. Each morning we would get up singing, "*De Colores! De Colores se visten los pajaros en la primavera . . .*" This wasn't my cup of tea any more than belonging to service clubs has ever been. But I saw it renewing the faith of many people who were lukewarm or indifferent, and that was alright by me. On Sunday morning the old Cursillistas (who had done the Cursillo before), and relatives and friends came into the "barracks" with a Mariachi band and woke us up singing "De Colores." It was like experiencing a thousand trumpet calls storming Jericho. Eventually, for the next month, and for a year thereafter, I was one of the old Cursillistas, teaching courses in both English and Spanish and waking up the new ones on Sunday mornings. Many friendships were made in the process (the Cecchinis, the Brewers, the Canepas, the Marianis, and so on); most of them have lasted a long time.

Following the Cursillo weekend, all "graduates" were divided into groups and were supposed to meet once a week and discuss common problems in living the Faith. This never lasted more than a few months, for it was too much to ask people of this world! It is amazing how few of these lay-inspired movements last as compared to pontifically approved orders like the Jesuits, Carmelites, Benedictines, Cistercians, Redemptorists, Franciscans, Dominicans, and many others, all of whom have lasted for centuries. Could that be a sign of the validity of ordination as a sacrament, under the aegis and guidance of the Holy Spirit and the Universal Church? I am sure that this is the case, as proven by the permanence of all these religious orders.

•

CHAPTER 17

AN EYE FOR PRACTICE

During my early days of practice, I was studying to pass the American Board of Ophthalmology exams and had to pass a day-long written test before I could apply for the orals. I passed the written exams. Six months later I went for four days to San Francisco to undergo seven separate sessions of oral examinations, each time facing one or two expert specialists in seven branches of ophthalmology (optics and refraction, external eye disease, medical treatment, surgical techniques, eye muscles and strabismus, glaucoma, and neuro-ophthalmology). Each section was three hours long and it took three and a half days of grueling questions by experts to get it over with. It was harrowing, and even at this late stage of professional learning, there was no guarantee of passing. However, I succeeded in getting my specialty certificate and became a graduate of the American Board of Ophthalmology.

Next, I applied to become a member of the American Academy of Ophthalmology and was accepted. At that time Dr. A.D. Ruedeman, my former chief, was president. He was a good friend of Dr. Derrick Vail, publisher of the American Journal of Ophthalmology, and through that association I had several original professional papers published. It was exciting and encouraging to be able to publish many scientific papers in those days, with no delay. Two years later I applied and had to undergo interviews for the American College of Surgeons. I passed and became a Fellow of the American College of Surgeons, another title (F.A.C.S.) I could use following B.A. and M.D.

In the past few decades, I and the eye surgeons of my era had to learn and re-learn umpteen new surgical procedures many times over. I have always been a heavy-volume eye surgeon and had to constantly keep up with all the new advances in treatment and in eye surgery. At times I was the innovator who discovered and modified outworn techniques and procedures. Many of the surgeons who did two or three procedures a week didn't keep up to date, and stayed far behind the inevitable progress. These eventually dropped out of doing surgery altogether and became medical ophthalmologists. They treated eye diseases and pathology, and referred the patients who needed surgery to the super-specialists (the cataract, glaucoma, retina, and corneal transplant surgeons).

In the mid-1960s, my medical practice boomed. An incident occurred late in 1962 which helped my practice grow. I was sent a young patient with severe headaches by Joe Brice (a variation of Brais), a member of the extended family. After thorough examination of the patient's visual acuity, his visual fields and the inside of the eye, I arrived at the diagnosis of pituitary gland tumor at the base of the brain. A casual remark he made to me as he was leaving the office about how he was losing his sexual desire, led me to further narrow the pathological type of tumor to chromophobe adenoma of the pituitary gland (a special type of the tumor). So I sent him for an X-ray exam of the *sella tursica* (the "Turkish saddle" of bone which protects the pituitary at the very base of the skull). The report came back from the radiologists marked "slight enlargement of the *sella tursica*, but not diagnostic of the presence of tumor."

I questioned the report and sent the patient directly to a neurosurgeon, Dr. Don Lamond, a fellow Canadian, telling him that because of the typical bi-temporal loss of the visual fields, the report is a false negative. I suggested that he operate soon and find out. When he did, he removed an enlarged pituitary gland. The pathology report came back a few days later marked "chromophobe adenoma of the pituitary gland." I had hit a bull's eye. This unusual "case of the week" was presented at the weekly surgical-pathologic conference on Saturday morning at the hospital. There were about eighty doctors in the amphitheater, some of whom barely knew who I was. As a result of the case, I became a celebrity overnight. Chromophobe adenomas of the pituitary gland are rare and my diagnosis was on the mark. Physician referrals began to pour in, and I was happy that I had done right by the patient, who is still alive today.

CATARACTS MADE SIMPLE

Most eye operations are cataract extractions, though the average person has a hazy notion of what a cataract is. A cataract is nothing more than the hardened and scarred crystalline lens, the living optical lens in the eye behind the pupil that we all have, its function being to focus the light rays on the retina so that clear vision is possible. During my days in training we used the intra-capsular cataract extraction (removing the entire cataract with a so-called capsule forceps), but as time went on, this procedure gave way to the extra-capsular cataract extraction, where the capsule (compare it to the skin of a grape) is opened, followed by removal of the nucleus (the seed of the grape), and finally, the so-called cortex (the pulp of the grape) is slurped up by suction. So the opened capsule alone is left behind in order to receive the intra-ocular lens that would separate the vitreous jelly in the back part of the eye from the so-called anterior chamber in front of it. Then Charles Kelman, a surgeon inventor, and friend of mine for many years—he just passed away this year—invented the process called phaco-emulsification, in which the nucleus of the cataract is fragmented by ultrasound, and then the fragments are removed by suction. Contrary to a false public notion, lasers are not used at the initial removal of a cataract. They are sometimes used months later to open a residual opacified capsule, behind the intraocular lens; but never at the initial cataract surgery.

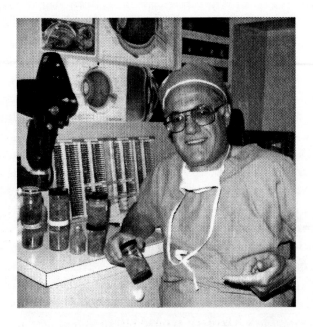

In the early days of practice I used to save the extracted intact cataracts in transparent jars and show them to patients needing surgery. The dozen or so jarful of cataracts I had in every examining room, were a potent visual evidence of my experience and credentials—much more effective than the degrees I had hanging on the wall. In spite of my still black hair and youthful appearance, when patients saw all these cataracts in a jar, they had living proof that I had done enough operations to satisfy their doubts if they had any. Of course, surgical success and word of mouth were equally helpful in increasing the patients' confidence.

Before 1970, the cataract patient had to wear "coke-bottle" thick glasses to replace the cataract-lens that was removed. Then, the intra-ocular lens was invented, first by Everett Ridley in England and then refined by many others. Ridley was an eye surgeon in London, England, who during the years following World War II treated many former RAF pilots with remnants of shattered airplane window panes in their eyes. Eventually, he figured out that the material of the shattered plastic was inert since its presence in the eye for a long time did not damage it. The plastic was PMMA (polymethylmetacrilate), a plastic material from which cockpit windows were made.

He got the idea of using a lens, made of this same material, inside the eye to replace the removed cataract. This was very ingenious on his part. The general idea was to put a plastic lens with the appropriate optical power in the original location of the removed cataract (in the residual capsule, behind the pupil), making the thick glasses on the face in front of the eye no longer necessary. I was one of the first half dozen surgeons (along with my friends Dennis Shepard, Harold Hand and a few others) to use the procedure in the United States. That was the beginning of a new era in eye surgery (around 1970-73). It was very exciting to me to be part of that evolution in medicine.

There were various stages of development in the intra-ocular lens (IOL) story. Dr. Ridley originally placed it behind the pupil. Then Peter Choyce in England, Tenant, Shepard, and Zeiter in the United States, started placing it in front of the pupil and behind the cornea, the clear window of the eye. However, the final consensus returned to placing it behind the pupil within the capsule of the original lens, because it proved to be the safer procedure, for various reasons which I will not go into here. At first, the lenses were of the hard plastic PMMA variety. Slowly, newer, softer, more malleable lenses were developed, so that now the lens can be folded like a taco and introduced into the eye through a very tiny needle-like hole, making it unnecessary to use sutures. Recently, Drs. Joe and John, my successors at Zeiter Eye Clinic, have started to experiment with soft *bifocal* intra-ocular lenses making the use of glasses for both near and distant vision obsolete.

In 1975, because of complaints by doctors who were not using intraocular lenses, there was an ill-advised moratorium placed by the State of California on their use. The rationalization given for this was that they were still experimental and could be harmful to the eye. Dr. Michaelis in Los Angeles, Dennis Shepard in Santa Monica, Henry Hirshman in Long Beach, and I, began a fight in the California legislature to lift this ban. We had to prove that intraocular lenses were safe. Just the same, all of us kept on doing the procedure at great risk to ourselves, even though the penalties were severe for doing it. Within weeks, intraocular lenses (IOLs) became unavailable in California, since the companies that manufactured them did not want to disobey the interdict proclaimed by the State, and they stopped selling them.

I recall flying to England with my wife Carol to visit Dr. Peter Choyce whose IOLs were still being used in England. We visited him at Chelsea-on-Sea, a delightful hamlet east of London. He had invited us to tea at his home one sunny Wednesday afternoon. In the midst of pleasantries, I bought from him thirty anterior chamber intra-ocular lenses and paid him on the spot the price he asked. Dr. and Mrs. Choyce were very charming and pleasant and we started to correspond with them. We flew back to California, bringing with us the IOLs, and continued cataract removal with IOL implantation, until the ban was lifted about a year later. The arbitrary interdict failed to stop the advance of medicine.

A SHORT-TERM PARTNERSHIP

When my medical practice began to grow, I started looking for a partner to relieve me of the routine procedures, so I could concentrate on the surgical side of the practice. Early in 1968, I obtained the name of a certain Dr. Arch Meredith, who wanted to come to California to practice. After we met and talked, he was anxious to work with me, and he signed the usual contract against competitive practice, in case he left me and went out on his own in our area.

Arch brought his family from West Virginia to visit Stockton and see what opportunities there were here. After he decided to join me, we helped him find a place to rent until he was established enough to buy a house. He had four children, one son and three daughters, who eventually became prominently employed in the community. Fran, his wife, was a southern belle, with the appropriate accent in speech and southern grace, and an exceptional sweetness towards everybody.

Arch had an uncle who practiced ophthalmology in West Virginia for many years, and who developed amyotrophic lateral sclerosis (ALS), the so-called Lou Gehrig's disease. The uncle had previously obtained an unusually generous disability insurance policy and after the onset of his ALS lived quite comfortably with his family on the proceeds from the policy, until he passed away from this debilitating neuromuscular disease several years later. Apparently, there was a previous history of this condition in other members of their family as well. So when Arch joined me in practice, he obtained on his own a large disability insurance policy in addition to the liberal one we bought for him. He just wanted to protect himself against the eventuality of ALS.

Three months before Arch finally moved to Stockton to work with us, we had a catered big welcoming dinner party for him in our backyard, and we invited about sixty physicians with their wives. It was in line with Aristotle's idea of *munificence* (a word coined by Aristotle) which the philosopher described as the highest form of magnificent generosity worthy of royalty. This was during the Merediths' visit to Stockton when they came to finalize matters with us.

He started in the practice, but unfortunately it wasn't long before Arch began to complain about the number of patients he had to see in the office and the many Hispanic laborers he found himself unable to communicate with, since he could not speak Spanish. Arch left my practice before the first year was up, and set up his own practice in a nearby medical building, about two miles from my office. This put me in a dilemma because he was violating the terms of our five-year agreement which specifically forbade him from opening a practice within a radius of ten miles from the office he left. I thought about the infraction for a few weeks and then realized that pursuing legal action would be a no-win situation for Carol and me. We reasoned that if we won, the medical community would say how could they do this to such a lovely young man starting out in practice? And if we lost, they would say it serves them right. So we decided to let it go, and it was one of the best decisions we ever made. It made a friend out of him, his family, and the medical community as a whole.

Sadly, within two years, Arch began to develop symptoms of ALS. It was not long before he could not practice at all. Thankfully, he began collecting the generous disability insurance that he had so prudently bought earlier on. At the same time, Fran had to leave the house and earn a living as a real estate agent. She took loving care of Arch like a ministering angel for over thirty years, and faced his paralyzed condition with exemplary equanimity, earning everyone's respect and admiration. Arch was paralyzed and couldn't take care of his own personal needs, nor could he even talk for the last fifteen years of his life. And Fran persevered through thick and thin. She remains in my mind a model of womanhood and a living saint, constant in her devotion to husband and family.

Every now and then I would visit Arch. He would be sitting in a motorized wheelchair in his home and he would communicate with me by writing on an electronic tablet he kept on his lap. Once he wrote, "Henry I appreciate your coming over to visit me. You know, I've learned many good things from you and I've always respected you. I want you to know that." I looked at his face and we both started to cry. In my heart I felt I had renewed our friendship and he gave me a chance to put away any resentful feelings I might have had. I told him I loved him because his infirmity reminded me of Christ, the long suffering servant—patient, accepting, and meek. He started crying all the more and we hugged each other.

He passed away in 2002 and had one of those extremely well-attended funeral services at which the love and accolades from family and friends were overwhelming. We all had tears in our eyes during a slide presentation on his life. Our community, and particularly his family, had lost a good, patiently suffering man.

The mention of hugging Arch reminds me of one of the points I used to make when speaking at medical conferences on the prevention of medical lawsuits. I would start the conference by telling an audience of eye surgeons, that after doing umpteen surgical procedures, I had never been sued. Then I would list items such as paying attention to what the patient says and feels, never discounting the patient's complaints, but investigating them thoroughly, and being honest and informaing the patient and his relatives of any untoward complication that might have arisen. I would always add that hugging the old patient at the proper moment was a very soothing practice and a sure prevention against law suits. In my practice, after the exam was completed and the elderly patient stood up to be taken back home (possibly to a rest home), I routinely asked them if there was anything they forgot to do? They would stop and look at me quizzically. "Well, aren't you going to hug your doctor before you go home?" I would ask them, thus giving them the liberty of doing it or not. In forty years of practice I have never seen a single case where an elderly patient refused to hug me; and they would often tell me, with tears in their eyes, that it was the first time anybody had offered to hug them in ten, twenty, or thirty years.

ONE OF MY FASTEST CURES

In those days, emergency rooms were not staffed with ER doctors as they are now. Such a specialty had not yet come into being. When a patient came in with an urgent problem into an emergency room, his own doctor (or a doctor taking calls for him) would be called in to see him. In Stockton, we had a solitary white building on San Joaquin Street that was used as an Emergency Care Center. I used to be called often to examine eye injuries, because I was the eager young eye doctor in town. I recall seeing many industrial injuries there, until the Center closed down because it was no longer profitable enough to compete with the hospital emergency rooms that were staffed with ER physicians at all times of day and night.

One evening, Evelyn Swanson, an elderly, friendly nurse who always took night duty, called me in to see a six-year-old girl who was brought in by her mother because of a sudden loss of vision. I rushed from home to the ER center downtown, figuring it was a sudden attack of acute glaucoma, or a retinal detachment—something really serious. I examined the girl, and found her eyes to be perfectly normal. When her vision was taken, she read the chart down to the 20/20 line with each eye with no difficulty whatever.

"When did this happen?" I inquired of the mother.

"About an hour ago, she was watching TV when all of a sudden everything went dark for her, and she could not see the screen," said the mother.

"So, what did you do?" I asked the mother.

"I panicked! I grabbed her, put her in the car, and immediately brought her here to have her eyes checked."

"But your daughter is seeing everything now, and the eye exam has revealed a perfectly normal pair of eyes."

Upon further inquiry, the story unraveled. Apparently, the child was watching television when the TV screen went blank. The old television had lived its allotted earthly life. At that point the girl screamed and told her mother that she couldn't see anything. The mother immediately brought her to the ER without realizing it was a mechanical problem with the TV. That case turned out to be one of my fastest cures!

MEDICAL ANECDOTES

Once I had a fifty-year-old woman from Mexico City who was referred to me by her relatives in Stockton. After examining her, I fitted her with minus-ten-diopters myopic glasses. (These are coke-bottle lenses with a high power of refraction, needed to see distant objects clearly in cases of severe near-sightedness.) She had lived her entire life in Mexico seeing the world blurrier than a Renoir painting. When she picked up the glasses she was happy at first with her new clear vision, reading everything on the chart at twenty feet away in the examining room. But a week later, she came back, very angry, complaining that she was seeing every tiny piece of dust on her furniture, and had to keep cleaning the house; and, "Besides," she said, "these horrible glasses make everything seem to be coming right at me." I told my optician to cut down the power of the lenses by half. When she picked up her new glasses, she was much happier even though she saw half as much as with the full prescription. She just couldn't tolerate full clarity. At the time I thought the whole episode had the aura of an Aesop's fable—the moral being that some people can handle half truths much better than the whole truth!

A few months later, the head of the Spanish Department at the University of the Pacific came to me for a routine eye exam. He was a true Spaniard who pronounced the Zs in Zaragoza in perfect Castilian (with his tongue between his teeth). He was in need of a change of glasses, and when he picked up the new glasses, he asked me, what would be the best way to keep the lenses clean. I made a slip of the tongue and told him *"con sopa y agua,"* i.e. with *soup* and water. I should have said *"con jabon y agua."* It had slipped my mind that *soap* in Spanish is *jabon,* and not *sopa.* He looked at me disconcerted and said, *"Sopa y agua! Sopa y agua! Doctor, como puede ser eso?"* (i.e. "Soup and water! Soup and water! Doctor, how can that be?") We laughed heartily when we realized my mistake. I can still picture him going home and asking his wife to make some soup so he can clean his glasses!

A decade earlier, when I was an intern at Harper Hospital, a boy with a club-foot was brought in by his parents two hours after midnight. A club-foot is a congenital defect one has since birth. The boy was seven years old. I asked the parents why they were bringing him in at 2:00 a.m. seven years after discovering the condition. They simply replied, "We couldn't sleep tonight. We thought it was time to bring him to see a doctor and find out if anything could be done for his foot."

Not all of my emergency room experiences were like these. Some were quite bizarre. I was called to the emergency room at Harper Hospital one night during my internship year. The patient was a three-hundred-pound African-American female who was pushed by her husband during a hassle at a New Year's Eve party at the Gotham Hotel, right across the street from the hospital. The funny thing was that she went backwards bottom first into the party's punch bowl. I spent all night picking out glass splinters from her huge backyard. That was strange enough, but nothing compared to the following week when I was called on to treat a skinny African-American male. He had a punch bowl filled with lye poured over his genitalia while he was asleep. It turned out that he was the unlucky husband of the obese woman he had pushed into the party's punch bowl seven days before.

A DEEP FRIENDSHIP

In Stockton, I had set Wednesdays and Fridays as my surgical days. For years I used other ophthalmologists as assistants, but much of the time they would be busy in their own offices and could not assist. So I started using a general practitioner as my assistant, Dr. Virgilio Solis. With a moderate on-the-spot training, he became a very efficient surgical assistant, and would always take time out from his office hours to come to the hospital and assist me. When my nephew Joe, came into the practice and became my assistant, Dr. Solis began assisting other doctors with their surgeries (orthopedic, cardiovascular, abdominal, or whatever he was called to do). He loved to assist and enjoyed the camaraderie that the ambience of the operating room provided.

Virgilio became a close friend as well. Since he was Hispanic, we talked in Spanish during surgery and the patients weren't alarmed by what we were saying. He would routinely accompany the patients back to the recovery room, giving them instructions in either English or Spanish. After surgery, about 1:00 p.m., we would sit for a few minutes in the doctor's room listening to Dr. Luis Arismendi and Dr. Spraecher and their entourage, discuss with gusto the politics of medical practice and/or administrative matters. At times they would get into heated arguments about germane subjects, which to the rest of us was very entertaining.

After joking with the other physicians, Dr. Solis and I would drive to a Basque restaurant downtown and have lunch before we went home. We particularly liked Villa Basque, which was run by the Ospital brothers, Jean and Pierre. They used to welcome us with open arms. The restaurant was always packed with a hungry clientele, especially on Wednesday, one of our surgical days. At the bar, where Pierre would insist on serving us *picons*, the Basque national drink, we would trade barbs and jokes with the bartenders and waitresses.

The salad was served family style, followed by a stew of boiled pig's feet as an appetizer and then a huge T-bone steak or prime-rib with all the trimmings. We were young, virile, and always hungry in those days. We would have plenty of camaraderie and lots of loud conversation with people at the other tables. Everybody knew everybody else since most of them worked downtown.

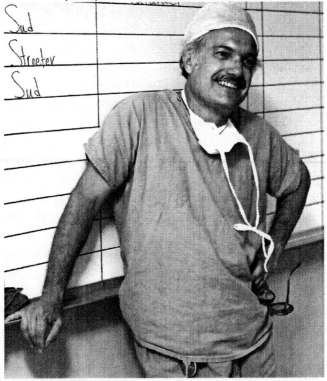

Surgery days; I am waiting in my scrubs to go in the OR; the wait between cases was long, until we built our own surgical center where we could do up to twenty operations a day.

Every first Thursday evening of the month the San Joaquin County Medical Society held its social monthly meetings. These get-togethers were extremely well attended, with drinks, dinner, and cards afterwards. I can picture with nostalgia Drs. Jack Williams, Gene Northcott, Art Chimiklis, and Stanley

Clark sitting around the poker table, smoking and betting until midnight. Now the meetings are held quarterly and the only way to get the young doctors to come is to invite their wives also.

Not all the doctors were extroverts, but at least most of them showed up. There were about five of us who told all the jokes and kept these evenings exciting. At rare times during the year, Dr. Edwin Roeser—a very serious and perfect fellow for the role—would stand up and give a short eulogy for one of our old colleagues who had just passed away, and we all wondered who would be next. But the party would go on after a minute of silence, and the drinking and joking would continue full blast. However, the scene has quieted down considerably since then. Now the society can't even fill a small room. The new doctors stay home with their families and most of the old doctors have passed away. The few old ones still living have lost interest.

Dr. Virgilio Solis was quite outgoing when he was alone with me, but he was always quiet at these socials. It seemed as though his happy moments were invariably followed by sadness or even tragedy, whether financial or personal. He finally passed away a few years ago.

I saw two of his children, Patty, an architect, and Carlos, a psychiatrist, at their father's memorial service at the huge Annunciation Cathedral in Stockton in July 2003. There were only three doctors present, Dr. Bernadino, an old friend of his who is now paralyzed, Dr. Nosce, an ophthalmologist, and myself. Most of the other attendees were relatives. So at the funeral of a very religious man, who had suffered several reverses, and bore adversity like a true Christian, there were no more than fifty people in attendance. I was sick at heart when I saw this, though my consolation was that Mozart, the incarnate god of melody and beauty, actually had only his wife and a handful of friends present at his funeral. Sitting in the pew next to Carol, I reflected on my friendship with the deceased.

Aristotle spent the last two chapters of his *Nichomachean Ethics* discussing friendship. After brilliantly expounding in the first eight chapters on the cardinal virtues of prudence, temperance, justice, and fortitude, he ended with a treatise on friendship, because he considered it essential to a virtuous life. "True friendship is the greatest of the joys of one's life," he wrote, "Harmonious close friendships can only be with a few and are difficult to maintain, but when they last, they are man's greatest treasure."

Dr. Solis's funeral had a profound effect on my thoughts and emotions. It was one of several experiences that have led me to a time of introspection. At Virgilio's funeral, I felt that a certain amount of solitude and quiet at this time was necessary for me to take stock of my life.

CHAPTER 18

SETTLING INTO FAMILY LIFE

When we first came to Stockton, we rented a house on Inman Street not far from the medical office. Hank and Elsie Ratto lived three houses away from us, down the street. One hot summer weekend, they invited us to go up to the mountains with them to spend a few days at their cabin. During that momentous excursion we fell in love with the Sierra Nevada Mountains. It was a *déjà vu* experience of my childhood's summer vacations in the mountains of Lebanon. That weekend I felt I was in Serhel again. It wasn't long before Hank asked us if we would like to buy his brother Warren's half share in the cabin, since Warren's kids no longer wanted to leave their friends in Stockton and go up to the mountain. We accepted immediately.

The large cabin overlooked the South Fork of the American River. It was 5,500 feet up, on a forested mountain, off Highway 50, and twenty miles from Lake Tahoe. Every Thursday during the summer, the Fish and Game truck would pass by our cabin on its way to dump a load of trout in the river, a quarter mile higher up. We would wait half an hour for the anaesthetized fish to wake up before we set out to the pool beneath the Strawberry Bridge where the fish were planted. We would catch our limit every time, and the children became expert trout fishermen. The nearby meadows were full of wild flowers as at that elevation summer was like the spring season. We started spending the two months of school vacation at that heavenly cabin.

I would come up on weekends and sometimes for a whole week and spend time with the family, away from the office and the hustle and bustle of the city. It was Serhel revisited. Eventually the Rattos stopped coming up because their kids wanted to stay in the city. Shortly after, we bought their share and had the cabin all to ourselves. The few neighbors around called our tract of homes "The Happy Valley." It all reminded me of the happy times spent in Serhel before my five brothers and one sister left the nest years ago.

THE AMERICAN RIVER

The American River ran along the edge of the property providing many different opportunities for summer fun. Early in the summer we would build a rudimentary dam on the river. The annual project was exciting for the whole family. We would choose a shallow spot and start building the dam by moving rocks around from the river bed itself and piling them high on top of each other. The water was freezing because it came from the melting snows of the Sierras. It was so cold that our hands and fingers would become half frozen and would lose feeling. It was actually pretty dangerous because if we banged a hand or a finger between two heavy rocks we wouldn't feel much pain, even if we were to fracture a bone; and we would continue moving rocks around, thus aggravating the injury. As a matter of fact, once I walked out of the freezing water and felt some discomfort in my right hand, which in a very short time turned to severe pain. X-rays at the hospital revealed a broken index finger of the right hand. I was unable to do eye surgery for two months.

I would return to Stockton in the middle of the week to work in the office, but before long I started taking off the whole month of August and driving up to where the weather was cooler. The children loved to see me take time off. They enjoyed the mountain air and learned how to fish for trout and climb rocks, just as I used to do in Lebanon as a child. At Strawberry Lodge there was a makeshift tennis court where we taught the children the rudiments of the game. It was a perfect time of leisure. We had decided earlier not to have a telephone or a television, so that the family fun could be generated internally. I think we owned every board game that was in existence.

At times the absence of a telephone presented difficulties for a busy eye surgeon. Carol reminds me of the many times the Highway Patrol would come knocking on the door to tell us that they're relaying a call from our office that eyes were available for corneal transplantation. At such times I would drive down to Stockton to perform the surgery. Once the H.P. offered to drive me down to Stockton 150 miles away when an emergency arose!

During the winter, we would frequently visit Carol's sister in Sunnyvale. My brother-in-law, Bob had accepted a job as assistant principal in that California city, and we became the best of friends. One Sunday afternoon we sat all the children in the back of our station wagon and drove to Carmel by-the-Sea. As we were driving along I pointed out a prickly pear plant on the side of the road. They all wondered about the taste of that fruit. So we backed up the car and I got out and proceeded gingerly to fill a brown paper bag with prickly pears, picking the fruit very carefully, as I used to do in Lebanon. I came back to the car and placed the paper bag in the back of the station wagon and told the children to leave the bag alone. I should have known better. Within fifteen minutes, all the kids started screaming and yelling in pain. They had taken the prickly pears out of the bag and were handing them around to each other. I spent the whole evening picking small thorns off little fingers. Their poor little hands were sore for days.

We spent a wonderful year with the in-laws, visiting back and forth, until they returned to Detroit for good. Bob had received and accepted a job offer as a principal there. A contributing factor may have been that his wife Camille wanted to go back to Michigan, as she missed Detroit and her parents. Since then, the parents have passed away, but Camille and Bob still live there. The distance has never stopped us from seeing each other frequently.

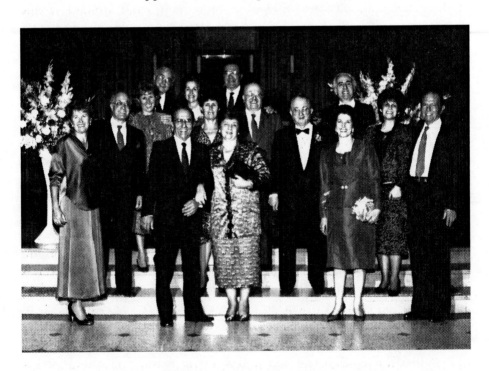

The seven Zeiter siblings with their spouses in 1992 (l. to r.):
Carol and I, Irene and Mike, Philip and Lydia (in front), Yvonne

and Edmond (in middle), Mary and Michel (behind), then Tony and Madelyn, Johnny and Irene, and Uncle Paul, who at age 82 was still tall and handsome (on the right).

After two years of renting a home, Carol and I started looking to buy. We looked for ten months and even explored the option of building on a lot, but we finally spotted an ad for a house in a section out of town that we had seen before and liked. It was in an area outside the city limits then, consisting of two streets with no sidewalks and large, estate-like front and back yards. It looked to us like an English country estate at the time. We fell in love with it and bought it.

It had a white wooden frame with dark blue shutters and a white corral fence. We lived in it for thirty years. We always loved the backyard for its peace, tranquility, and spaciousness. Some days, I would just sit there for hours, especially on my afternoons off, relaxing in the shade of the twenty-four poplars which lined the western edge of the yard. Carol loved the house because of the large bedrooms and kitchen. As they grew up in that house, the children would play tag football or baseball in the yard with their cousins and friends. It helped them to become great little league baseball players as they grew up. Our son John's interest in Little League baseball has lasted all these years. He has managed and coached his children's teams for twelve years now.

Taking the children often on fishing trips was another activity—a most enjoyable experience, that the boys still remind me of. During one of those trips, we caught *the* big fish. We were fishing off a lagoon with Pablo, our cousin, not far from Jackson, California, when I felt a huge bite and then an extraordinary pull that almost took the fishing-pole right out of my hands. I decided to bring it in slowly because it felt too heavy for my 8-pound fishing line. It gave us a good fight for about ten minutes as we brought it close to shore. We had taken turns allowing the fish to play the line. Suddenly, it leapt out of the water and landed right at my feet, with the hook still in its mouth. It was the silliest thing, for we didn't even have to use a net to bring it in. It was an eleven-pound, twenty-four-inch long, large-mouth, freshwater black bass, as we found out later at the bait shop.

I was going to take it home, clean it, and cook it, but Pablo was shocked and said to me, "Do you know what you have just caught." I said, "Yah, a big fish." "You're crazy?" he said to me. ("You're crazy" is one of Pablo's favorite expressions.) "This fish is probably the biggest freshwater large-mouth caught anywhere in California this year." Pablo insisted on taking us to the fish and bait shop to have our picture taken for the sporting section of the paper. And sure enough, the next day we appeared in the sports section of the *Stockton Record,* proudly holding our fish—the largest. It was the biggest catch of its kind that year! The fish is preserved and mounted on a captioned board and is hanging in John Henry's office with the newspaper article next to it.

THE CHILDREN

It would be a remarkable parent, indeed, who could write about his children dispassionately. I am not that parent. Moreover, in writing one's memoirs, one must take into account the particular sensitivities of those closest to him. It is one thing to share one's private facts with the world; it's quite another to share the private facts of another with the world, too. I do not wish to do that here with respect to my own children. But I would like to tell a bit about them, at the risk of being an indulgent parent.

JOHN HENRY

Our son, John Henry, our oldest child, is a classic Type A personality. He has always been driven to success; a leader in his field. He was president of his class in grade school, president of the student body in high school, and president of his fraternity in college. He loved his studies, held a 4.0 average through four years, and was valedictorian at St. Mary's High School in Stockton.

He had his mother's talent for sports and was a formidable baseball player in high school. Indeed, while in medical school in Houston, he assembled his medical school classmates and led them in the City of Houston baseball league, where he hit eleven homeruns in fourteen games, and helped his team win the title over a bunch of tough teams filled with brawny blue-collared players. Currently his four children are each involved in different sports.

He had wanted to be an ophthalmologist since he was six. He was always one of those kids who was dutiful and responsible with everything he did, no worry whatsoever to a parent. He is well-adjusted, through and through, and retains close friendships with classmates going back to grammar school. He is a business genius, a tireless worker, a dedicated player, constant and straight as an arrow. As the classical description goes, "In him all the humors are mixed in the rightful proportions." He loves the intellectual life, apart from medical practice, and bears a cultured good bearing, capable of strolling through a museum and identifying paintings and periods of art. He even likes classical music! (But alas, he listens to country music most of the time.) And finally, and most importantly to Carol and me, he is a model in his Catholic faith and lives a life of piety and humility. Lynette, his college sweetheart, whom he married, is equally capable and devoted.

I don't believe in horoscopes, of course—they offend the providence of God—but I did encounter a strange experience when John Henry was in high school. Chung Ja, the elderly Korean mother-in-law of our past Stockton Symphony conductor, told Carol and me in 1978, without ever seeing him or knowing him, that, according to the day, month, and hour of his birth, John Henry would have all of the above mentioned characteristics.

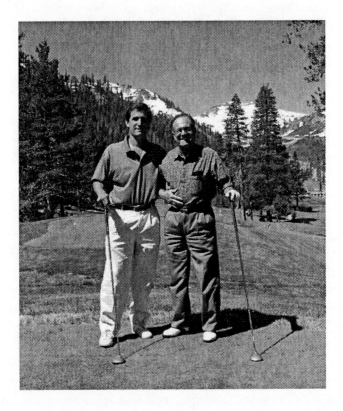

John Henry and I enjoying a round of golf at Tahoe Donner, close to our summer home in the Sierra Nevada mountains of California.

PHILIP

The womb delivers children differently and Philip, our second son, came out markedly different from his brother John Henry. This is not a disparagement—just a description. Born a year-and-a-half after him, Philip is a classic Type B personality. He is, as they say, "laid back," not driven, mostly contemplative. Unlike his Type A, left-brained brother, Philip is extraordinarily artistic, and right-brained.

The summer prior to his last year in high school, I traveled with him to Venezuela. We visited my brother and sister in Caracas and then went south to the Orinoco River jungle and saw Angel falls, the highest in the world. He came back motivated and had nothing but As in his fourth year. It helped him get into California Polytechnic University's architectural school, one of the best in the country. Yet shortly afterwards he went into a difficult period in which he was trying to "find himself," to discover who he was and what he should do with his life. I used to call him Siegfried—he was fearless, but rash.

After graduating, he experienced a crisis of faith and abandoned the Catholicism of his childhood. But a trip to China, and a stay in a hotel there, changed his life for ever. He picked up a Gideon Bible and started reading it. He read through the Bible twice from cover to cover. Within that year, he had several deep spiritual experiences and began to understand the message of the Good News.

Throughout this period, after having studied Sacred Scripture Philip began to realize the importance of spiritual growth. In his professional life as an architect, he observed that people gave little attention to their moral and spiritual well-being. He was perplexed by the "let's keep up with the Joneses" attitude, and by the indifference of people toward God. The afterlife was of no concern to most people he met, and, if they had any concern, it was belied by their lifestyle. Their fleeting happiness, he saw, depended on the accumulation of possessions and the attachment to the passing pleasures of the moment.

During our discussions he mentioned to me that he was writing a book on the subject of religious indifference, which eventually was published under the title of *What's Love got to Do with It?* I told him to read the *Pensées* of Blaise Pascal, the seventeenth-century physicist, mathematician and philosophic thinker who once wrote the following regarding religious indifference:

> The immortality of the soul is a matter of so great consequence to us and which touches us so profoundly that we must have lost all feeling, to be indifferent to knowing what it is and whether it is real . . . This carelessness of people towards a matter which

concerns themselves, their eternity, their all, drives me more to irritation than to pity; it astonishes and shocks me; to me it is monstrous. I do not say this out of the pious zeal of spiritual devotion. On the contrary, I expect that we ought to have this feeling from principles of human interest and self-love; for this we need to see what the least enlightened person sees . . . It does not require great education of mind to see that death, which threatens us at every moment, must infallibly place us within a few years under the dreadful necessity of being either forever annihilated or eternally happy . . . And thus it is unnatural that there should be men indifferent to the loss of their existence, their all, and to the perils of eternal suffering . . . They are quite different in regard to all other things. They are afraid of mere trifles . . . The same man will spend days and nights in rage and despair over the loss of office, or for some imaginary insult to his pride, and yet he is the very one who knows without anxiety that he will lose all by death.

—Pascal, *Pensées*, 194, 427.

I explained to my son that Blaise Pascal (1623-1662) had previously formulated the theory of probability in the process of developing statistics into a science. He was interested in gambling and worked out calculations for wagering. He was one of the first to enunciate exact rules as to what would be an appropriate risk to take in order to win a particular amount of expected reward. This led to his famous rule called Pascal's Wager. He stated that even for those who believe the probability of there being an after life is very small or nil, it is better to err on the side of caution and do one's duty towards God, and prepare oneself for the possibility of eternal life than to be indifferent and lax and lose eternal bliss. He reasoned that if one practices devotion and it turns out that there is no eternal life, one has lost little or nothing—an infinitesimal amount—compared to the loss of eternal happiness—an immeasurably infinite amount—if it turns out that there is an afterlife. He based his thinking on the fact that only a fool can claim to be absolutely sure there is no afterlife; and to live as if there weren't any, would be to make the worst wager ever, when comparing the small bet with the infinite reward.

After the publication of his book, Alicia, Philip's wife, read it. She told me recently that after her husband's conversion she was still in doubt, until she decided to wager for belief in God. And then it took her one year of practicing her faith to become certain that her choice to wager was the right one. I was not surprised at what she said, because that was precisely Pascal's intent when he advised the indifferent to make a decision to believe, knowing that not through wagering, but through an experience of faith, one grows in devotion and depth of belief.

While continuing work as an architect, Philip continued to read, study, and pray much on the side. He became concerned about the dangers of raising his children in a secular environment, and has sought to keep them far from television, irresponsible movies, immodesty, and immorality. He and Alicia live on a 174-acre ranch outside of Sacramento, where they raise their six children, isolated from the world. Philip is as sensitive as an artist and as spiritual as a monk; he is a devoted father and spouse, and a loving son. I am more comfortable talking philosophy, theology, life, and family with him than with any of the other children. He is a different son, but cherished all the more for that difference.

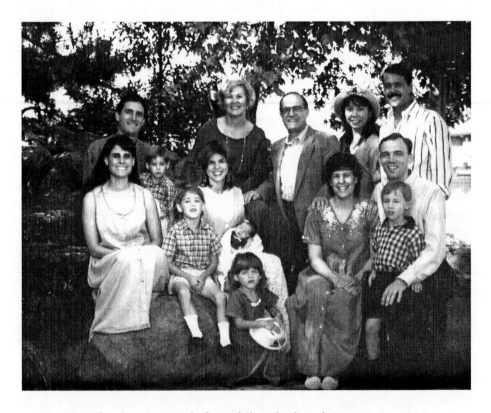

Our family in 1995, before Phil and Alicia begot us six more grandchildren, and Suzie one more; clockwise from the top left are John Henry, Carol, Henry, Alicia, Phil, Tony, Joseph, Suzie, Danielle, baby Sierra in Lynette's arms, John Henry Jr., Paul and Camille.

SUZIE

With alpha-numeric significance, Suzie was our Type C child, sweet, kind, non-confrontational, empathetic. She would often spend time with the elderly, especially elderly priests and nuns, talking with them, helping them. As a little girl, she was always the first to greet me coming home from work and would jump into my arms for a hug.

She wanted to be a movie actress at one time. She participated in school plays and musicals, and I still feel like crying when I picture how pretty she looked as Sharon in *Finian's Rainbow*. She had gotten the lead in her last year of high school. She was an accomplished pianist (especially of Mozart sonatas), and was an excellent student, using her natural intelligence to full capacity. She has always had a natural tendency for learning, and is the kind of person who will pick up an encyclopedia and read it for fun.

When she was considering which college to attend in high school, I had a parent's miracle beyond measure. I came home early from work one day and saw an informational packet of college materials for her from a school I had never heard of before—Thomas Aquinas College in Santa Paula, California. I couldn't resist looking at it and, lo and behold, it was a school of my dreams. Founded in 1971, it offered a classical liberal education based exclusively on the Great Books of Western Civilization and the Socratic seminar method of instruction. The school offered a four-year program of philosophy, theology, mathematics, experimental science, literature, history, language, and even music theory. All the classes were mandatory—no electives—and were integrated to provide a complete exposure to the greatest minds in history. The school had modeled its program after the successful St. John's Colleges (in Annapolis and Santa Fe), but with the distinctive mark of being Roman Catholic, that is, the curriculum was centered on the theology and philosophy of the Roman Catholic Church, namely, that of St. Thomas Aquinas, the theologian, and Aristotle, the philosopher.

Well, this was a school after my own heart—one whose curriculum I had tried to pursue in some small measure before entering medical school. Naturally, it would be my earnest wish for a child of mine to attend it. But I was also smart enough to know that any pushing I might do for it would propel a child in the opposite direction. So, I decided not to say anything. I put the materials back in the envelope and left them for Suzie when she came home. And then I prayed.

A couple of days later, Suzie said, "You know, Dad, I was looking at this school called Thomas Aquinas College."

"Oh?" I said, trying to sound nonchalant.

"Yah, it looks kinda interesting. Original works, integrated program, small classes, intimate environment."

"Maybe we should go visit it?"

And that we did. The visit confirmed everything I thought about the program and I was ecstatic beyond measure when Suzie decided to apply and eventually attend.

I got vicarious satisfaction over the years to see her studying philosophy with Plato, Aristotle, and Aquinas; learning mathematics through Euclid, Apollonius, Ptolemy, Copernicus, Galileo, Descartes, Newton, and Einstein; reading the best in literature from Homer, Virgil, Aeschylus, Dante, and Chaucer to Austin, Tolstoy and Dostoyevsky; studying political theory through Locke, Hume, Rousseau, Tocqueville, and the Federalists; and learning about God through Augustine, Aquinas, Anselm, and Athanasius, and many others.

I was so taken by the education there that the College eventually became a large beneficiary of our charitable contributions and I even joined the Board of Governors where I have been a member for over 20 years. Some of my most lasting friendships have been with my fellow governors, and some of my most enjoyable experiences have taken place through my impromptu visits with both students and faculty members.

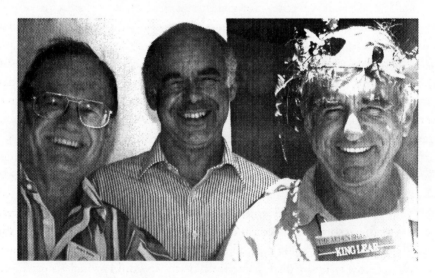

Photo taken at the 1995 Thomas Aquinas College Summer Seminar, when Shakespeare's *King Lear* was one of the works discussed—Shown are three "philosophers" (l. to r.): Aristotle (me), Plato (President Tom Dillon), and King Lear (friend and fellow board member, Jim Barrett).

Suzie met her husband, Tony Andres, there—a tall, athletic, gentle soul like her, with a passion for the intellectual life. Tony obtained a doctorate in philosophy at Notre Dame University and he is now the chairman of philosophy at Christendom College in Front Royal, Virginia, a small Catholic college that aims to offer a program based on faith and reason. He has written several essays and two books on the subject of logic.

Suzie is a stay-at-home mother of two children, who keeps up her reading life on the side. She homeschools her children and recently published a book on home schooling. In the past she has had the uncanny knack for sending me *the* book I am somehow looking for at the time.

CAMILLE

Camille, the youngest of our four children, is unlike all the others. Yet she is similar to them all, too—a veritable blend of personalities and tendencies.

Growing up, Camille was a model, deferential, respectful child with proper manners. It was as if she was bred by Emily Post. She was also intense, athletic, and perpetually bronzed. She loved, and still loves, rock climbing, which I can't help but think is a natural metaphor for her own life, given the obstacles she has had, and will have, to overcome.

Much to my great pleasure, she followed her sister, Suzie, to Thomas Aquinas College. But much to my displeasure, she became rebellious and dropped out. She did manage to keep good grades and was able to transfer to UC San Diego, where she was on the women's basketball team. She learned water-skiing and surfing while in balmy Southern California and is an avid rock and mountain climber now. The years ahead proved to be tumultuous ones; but she eventually graduated with a major in biochemistry and biology.

Then she had a breakdown that led her to her own Mount of Calvary, which she must spend the rest of her life ascending. She was hospitalized and diagnosed as having bipolar disorder, because of the extreme mood swings she experienced. After several rough episodes, she committed herself to treatment and has been meticulous about taking her medication. She eventually earned a master's degree in social work from Walla Walla State University in Washington State and has been working as a therapist at a large clinic in Washington. Her work is extremely demanding, but she is up to the challenge and loves the psychological aspect of it.

She has remained the same responsible and dutiful individual she was as a child, Kantian-Germanic like. And through her dogged independence and determination, she has overcome a crippling disability and will succeed in whatever she does. For this, we are exceedingly grateful.

III

CLEANSING OF BODY AND SOUL

CHAPTER 19

CRISIS AND TURMOIL

Between 1962 and 1968, life in Stockton was pleasant and enjoyable, and we became friends with many members of our extended family. I'm referring in particular to Nadim and Renee Malcoun, Joe and Marie Barkett, and George and Emily Rishwain. We used to get together most Sunday afternoons to play bridge (as two foursomes), or would just pile up into one or two station wagons and go picnicking in some park or just plain drive out into the country sight-seeing. On Tuesday evenings, we played nine-hole twilight golf with George and Emily at the Stockton Golf and Country Club. Sometimes we were joined at golf by Bob and Joan Rishwain or by Marie and Ed Rishwain, all cousins of ours.

The Country Club provided an interesting study of the habits that people develop. There were serious golfers who played three or four times a week and even a few who played every day. I was becoming an avid golfer, even though I rarely scored below ninety in eighteen holes. Yet, the habit was forcing me to be away from my growing family on weekends and Wednesday afternoons. After a while, I realized that this routine could become damaging to my home life. Initially, I began to join the domino and card players who hung around the club house on most afternoons. They were wealthy men, in general, who had their enterprises taken care of by managers, assistants, and overseers and their home life appeared to take second place to their daily country club routine. I soon found that I couldn't reconcile these habits with my cultural and philosophical bent, and dropped out of the club.

Then there were those who were suspected of carrying on with other members' spouses. These Don Juans were invariably tall, good-looking men who always appeared debonair and kept their hair well-combed and pressed down with brilliantine. At that time there was a story making the rounds about the male golfer who accidentally entered the women's locker room to shower after a round of golf. Hearing female voices upon coming out of the shower, he knew he was in the wrong place. What was he to do? He wrapped a towel around his head and walked right out completely naked, so no one was able to recognize his covered face. Well, after a few giggles, the first female club member said to the others, "I *know* he is not my husband." The second one said, "I *know* he's not my boyfriend." And the third one said, "I *know for sure* he doesn't even belong to the club!"

One of the closest friendships I had in those days was with Bob Rishwain, an attorney who was my second cousin. Bob was, and still is, one of those avid golf club members with a low handicap, and after-hours would often sit with the card-playing group for hours at a time. I met Bob on my first trip to California in 1957, when I came to take an externship at the UC San Francisco Medical Center. I was first introduced to his father, Ben, who was one of the sons of my deceased Aunt Laura (Ziara), my father's sister. Ben was a prominent man in town—the owner and manager of the Ambassador Hotel, also the head of the San Joaquin County Republican Committee—and quite debonair in bearing. We took a liking to each other immediately. In short order he introduced me to all his influential friends. I would go to the Ambassador Lounge and Restaurant for lunch or dinner often and visit with Ben.

It was inspiring to see Ben at work in his own restaurant for he was the ultimate owner host. He would go from table to table, asking people, "What else can I do for you? Is the food to your liking today? Can I bring you anything else? My name is Ben and it's my honor to be your host." That's how he was around the tables, even with people he had never seen before; in fact, especially with them. He was sincerely interested in people. It was a practical, personal gift he had that brought people back to his restaurant and hotel time and again. Unfortunately, he had bad kidneys with subsequent high blood pressure, and he died less than ten years after I first met him.

Ben and Mary had two sons. The younger one, Tony, had inherited his father's kidney problems, but nonetheless he went to medical school and eventually became a good physician. I am told that when he was only a child he used to go around the neighborhood carrying a toy medical bag and asking people if they were in need of medical attention. Several years ago he underwent a kidney transplant and is doing very well now, following the surgery. The older son, Bob, became my friend the day he came back from law school to practice in Stockton (1965). He opened his office in the same building as mine, and that was our mutual cousin Dr. Barkett's building.

I had met Bob several years before at his engagement party in 1957. Bob was attending Stanford University as an undergraduate at the time I was in California for my UC externship. He once told me that he went there from high school where he had all As with a big head, but was soon humbled when he found out that the other kids at Stanford had even bigger heads for study and competition. He soon buckled down and within three months was close to the top of the class. However, his father was a tough customer with high expectations. "There were times," Bob once told me, "when I would enter the house in the evening not knowing whether Dad was going to hug me or slap me."

Bob's engagement party was at his father's Ambassador Hotel. A year later, I attended his college graduation at Stanford University and he subsequently went to law school at Santa Clara University near San Jose. When he came back to Stockton, I adopted him as my lawyer and welcomed him as a family member. His wife, Joan, became Carol's best friend—and still is forty years later. Their attraction to each other was immediate, as Joan was a green-eyed Swede with blonde hair like Carol and similarly had married a type-A Lebanese.

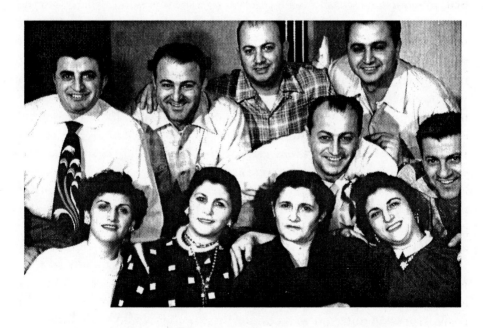

Aunt Ziara's ten children: (front row, l. to r.): Isabel Mas'ad (the youngest), Bernice Michaels, Sadi'a Barkett (my godmother), and Mary Jacobs; (second row, l. to r.): Ben and Shiben (Joe Sr) (crouching); (back row, l. to r.): Peter, George, Mike, and Edmond. Between them they have thirty-seven children (second cousins to me), who in turn have about one hundred and fifty progeny (third cousins to me), some of whom are beginning to marry and have children of their own, endowing me with even more cousins. And the Rishwains are only aunt Ziara's progeny. In Stockton, we have other cousins and second cousins, who are the progeny of Dad's brothers, Ass'ad, Anthony, and Pablo.

ERRONEOUS ZONES

The 1970s were the beginning of what I call "solipsism," or the "me" generation. It appeared that Bob, Joan, and Carol were undergoing a midlife crisis, but so was everybody else. It became difficult to tell whether the revolt was due to an individual's hormonal imbalance, or a product of the generation (we were living in the notorious 1960s and '70s). As to Carol, she had not practiced nursing for over fifteen years because she was working hard at home raising four children. That has always been harder than working in the world outside the home. Yet she decided now to return to school at the University of the Pacific to become a psychologist-marriage-counselor. In those days, it seemed every time I turned around some wife or another was leaving the home to work in an office as a psychologist or to sell houses as a real estate agent. It was the era when women began to hit the workplace in force. By then, we were out of the Country Club, thank God (it had become a den of divorcees), but we still spent social time with several members of the club, both those who were our relatives and those who were acquaintances.

The 1970s saw a plethora of groupies following this or that author psychologist's theories. Worse yet, many were following self-styled gurus who promised nirvana. These people were springing up all over the landscape. Though Carol never belonged to any particular group, nonetheless she was involved with several like-minded friends who would one month take up yoga, the next Tai Chi, and the month after go to gatherings such as EST (a psychic fad at the time), or any of the other fads of emotive therapy, transactional analysis, or what not. And all the while, these friends would be suggesting to one another all kinds of new self-help books by Eric Berne, Wayne Dyer, Daniel Goldstine, Shirley Zukerman, Erica Jong, etc. I made it my business to read most of these books to know how to protect my family from the onslaught of confusion I foresaw coming. It was difficult to keep up with the reading material and at the same time work for a living at the office!

Every time I saw a book on the shelf after Carol had read it, I would pick it up and start reading: Dyer's *Your Erroneous Zones*; Hendrix's *Getting the Love You Want*; R.A. Johnson's *I, You and We*; Steere's *Bodily Expressions in Psychology*; Turko and Tosi's *Sports Psyching*; Goldstine et al's *The Dance Away Lover*; and on and on. The titles themselves often gave a hint of the pseudo-psychological advice being put out for popular consumption. I laugh now when I recall some of the other titles, like *How to Take Care of Number One*; *What Do You Say When Someone Says Hello?*; *Where and How to Find Yourself*; *Where Are you Going Now?*; etc . . . Similar books are still flooding the market such as Gray's *Men are from Mars and Women from Venus*, and there is no end in sight, given the unhappy lot of people we are and the great number of writers offering popular advice.

I am certain that the authors of all these popular publications made out very well financially at a time when family cohesion was becoming weak. They most certainly helped push it to greater morbidity. I was not surprised when many of them (for example, Dr. Spock, Erica Jong, Rogers and his group) began to see, as time went on, the disastrous results from their preaching and writing and began to strike their breasts with their *mea culpas*, in *Time*, *Newsweek* and *Psychology Today*, admitting publicly that their ideas and their books have ruined a whole generation.

In all fairness, however, there were many novel psychological insights ably presented by many of these authors within their texts. A salient example was Eric Berne's descriptions of the various games people play with themselves and each other. His psychological descriptions were enlightening on a subject of great behavioral importance. So was Goldstine's classification of personality types (victim, rescuer, passive aggressive, tough-fragile and so on), describing them from his own therapeutic experience and from the records of both his patients and his colleagues'. R.A. Johnson's penetrating analysis of male, female and combined traits (anima, animus, etc.) was Wagnerian in concept as he used the opera master's character types for illustration. These authors' insights were on the mark—and not only for persons seeking therapy. Their descriptions of behavior can be witnessed daily in supposedly "normal" people. Charles Baudelaire's verse in *Les Fleurs du Mal* is appropriate here: "*Hypocrite lecteur, mon semblable, mon frère*" ("You, my hypocrite reader, my same self, my brother").

The problem, though, was that most people didn't have the psychological and philosophical insight to wean the huge amount of trash from the few pearls present in the publications of most of these authors. It was a situation quite similar to reading Darwin, or Freud, or Nietzsche. Whatever truth there was in their thoughts gets lost—if not in their own extrapolations, at least in the misinterpretations and exaggerations of their followers and apologists.

It was the decade of solipsism; the decade of the "me" generation; the decade of the "I have to find myself"; the decade of "there must be something better out there!" The continuing result is the present decade of total sexual and behavioral permissiveness, the trashing of modesty, the relativistic outlook in religion, thought and morals—in one word, the evident bankruptcy of this MTV generation.

Originally, the rationalization for permissive behavior in marriage was that "the other spouse was rude, crude, and overbearing." I would be the first to admit the validity of these accusations. None of us had taken courses on marriage etiquette or spousal behavior. These courses were not taught in schools and still aren't. And looking back now, I am aware that the 1970s was definitely the wrong decade for me or for anyone else to *even think* of contradicting the other spouse, or to show any verbal disrespect or to make any faux-pas— especially in view of the endemic of *hormonal hurricanes* everybody was going through. I now admit that if these things were sins, I must have committed plenty of them, but hardly ever deliberately or with malignant intent. In any case, spousal relationship becomes better with experience, not by taking a course, even if such were available, but by conscious and loving practice. Patience and compassion are still the required virtues when it comes to marital disagreement and/or imagined misdeeds on the part of one or the other of the spouses. Unfortunately, such pristine virtues seem to be in short supply when the person in question is undergoing a *midlife crisis*. When I discuss it with other doctors, I call it the "hormonal hurricane."

OUR TURN

Everybody in the various psychotherapy groups at the time was close to the dangerous age of forty, but the leaders of the groups were invariably quite a bit older and should have known better. As a result of all this, Bob and Joan separated, and then divorced; Jack and Peggy, not relatives, but close friends, ended up leaving each other. Neither remarried which I take as a sign of their maturity. Max left Joann, just as he had left a previous marriage; and the story goes on and on. The social fabric was being torn apart and people were becoming more and more indiscrete, psychologically "pseudo-free." They were all openly exhibiting their infidelities, just as problematic adolescents tend to attempt unsuccessful suicide as a signal for help.

Little was I to know that the same tragedies striking those around Carol and me were to imperil our relationship also. Carol says that for two or three years before our particular hurricane struck, she was sending me various signals that she was unhappy with our relationship. But I was blind to it all, until the evening when she said to me, "I would like to move out to find myself." I discouraged her at first with whatever logic I had at hand, and she calmed down. When a few months later she made the same request, I woke up to the danger, enough to be more solicitous and caring, both because I loved her dearly and for the protection of the family and the marriage. She acquiesced again, but more months of "hate-looks" followed, without intermission.

Finally, one morning she called me at the office to invite me to lunch at a Black Angus Restaurant. I was happily surprised and looked forward to lunch with her, not realizing the news to come. As we sat down she told me that she had already moved out with Camille, our youngest, that very morning, with the help of one of her female friends who was acting as her confessor and sounding board at the time. I sat at the lunch table, miserable and depressed. I never thought Carol would go through this and put us all through it, as I always believed that she was more practical and stable than others in our circle. I didn't realize that counsels of patience were anathema, and that this disease was virulently contagious. I should have remembered the beginning verses of Dante's Inferno, by now my favorite quote:

> Nel mezzo del cammin di nostra vita,
>   Mi ritrovai per una selva oscura,
>   Che la diritta via era smarrita.
> Ah quanto a dir qual era è cosa dura
>   Esta selva selvaggia e aspra e forte
>   Che nel pensier rinnova la paura!
> Tant'è amara che poco è più morte . . .
> —Dante, Inferno, Canto Primo, 1-7

> ("Midway upon the journey of our life
>   I found myself within a forest dark,
>   For the straightforward pathway had been lost.
> Ah me! How hard a thing it is to say
>   What was this forest, savage, rough and stern,
>   Which in the very thought renews the fear.
> So bitter is it, death is little more . . .")
> —Longfellow's translation

Dante's excellent seven-verse description of midlife turmoil and crisis—which begins the greatest epical poem in Christendom—shows how long the phenomenon has plagued mankind and the difficulty of finding a solution to it. In his allegorical epic poem, Dante had to pass through Hell and Purgatory, before reaching Paradise. There is nothing new under the sun and no other way around the crosses of living.

Carol and I had to pass through the fire that heals. We had to inform John Henry, Philip, and Suzie, who had observed the whole thing developing, because of the disordered life style of the crowd Carol was hanging around with. I decided to play house father for a while, since I had no other choice in the matter, all along hoping that the situation might turn out to be a passing fad. I phoned Dad in Lebanon and asked him to come over and help me with the children, as I had a medical practice to run and plenty of business ventures to worry about. When he heard the news he was devastated, for he always liked Carol, yet he left Lebanon immediately and came to Stockton to see what was going on. The old man had his own problems too. The civil war was devastating Lebanon and the world he loved so much was collapsing.

As summer approached and Carol hadn't come back, I started building a swimming pool in our huge back yard to keep the children happy or at least content. I asked Teresa Capps, one of my office employees, to baby sit sometimes and to drive the children to school, or otherwise keep them occupied. She was young, barely out of her teens, and could relate to them. I started reading all the pop psychology books that Carol had left behind, so I could understand where she was coming from (and not in order "to find myself," or her, as I knew very well where she was!). Carol left home on April 21, 1978, and I kept in contact with her as much as possible.

She had her condominium furnished by an interior decorator, Joe Jacobs, a relative of mine who did a fine job. At that time, he informed me that she had asked him to choose colors that would go with our house on El Camino, in case she returned. That gave me some comfort, but, more important, it was a valuable tip for the future that I did not miss. In those lonely and interminable days of mental pain, I was looking for any sign that would give me hope of Carol's return. My love for her sustained me in my darkest moments, and besides I refused to consider any alternative other than her return. I was certain that Carol was suffering as well. St. Paul in his Epistle to the Romans sums it up this way, "We glory in tribulations also: knowing that tribulation works patience; and patience, experience; and experience, hope." (Romans 5:3-4).

Five weeks later, on Memorial Day, when all my relatives were picnicking with their families, I lay in bed face down, lonely and disillusioned. I got up and called Carol on the telephone. I told her that I had learned my lesson and that she had proved her point to me, and that the children and I would like her back home. I added that we all loved her very much and missed her. She answered me, "Good for you! I am glad you're learning. You'll have a chance to practice all this on your next wife!" and hung up the telephone. I felt as if a sharp knife had just penetrated my belly. I was disconsolate. I went back to my room and threw myself on my bed, now really depressed and forlorn and not caring whether I suffocated or not. I cried my heart out, and prayed for God's help. The pillow was soaked with my tears. When I got up, I thought of what John Graham, our English teacher in London, Ontario, had told us when studying the *Iliad*—that we should never be ashamed to cry, because Achilles, the greatest of Athenian heroes, cried inconsolably when his friend Patroclus was killed by Hector, the Trojan.

To keep from suffocating in my soaked pillow after the good cry, I got up and wrote the following,

> *O Dear Lord, life is lots of suffering interspersed with a few smiles! When will I find peace and happiness, the Promised Land? How can I survive with toil and my own effort when all is a heavy burden and utter spoil? Please, dear God, have mercy on me! Oftentimes I feel like King Lear must have felt: "As flies are to wantom boys, so are we to the gods; they kill us for their sport" (Shakespeare). Have pity on me, Lord, for mercy's sake; Spare me now these painful moments of my life, and revive in me the good and happy times I spent in your presence in my life. I remember much happiness in my past and that is the worst of all existential states. My happiest moments are remembering my happy times of childhood, which I experience less often now. Help me to recall only the sunny days of my life; to remember the days of levity and of freshness, while everything now is old, dull and falling apart.*

My "Lamentations" continued, like Jeremiah, Ezekiel, and Isaiah long ago, as for weeks I filled a notebook with wailing and the gnashing of teeth. But that day, after I finished writing, I got up and walked across the street to our neighbors, who were having a Memorial Day picnic in their back yard. I was hearing their festive music from across the street. The jubilant noise was actually what got me out of bed. I was astonished to see, of all people, Carol, already there. She was smiling at me as if we never had a miserable phone conversation half an hour before. Was I going crazy, or rather was she? Her behavior seemed a little strange, and she appeared to be both self-possessed and yet confused, smiling and yet unhappy. On her face I could read her indecision as to what ring she ought to throw her hat in: whether she wanted to abandon her future to the wind on a whim, or wisely salvage her life. What I was intuiting seemed to contradict the assuredness she had exhibited earlier on the phone.

Later that night I thought about what my wife's face had revealed, and I had trouble sleeping. I guess she had the same problem, because she called me at midnight, sounding as if she was in some sort of pain. She sounded forlorn and confused; her voice was distant and barely audible. She mumbled that she had taken several sleeping pills and still couldn't sleep. "Oh! My God! She could die," I said to myself. "No wonder she sounds out of it."

"I'm coming over," I said

"Don't you dare," was her reply. "I am okay. I'm not going to harm myself. I just wanted to talk to you."

Was that another sign of her reaching out, but trying to hide it from me? Tough-fragile behavior is often a sign begging for help, difficult to hide. I went over to her place anyway, and knocked on the door. She said to me from the window, "I'm okay. Go back home and get some sleep. Please stop worrying about me!"

The next morning on my way to the office, I passed by and left her two bottles of her favorite wine by the door, without a note.

She called me several days later, wanting to buy the condo she was renting. It was on the lake in Lincoln Village West, the hub of the 1970s hormonal hurricane. I didn't want this situation to become permanent, so I felt my heart drop. And yet I was beginning to become callous out of desperation with her taunts; and I was beginning to feel ready to accept the inevitable, a dangerous state of mind that would have sunk *both of us*. I forcibly stopped this destructive chain of thought realizing that one of us had to stay sane, strong and resilient. The next day I called the Lincoln Village association about the condo transaction.

DEATH INTERVENES

Buying the condo for Carol kept her friendly to me, at least for a few weeks. Then she got a call from her family in Detroit informing her that her father was not doing so well, in fact, that he might be close to death. He had terminal prostatic cancer with metastases in the vertebrae. Carol's father, George Schooff, was the nicest person in the family—God-fearing, "humble and meek," a Christian after Jesus' heart. He had retired from teaching athletics several years before, only to have a heart attack and then go into a severe involutional melancholia that required electric shock therapy over a period of several months. Shortly after the heart problem was treated successfully he was diagnosed with prostate cancer. At first the doctors thought they had removed all the cancer from him; yet, he didn't even live beyond the period of provisional cure (five years), when they found he had metastases. He was close to the end and Carol had to be there. She took little Camille with her to Detroit and stayed there for about six weeks.

In the past, George and Harriet Schooff used to visit us often in California. On one of their visits, I had taken my father-in-law to play golf at Pebble Beach; we even had a caddy all to ourselves. He was a golf instructor once, so he loved the famous California golf course and never forgot that event. Another year, we met George and Harriet at the Broadmoor Hotel in Colorado Springs, a magnificent resort with great restaurants and spectacular views. We played their manicured 27-hole golf course several times. George was in his element. One day we were playing behind a slow foursome. We saw a marshal's cart speeding towards us; he stopped and asked us to please stay a full link behind the couple in front of us. He continued, "I'm sorry, but the Maytags don't like anybody pushing them." When I asked the marshal who they were, he informed us that the Maytags were the scions of Colorado Springs and had been generous enough to build the 27-hole golf course that we were playing on. What an experience! It was only when George began rambling about the quality of the Maytag washer and dryer he had at home in Detroit that I realized who these Maytags were. No wonder the marshal was deferential to them!

Every so often, Carol and I would go back to Detroit to visit her parents and sisters, and at the same time would see my brother Mike and his family in Windsor. We always slept in the finished basement at Carol's parents' home. It was cool down there even on hot summer days; it was painted pale yellow and had its own bathroom. At various times during the day it was our refuge, as one could visit only so much.

I recall with fondness the evenings when at happy hour I would fix three old-fashioneds, one for George, one for Harriet, and another for me. Carol always wanted a glass of wine. I rarely have an old-fashioned anymore, but whenever I do I recall those happy days when her parents were still alive. These memories always remind me of how short and fleeting life is. We hear people say, "You're as young as you feel," as if feeling young is going to decrease one's age and take away the fear of death. "Of all the wonders I yet have heard, it seems to me most strange that men should fear, seeing that death, a necessary end, will come when it will come." To me these are the most memorable verses in Shakespeare's *Julius Caesar*.

I remember well George and Harriet's many visits from Detroit. We always took them sight-seeing to Yosemite or San Francisco. In the city, their favorite spot was the "crookedest street in the world," Lombard Street, as it wound down in a serpentine way, before going up again towards Coyt Tower by the Embarcadero. They loved the beautiful plants and flowers on both sides of that street and the sight of all the automobiles meandering slowly down its multi-curved contour. They fell in love with California's climate, but unfortunately they were too long established in the Midwest to make a final move here.

When Carol went back to see her father, I would lie in bed alone (in Stockton) and imagine us staying in the same basement that used to be our quarters when we visited Detroit, and I would picture her sleeping in the same bed which supported much of our intimacy. During her absence, I heard that she had seen an attorney in Stockton, Mr. Nat Brown, Esq., a man known by everyone in the county as the most vicious divorce lawyer in California. Yet I was glad that Carol was taking care of her father in his dying days; at least she wouldn't be here in Stockton taking any action.

One day, Jimmy, a distant relative of mine came to see me at home. I had not seen him for years. He was a former mayor of Stockton who was recalled a few years before. Shortly after that, as misfortune would have it, his wife left him for another man. So he came to tell me that he had heard about my plight, and wanted to give me some advice.

"Henry, my wife left the home and ran away with her lover," he said to me. "The children stayed with me. She came back several weeks later and told me that she was sorry for what she did and wanted to return home. I was very glad that she had come to her senses and I welcomed her back with open arms. A week later she asked me if I wouldn't mind leaving the house for a few days as she needed some time alone to recollect herself and think things out, but that I shouldn't worry about her because she was happy being home now."

Continuing with his story, he said, "She was happy being home, alright! Like a fool, I left. A few days later, I returned home only to find out that all the locks had been changed. When I knocked on the door, she started yelling at me from the inside. Henry, would you believe she had her paramour with her, in front of my kids, inside the house that I slaved to save enough money to build. And now it is for her and her lover's enjoyment and pleasure!" I wondered what to believe or not to believe, and whether I was in for a similar sad ending.

Well, I didn't have a chance to think about it more because Carol called me to say that her father was in the hospital on his death bed. "Do you want to come?" she asked.

"Of course, I want to come" I said, "I love your dad and, besides, I want to be near you and the family in their bereavement."

But the boys refused to go with me. I was mad at them, and to this day I regret not having forced them to go with me. I boarded a plane with our daughter Suzie and was in Detroit in no time at all. Bob Peterson, my friend and brother-in-law, picked us up at the airport. While Suzie slept in the back of the car, he brought me abreast of all the news: Carol's feelings towards me, or against me; how the rest of the family feels about her and me, and so on. We got to the hospital and rushed to George's room.

I had barely gotten to the foot of his bed, (with the wife, the son and all three daughters on either side of him), when he opened his eyes, lifted his head slightly, looked at me and said in a pitifully weak voice: "Henry, you've come! I am so glad." And with that, he laid his head back and took his last breath. The family was in dismay as to what to do. I was at the foot of the bed. I put my hands out and grabbed Bob's hand on one side and Camille's on the other and began with: Our Father who art in heaven, hallowed be Thy name . . . . The whole family took the cue and joined in. It was a spontaneous intuitive gesture, because I loved George and wanted very much to remain a part of the family that I also loved.

George had a beautiful funeral. Ken's son, George Jr., recited "Casey at the Bat," which George Sr. had always loved. I flew back to California with both Suzie and little Camille. Carol allowed the little one to come with us so she could be together with her brothers and sister a while longer. Carol stayed another week before she returned to California. Prior to going to George's funeral, I had promised the kids that I would take them to the beach at Santa Cruz. So when I got back we set out immediately for Santa Cruz as I had promised them. All four of them were together now, for the first time since their mother left the nest.

The children had a great time in Santa Cruz. Jiddu (grandpa, my Dad) came along and was of great help. I was very sad and worried about Carol not being with us, but I didn't allow it to show in front of the children. They were having a good time and I wasn't going to spoil it. It so happened that for years it was our family's custom to vacation in Santa Cruz, by the ocean.

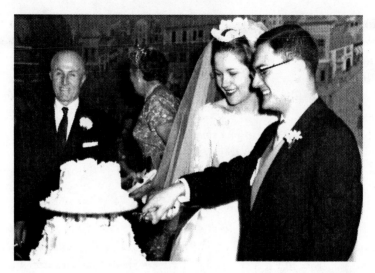

Cutting the Cake - During my times of trial I kept the happy memories of our wedding day in front of me, as if both to torture and sustain myself during my ongoing grief. In the photo Dad is seen very happy for me; and Carol's Mom is seen moving away, as if mourning our future trials. The symbolism in this photo is uncanny.

I learned during that trip that children can never replace a spouse—the one irreplaceable companion for life. I also felt sorry for the children of a divorce, for they don't deserve to see their parents apart. I could see already that life without Carol would be miserable for me, as I could not stop thinking of her the whole time and imagined her at my side, enjoying the ocean views with us.

On the way back to Stockton, when the seven-day vacation was over, one of the boys in the back of the station wagon (I don't remember which one) asked me, "Dad, do you think mom will ever come back?"

With tears in my eyes that he couldn't see, I said, "Son, there is an old Lebanese proverb that says, when things look their worst and the clouds hover over the earth causing utter darkness; it is then that the wind blows and chases the clouds away, and the sunshine returns."

That was exactly how I phrased it, but I wasn't sure if there was such a Lebanese or Chinese or Zulu proverb. It was the inextinguishable hope in my heart that made me utter those words. We got home, and as I opened the door I heard the phone ringing. I went all the way to our bedroom and picked it up. It was Carol. She informed me she was back from Detroit and was wondering if "I would take her back."—But only for the children's sake, she said. That was fine with me. First things first!

Two days later the children received a letter addressed to them from a well-meaning relative. It was almost ten pages long. I read it with them and the gist of it was:

Your mother and father don't love each other anymore. These things happen in life. When love dies, it dies forever. It's like a glass that shatters. It cannot be put back together. Love is the cement that keeps people together, but now that love is gone . . . .

The letter continued:

Accept what has happened; it's part of life. Your mother and father had problems which proved to be insoluble. They're incompatible with each other. They're better off without each other and you're the better off for it too. Learn to live with it. Don't be forlorn, we all love you and we will support you.

I guess it meant that we will support you provided your dad stays in the dog house! What trash! I looked at the children and asked them what they thought of the letter. John Henry, seventeen years old at the time, said, "Only people who don't know how to compromise are incompatible. You and Mom are not like that, you've always known how to give and take." I was impressed by what he said and thought to myself that he would surely become a success some day.

Philip and Suzie then said, with one voice, "We don't believe a word of this letter. Please keep working to bring Mom back." All of them were upset for several days by this letter, but together, with God's grace, we remained hopeful.

No child wants to accept, let alone be informed of, the demise of his family. I was impressed by their maturity. They were not ready to give up and neither was I. We all thought very poorly of divorce, any kind of divorce. For me, this aversion stemmed both from my family's history, my Catholic upbringing, and my Lebanese culture.

THE BEST SLEEP I HAD IN MONTHS

A week later, Philip and I were invited to Carol's condominium. She took us to the patio, where she was barbequing steaks for us. "I want only Philip and you to come," she had said to me the day before. She told Philip, "I am coming back for you and your brother and sisters, not necessarily for Dad, but I want you to know that I still love your Dad, even though I feel unable to like him yet."

A few days later, Carol came over to see us with a well-prepared supper. This continued for several months, even though she was unable to pull the plug and return for good. I guess she still needed a little time to mull things over in her mind. In December, Carol suggested that we all go to Hawaii for Christmas. The first afternoon of our arrival there, she took a shower, put on a red negligee, and started to paint her fingernails and toenails on the bed next to me.

"What color would you like," she said to me, "I want to look good for you." I almost fell off my side of the bed. It was the first time in over a year that she wanted to be anywhere close to me. I said to her,

"I like any color you like, Darling."

"I know you've always preferred red," she said.

I told her that she was quite right. After she finished painting her nails, we reunited with one another. It seemed for a moment that nothing ever happened between us. She looked happy, but I have no idea how she really felt. But I do know that I felt I was in heaven.

After a week in Hawaii, we flew back to Stockton and got in late at night. I asked Carol if she wanted me to drive her to her condo. She said, "No, I think I'll stay here tonight." She slipped into a nightgown and got into our marital bed of seventeen years. We slept right next to each other all night. In the morning, I woke up early to find my arm under her head and hurting badly. We must have slept like that all night, so my arm was stiff and killing me with pain. I did not want to remove it from under her head lest I wake her up. One hour passed and then another and she was still asleep. I didn't want to move my arm even though the pain was getting unbearable. She finally opened her eyes and asked me if I had a good sleep. I told her I slept like a log. "What about you?" I asked her. "I had the best sleep I've had in over six months," she dolefully admitted. She never left our home again. It took more than a year for her to both "love me and like me," but she was actually very happy during the whole healing process. We had both suffered much but we were chastised and purified. I knew that prior to the separation I was just as bereft of consideration towards her as she became toward me. But following her return, we slowly grew in love for each other so that now, twenty-seven years later (and forty-five years into the marriage), neither one of us can fully describe the depth of our love and the devotion we have for each other.

Who can put it better than the old bard?

> Let me not to the marriage of true minds
> Admit impediments. Love is not love
> Which alters when it alteration finds,
> Or bends with the remover to remove;
> O, no! it is an ever-fixed mark,
> That looks on tempests and is never shaken;
> It is the star to every wandering bark,
> Whose worth's unknown, although his height be taken.
> Love's not Time's fool, though rosy lips and cheeks
> Within his bending sickle's compass come;
> Love alters not with his brief hours and weeks,
> But bears it out even to the edge of doom.
> If this be error and upon me proved,
> I never writ, nor no man ever loved.
>
> —Shakespeare, *Sonnet CXVI*

CHAPTER 20

PSYCHOANALYSIS

During the early 1970s I was involved in too many activities: developing real estate; experimenting with new and more daring surgical procedures; being elected to the presidency of the Stockton Symphony Association; taking courses in conducting from my friend, Maestro Kyung Soo Won; taking piano lessons at Delta College from June Church; watercolor painting lessons from Dr. Charles Hess at Delta; oil painting instruction from Raul Mora; painting assiduously; taking part in umpteen social functions (medical and family occasions), and waking up routinely at four in the morning, then for half an hour having a hard time going back to sleep.

I was also auditing several courses at the University of the Pacific: metaphysics and anthropology under Dr. Herbert Reinelt (chair of the philosophy department), ethics and symbolic logic from Dr. Gwenneth Browne, and natural philosophy and modern scientific thought from Dr. Jim Heffernan. The classes were demanding mental exercise, but, oh, for me they were gourmet dinners to feed a gnawing hunger. For several months after having taken the symbolic logic class, very little of what people said made any logical sense to me. I began to think there was little connection between what people expressed in their speech and the premises that motivated what they said. I started to forget about logical thinking altogether and felt I was living a parable in one of my countryman Gibran's books.

As the parable goes, once upon a time, a spring of fresh water suddenly erupted next to the king's palace in a faraway desert kingdom. People ran to the new spring and began to drink from it to quench their thirst. But the water was poisoned and they all went mad. The king and his family, however, had their own fresh water spring and retained their sanity. But when the people went mad, they lost their ability to understand the sane laws of the king, and they rose in rebellion seeking to kill the king and his family. The king, being wise, ordered his family to follow him and drink from the same spring that the people were drinking from. Consequently, the king and the royal family went mad also. And thus they came to understand the people, and the people were able to understand them, since all parties spoke the same mad language now, and the revolution was aborted, and all lived happily mad forever after.

I was beginning to think that I should have to drink from some poisoned spring to be able to communicate with others, in the world's customary illogical manner! So I decided not to expect to hear logical reasoning from anybody, and I began to understand everybody, and they once again started to understand me.

At the same time, in taking stock of my sundry activities, none of them seemed intrinsically damaging or painful; indeed, they were exhilarating. I thought this was normal activity for a man in his late thirties: loving life, contributing to the community, and at the height of virility in business and at home. Still, the whirl of activities was enough to make Carol wonder whether I was in some sort of manic phase. Indeed, the four-in-the-morning routine alone seemed to be crying for some psychological exploration.

Both Carol and I had always been interested in psychology. So when her psychiatrist brother Ken was visiting us in Stockton, in the fall of 1971, she asked him a simple question: "You've known Henry for over ten years. He is active and productive, yet there is this waking up at four o'clock in the morning and this extreme flurry of activity he appears to thrive on? What is behind all this?"

He could have said simply that I was a hypomanic Type A personality, and dismissed the whole thing. But Ken went further by making a suggestion that helped change a part of my life. He suggested a trial of psychotherapy to find out what's going on; but not just routine psychotherapy. He suggested that Carol invite a group of the most prominent psychiatrists in the area for a party. "Let me suggest the doctor that I find to be the best for Henry," he said to her privately.

I wasn't aware of what Carol and her brother were up to. As Carol prepared a party, I thought it was solely for the purpose of introducing Ken to psychiatric colleagues. At the party, Ken talked and socialized with Drs. Bob Hill, Bob Brendmeyer, Bob Austin, Arnold Scheuerman, and several others. They were all friends or acquaintances of ours. But there was one among them, whom I had never heard of or seen before, who struck Ken's fancy. When the party was over, he told Carol that Dr. Henry Brewster was the one, and only one, for Henry.

Dr. Henry Hodge Brewster was a portly, elegant, well-trained psychoanalyst of the pure Freudian tradition. He was a descendent of a May Flower family in Boston. He graduated "summa cum laude" from Harvard, had gone on to psychiatric residency also at Harvard, and eventually into psychoanalysis under none other than Anna Freud (Sigmund Freud's own daughter) in both Boston and Vienna. The psychoanalytic tradition could not have come down from its discoverer in a more direct line than this one. Ken told Carol that he had told Dr. Brewster a little about me at the party, and that Dr. Brewster thought that we would both understand and enjoy each other. Ken emphasized to his sister that I would surely benefit, since he had undergone analysis himself, not because of a psychological crisis, but because he knew it would be of great help to him professionally to explore his own mental makeup, and would open up a whole world of new experience in his life. "It would be the same for Henry as it was for me, a sort of know-thyself experience, a pilgrimage into the mind, and I know that Henry would like it," he told her.

It took Carol another week to break the news to me. She thought I'd be shocked and defensive. Well, to put it succinctly, I was delighted. She couldn't believe it. My reply to her was, "What a great idea!" Ever since medical school, I had been interested in psychiatry and particularly in Freudian theory and psychoanalysis. Here was an opportunity being offered to me to turn all my frantic activity into knowledge of self that might lead me to greater self-actualization. "Man, know thyself!" has been my quest since my teenage years.

At Western Ontario Medical School, our dean was Dr. Hobbs, a psychiatrist. He made sure we all took a semester of psychiatry each year for the four years we were in medical school. No other school in North America had such an ambitious psychiatric program for its medical students. I loved the subject. At one time I wanted to make it my lifetime occupation. In fact, I had decided to go into ophthalmology mainly because I figured that a limited specialty would allow me plenty of time to explore the psychological implications of the works of my favorite authors: Sophocles, Shakespeare, Dante, Dostoyevsky, Kierkegaard, and especially the mystics, Teresa of Avila and John of the Cross, as well as the Muslim Sufis that I was reading on and off, Al-Hallaj, al-Ghazali, and al-Rumi. It was quite a list I had prepared for myself. I wanted to master a circumscribed field such as ophthalmology, and become financially independent so I could spend time being a dilettante, a *bon vivant*, a psychologist, and a philosopher all in one. Yet like the Martha of the New Testament, I was still anxious about too many things. Now with analysis I would have the perfect opportunity to find out what made me tick.

I had also known and read much about Freud's life, and particularly his *Psychopathology of Everyday Life* and his *Interpretation of Dreams*. I had even visited his old office in Vienna. I knew that, as far as Freud was concerned, to become a psychoanalyst the student had to be a medical graduate, (preferably with an interest in neurological disciplines), and had to undergo four years of psychoanalysis under him or one of his trainees, then presto—he would become a psychoanalyst. Well, Hank Brewster was Anna Freud's student, who in turn, was trained by her father. I was a medical graduate and was practicing a semi-neurological specialty and, come to think of it, had obtained the neuroanatomy prize in medical school. All I needed now was four years of psychoanalysis under Dr. Brewster and I'd be a *de facto* psychoanalyst myself according to Freud's own dictum. What a trip for me that would be, I thought! This would be a new adventure, much more appealing than making and fretting over more money than I'd ever spend.

So I accepted Carol's suggestion gladly and went on to both enjoy and suffer through, not just four, but twelve full years of one-hour daily sessions, five days a week, and fifty-two weeks a year of psychoanalysis. Any vacation was discouraged by Dr. Brewster. He would say to me, "What? Now that we are getting close to solving an impasse, you're going to run away from it? How could you possibly think of doing such a thing?" The psychoanalytic sessions went on for a first course of nine years, then one year off, followed by another three years for a total of twelve years. Then, and only then, did Dr. Brewster and I believe that the end of my analytic quest had been reached. We decided the work would suffice for a lifetime of introspection and self-analysis. He then suggested Karen Horney's book on *Self-Analysis,* which I proceeded to buy and read.

THE MOST DIFFICULT PATIENTS

What was psychoanalysis like? Why undergo it? Was it necessary or was it a mental luxury? Who does it benefit?

Dr. Robert Hill, a psychiatrist friend of ours, had told me several years before that the most difficult patients he's had to deal with were the driven rich and the extremely unlettered poor. The most impossible patients, however, he told me, were people of Middle Eastern origin. He confided that he's had a few distant relatives of mine as occasional patients, and that he now refuses to accept any of them, even if their lives depended on it. "It's too traumatic to me personally, to have a patient who won't respond, and who voluntarily avoids all inquiry into his behavior." He added, "They become defensive, even when they themselves have gotten close to cracking open the cover under which they are operating. It is at this crucial juncture that they leave treatment and never come back. I don't mind treating neurotics, but borderline personality disorder is normally unresponsive to analytic treatment."

He was correct because one of the tragic consequences of psychoanalytic theory in the United States was that in the 1940s, '50s, and '60s, most Jewish-German trained psychologists and psychoanalysts who had fled Hitler, immigrated to the United States and were using strictly Freudian methods to treat bipolar disease, with no success whatever. So they were committing all problematic patients who wouldn't respond to analysis into mental hospitals as schizophrenics, including those patients who were bipolar or borderline (because they did not respond to their treatment). Psychoanalysis may be effective with neurotics, but not with psychotics or borderline cases. Decades later, most of these bipolar patients were placed on lithium, tegretol or other medications, and released from mental hospitals. It became well known that their behavior, which was due to chemical imbalances, was responding to the newer drugs, when all the talking (psychotherapy) in the world wasn't helping them. It is unfortunate that for most psychoanalysts of those days, medications were anathema.

So why undergo psychoanalysis, (or any other form of psychotherapy), when a daily dose of Wellbutrin, Zoloft or Prozac could alleviate the problem? Well, medically speaking, that would be like taking aspirin or Motrin for a brain tumor. It helps alleviate the pain, but is not a long-term solution. The psyche has to be plowed much deeper than that. I suppose a person has to be psychologically motivated and have the courage to dig in and wash out the repressions, obsessions, and compulsions out of his or her mind.

PHILOSOPHICAL BASIS OF PSYCHOTHERAPY

I wanted to understand the inner workings of my own mind in a more particular way than Socrates, Descartes, Kant, and the philosophers had understood theirs. I say this because philosophers generally deal with universal and abstract concepts that apply to everybody and to all things. They do not necessarily delve into the depths of their own individual psyches, or anyone else's, because that would be a matter of particular concern, in contrast to universal concepts—though some of them may have understood their psyches during their life, like William James or Kierkegaard, philosophers who were interested in personal psychological questions.

A big question in philosophy, for instance, is why did Socrates decide to drink hemlock, even though a way to escape was offered to him by his Athenian pupils? Did he really want to give the youth of Athens a lesson in obeying the laws of their country, as he claimed in Plato's dialogue, *The Crito*? Or did he have a martyr complex? Or did he want to get away from his nagging wife, which situation drove him to downtown Athens every day (with no pay) to talk to the boys in the agora? What other considerations entered his extremely logical, mature, and complex mind? In his *Dialogues*, Plato mentions only one reason behind Socrates' behavior, that of giving an example to the young about obeying the law. I doubt that it was that simple. After years of psychoanalysis, I realize that there are usually many reasons for any one act. The reasons for a certain behavior, or for man's innate search for happiness, or even for putting up with life altogether, are complicated and difficult issues in a mature and educated person, like Socrates. Too much knowledge (if there could be such a thing) and great intelligence do not necessarily lead to bliss. As a matter of fact, in some people the amount of knowledge they possess is in inverse proportion to the happiness they experience.

Psychoanalysis is not a panacea. It is, however, a beacon of light into the depths of the soul. Even the mystics, St. John of the Cross for one, wrote about the dark night of the soul, the period one has to undergo to reach the highest illumination. St. John was a great psychologist as well as a mystic, steeped in Aristotle's *De Anima* and St. Thomas's psychological treatises. In his own way he described the effects of the analytic procedure, long before Freud made the term psychoanalysis popular.

St. John of the Cross described in exact language and detailed steps what it means to go through hell and purgatory before reaching heaven. Dante did the same in his *Divine Comedy*. My experience was that at times analysis was unsettling, but I expected that. It was well-informed and embodied the very Socratic idea of *"Man, know thyself!"* It was my kind of thing intellectually and spiritually. It was the quintessential Henry; the *ME* I've known since childhood. "Men by nature desire to know," said Aristotle. I've used that quote ever since I was seventeen. After analysis I can now testify to the completion of Aristotle's dictum in my own words, "Men by nature desire to know—all kinds of things in the outside universe, but are afraid by nature and averse by temperament to get to know what makes them tick, their inner selves."

Sometimes I wonder if the mystics' desire to get to know God stems from their desire to understand themselves. Their wide existential experience (their intuition of being) led them to realize that it was in getting to know and love God that they were enlightened as to who they were. They knew through prayer, devotion, and suffering that they only existed in relation to Him and that without Him they were (existentially and truly) nothing. St. Augustine, St. Teresa of Avila, and St. John of the Cross, were supreme psychologists. This can be gleaned from their intuitive psychological writings. Besides, they had to deal with hundreds of novices, priests, and religious—and with municipal and royal personages every time they had to establish a new convent or monastery. They investigated their own psyches through both theoretical knowledge and agonizing physical and spiritual suffering.

Their writings are an open window into the breadth of their inner experiences. St. Augustine's *Confessions*, written in the fourth century, is to this day the supreme example of autobiographical search into the passionate desires of body and soul. And any reading of St. John of the Cross or St. Teresa of Avila will prove the same point. In her autobiography, *The Way of Perfection,* and in *The Interior Castle*, Saint Teresa shows herself to be one of the most astute psychological writers of all time. The very phrase "interior castle" gives a ready hint of what her search was all about.

In an oft-repeated anecdote in the Levant, Avicenna (*Ibn Sina*), the great physician-philosopher of the East, met with a great Sufi mystic. It was a meeting of intellect and intuition, of reason and faith, of inductive and deductive thought. After the meeting, Ibn Sina reportedly stated, "All that I know, he sees," and the Sufi master is said to have declared, "All that I see, he knows."

Unfortunately, the run-of-the-mill psychologists and psychiatrists do not read these kinds of texts, nor are they exposed to them in their training. Indeed, their avowed agnosticism or atheism keeps them away from reading such works. Their claim of open-minded freedom stops at the door of philosophy and religion, and that is because after years of devotion to their specialized field, its tenets become their religion. I once put my wrist watch on the table and asked one of my atheist sociology professors in college if he would tell me how many eons it took that particular watch to *make itself* out of the elements it contains. He said to me with emphasis: "Never!" Then I asked him why he would believe that an astronomically more complicated being such as man *formed himself* out of similar elements. In response, he tried to tell me that living things have evolved differently and have their own rules, which don't particularly obey the firm universal laws of nature. From a logical point of view, he was falling all over himself trying to explain his beliefs. It was soon obvious to the other students present that his logical argument was poorly developed (almost infantile) and that his rigid beliefs were less credible than belief in God.

The discussion proceeded with simple Thomistic logic that I had learned a year earlier in Father Dwyer's philosophy class, and logic which succeeded in obliterating his argument. My confrontation was purposeful, because I had been watching him poison the minds of my fellow pre-med students for months with his unfounded theories, flaunting his agnosticism and personal skepticism. None of these innocent students had ever taken a course in philosophy or theology, let alone logic. It turned out that he had no more training in logic than his students had, which in a way explains his own swallowing—hook, line, and sinker—all the usual pseudoscientific jargon and extrapolations that had been making the rounds of universities ever since the so-called Age of Enlightenment, over two hundred years ago. I still ended up getting an A in his course and his awareness and respect for the truths I had brought up during the year began to show in his changed attitude towards his students.

Now, St. Augustine, St. Teresa, and St. John of the Cross were not alone in their deep psychological knowledge, derived from personal experience rather than purely from books. There lived many other seers in the 11th, 12th, 13th, and 14th centuries (and still do now), belonging to different religious disciplines, who have described the same process of painful self-purgation leading to self-knowledge, and ultimately to reaching illumination by a higher spiritual force. I am sure that explanations of psychoanalysis along these philosophico-mystical lines have been proposed, but I have never seen them in print. The closest I know of is Maritain's *Les Degrés du Savoir* (*The Degrees of Knowledge*), a work in which he ascends through the various stages of knowing, from uneducated opinion, to logical, mathematical and scientific knowledge, to metaphysical, theological, and finally to mystical knowledge. His ascent through the various degrees, or stages, of knowing is masterfully done.

ME, A CASE STUDY

For twelve years, Dr. Brewster's wife Judy would open the door for me after I had rung the bell, and she would lead me to the office her husband had in their home where he would be sitting, waiting for me. During the fourth year, there was a period of time when I did not see Judy around. So, lying on the couch while Dr. Brewster was seated on a recliner to the rear left of me, I asked him in a friendly manner, "How is Mrs. Brewster?"

"Why do you ask me? Are you worried about her?" he said to me.

"Dr. Brewster," I said, "I asked because I haven't seen her for over a week."

"Do you miss seeing her?" he asked me.

I didn't have the heart to tell him, "Why would I miss the old hag?" So, I said nothing for about a minute.

He waited me out, but then said: "Are we going to proceed with our work today?"

"Yes, Dr. Brewster. I had a most unusual dream last night . . ."

So Henry Brewster would sit back in his recliner as I related the dream to him while I was lying down on the couch to his right.

"Well go on," he would prod.

"I dreamt there was a Christmas party at our office with many doctors and nurses drinking and laughing . . . My father came to the party uninvited and saw me in a compromising situation . . . Then he abruptly left without saying a word, etc . . ."

"How did you feel in the dream?" Dr. Brewster would ask me.

"I remember having the feeling in the dream that 'I was no longer the boy who has to worry about what Dad thinks.' After waking up, I wanted the dream to continue. I soon fell asleep and the dream started again where it had left off."

"So, you woke up even though your dad was not there? Did you feel ashamed?"

No way, I said to myself, but I didn't tell the doctor that. I said to him, "I guess when I saw my father, I had to wake up or be discovered by him in a situation not to his liking."

"But he did discover you, misbehaving. Any memories or incidents in childhood you care to talk about?"

"Not really; I had a very normal childhood, happy in all respects."

"Fiddlesticks," he would intuit, "Why are you talking nonsense, when you were free-associating so well before. Go on free-associating and maybe we'll get somewhere in our work!"

He always talked about "our work." Several years later, as I was reading the anonymously written mystical book, *The Cloud of Unknowing*, the author kept referring to "our work," meaning "loving God at all hours with one's mind and one's heart." I thought of Henry Brewster then and his "our work," a term he always used to refer to the prolonged labor of unearthing the repressions accumulated in the subconscious since childhood. I said to myself, how incredibly associative is the human mind and how circuitously it works—particularly within our dreams.

The rest of the session would go on with free associations, and the meaning of the dream took three or four sessions to unravel. It turned out that Dad, who was in Lebanon was a surrogate for Carol, who was gone to see her parents for a week, and I used Dad in the dream to stop me from carrying on to fruition any strong desires I had while she was gone, both in the dream and in real life. It was a protective mechanism at a time when I was at risk because of certain desires I had confessed to the analyst earlier. Dad was a stop sign for me in the past, and now he was a stop sign in the dream, a sort of surrogate conscience.

I ask my reader to be understanding of my skipping over the dream, since there was much, much more than I revealed here. I had to work the dreams out myself in session. Dr Brewster would often say to me, "It's your dream, not mine!" Without going into every detail of the analysis of that dream, it turned out that it contained minor issues of desire and libido, but significantly greater meaning concerning repressed fears of loss and failure, and a deep aversion to any absence of my wife from home. This was at a time when the marital crisis was slowly rearing its ugly head.

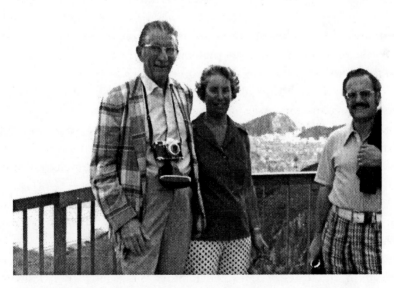

Dr. Henry Hodge Brewster and his wife Judy on a medical tour with us, to Rio de Janeiro in 1983—My analysis had ended a year earlier.

THE MEDIUM IS THE MESSAGE

Analysis often relies on dreams—the "*via reggia*," the royal road, as Freud called it. But in analysis, much more than dream interpretation is used. Events of the day; disagreements with people, children, or marriage; worries about stock market losses or gains; management problems in the office; situations with projects or people—all are fair game. In attempting to reach understanding of one or all of these factors, reliance is placed on language slips, free association, repression or withholding of information that could be of value to the analyst, loss of certain memories, active imagination, wish fulfillments, and many other factors. All are used to bring out repressions and feelings long forgotten. Normally, psychological defense mechanisms are necessary for the survival of the ego, and thus they are freely used in real life (as well as in analysis). Uncovering them through analysis is frequently of great help in discovering and solving problems of self-esteem, passive aggression, overt aggression, anxiety, obsession and compulsion.

Freud described the psychoanalytic process as a "talking cure" involving efforts in reminiscence, since the things that we have put out of mind, he wrote, "are hindered from becoming conscious, and are forced to remain in the unconscious by some sort of force," which he called "repression." This occurs when "a wish has been aroused, which was in sharp opposition to the other desires of the individual, and was not capable of being reconciled with the ethical, aesthetic, and personal pretensions of the patient's personality. The end of this inner struggle is the repression of the idea which presented itself to consciousness as the bearer of this irreconcilable wish [or deed]. This was repressed from consciousness and forgotten", but never entirely disposed of or erased. Freud applies his theory of the "*oblivion of what is disagreeable*" to everyday occurrences, such as the forgetting of familiar names, slips of the tongue, and the repression of memories that were emotionally traumatic in early life.

Quite often in analysis, single dreams or events may turn out to be not so significant, unless analyzed in relation to other dreams, in search of a pattern. Long-standing habits or addictions, recurring character flaws, unexplained motives of destructive behavior, are all taken into account as important factors. Add to all this the issues of transference, projection, or identification with the analyst that begin to occur as analysis is coming to a close. Yes, the human mind works in very circuitous ways, and most people are nowhere near understanding their motives or beliefs. That is why it may take years of psychoanalysis, particularly if it is undertaken not so much in response to an acute neurotic problem, but as part of psychoanalytic training, or as a method for a general inventory of the self. Analysis can be an intense inquiry to root out one's character flaws or to strengthen one's virtues and talents. It is an eclectic, protean discipline, in line with the ancient dictum of: "Man, know thyself!"

Another essential revelation that I learned in the process is that in certain circumstances there is neither a step-by-step plan, nor complete and thorough results. The very *undergoing* of the process *is* the *meaning* of the process. It is much like McLuhan's dictum: "The medium is the message." The medium of analysis itself, the very undergoing of it, is *the talking cure,* the liberating and enlightening process, and quite often it is the cause of the suffering and pain that precedes the liberation. Finding the truth about oneself and banishing the multiple masks that dreams represent is necessary for self-actualization. It is a salutary discipline, leading to personal emancipation. The most intuitive and selfless spirit ever, Christ, pointed this out when he said: "The truth shall make you free."

I know that psychoanalysis has come under scrutiny in the past few decades. It does have its faults, its critics, and there are questions as to its relevance in our time of effective psycho-pharmacological wonder drugs. Its detractors point to its cost, the length of time it takes, its uncertain cures and its reliance on questionable Freudian theory. Yet in my experience, for someone who has the means and the time, and a dose of common sense (and the ability to take things with a grain of salt), it is unequaled as a method for reaching awareness of the self, of one's flaws, of what makes one tick; it is a great aid in the progress towards knowledge of the self.

CHAPTER 21

TRAVELS

For years after I resigned from the Country Club, I felt free to play golf at any time and on any course I wanted; then I became more serious about snow skiing and tennis. I wanted to stay close to Carol, who was starting to play mixed doubles with all of her tennis friends. I started snow skiing, since both Carol and the children started doing that and I didn't want to be away from them. In those days we kept exploring the wonders of our central California surroundings. We would visit Columbia, the well-preserved "forty-niner" town with its reminiscences of California's wild gold rush days. In the springtime, we drove up to "Daffodil Hill," fully in bloom in the Sierra foothills. Every so often, we took one-day drives up to Yosemite Park, and sometimes stayed overnight at Camp Currey or ate at the Ahwahnee Hotel with the in-laws when they were visiting, which was almost every other summer.

In 1968 Carol and I took her parents, George and Harriet, to visit Lebanon. We had a grand time. We landed in Beirut, where Dad met us at the airport. We stayed one night at the Phoenicia Hotel and the very next morning drove up to Serhel. I had not seen it for twenty years. It was late afternoon in Serhel. We had gotten to Serhel a few hours before sunset, by way of Beirut. It was then that Dad took us for a short hike about a hundred yards from the main curve on the road, and showed us the magnificent view of the Kadisha Valley and Canyon where Serhel stood. The scene in front of me reminded me so much of Yosemite Park, near us in California. That evening, my mother-in-law came out to the porch and looking at the clear sky full of stars above us, she remarked on how beautiful and brilliant the heavens were. I pointed out to her that it was indeed heaven on earth, but that she was really looking at the lit villages above us, on top of the surrounding mountains, Arbeh, Beit Minzer, Haddad, and so on. These were small villages perched on the side and at the top of the cliffs and mountains. The houses could not be seen, but their lights were bright and mingled with the stars above.

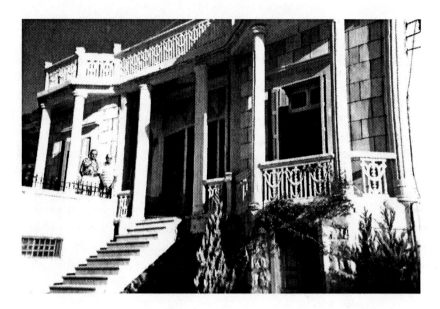

Our summer villa in Serhel as it appears at present. I was born in the room to the right, upstairs. On the balcony to the left are Bacchus Sessine and Antonio Ragi Sessine, the only cousins I have left in Lebanon. Antonio has been the caretaker of the house for 20 years.

Harriet recalled the awesome scenery she had witnessed along the coastline on our way from Beirut and now this dreamlike, ethereal sight of unseen villages mixed with the stars. "Lebanon is a well-watered rose surrounded by immense deserts all around," she observed. "Neither Syria nor Israel are ever going to leave the rose alone without plucking its petals and sepals." This intuitive remark of my mother-in-law proved prophetic, because a few months after we returned to America, the Israeli Air Force, in a show of military superiority, attacked and destroyed the entire Lebanese *civilian* national airline (MEA) in a surprise attack on the airport at Beirut in 1968. The reason given was that the Palestinian Liberation Organization is using Beirut as its headquarters. Fourteen years later, in 1982, Sharon's army invaded Lebanon and occupied part of it for twenty years. The Syrians were asked to come and defend Lebanon, but after the War ended they also refused to return home. It was another thirty years before they left. Like Costa Rica, Lebanon prides itself on having more teachers than soldiers and law enforcers. The 2005 mid-year statistical review put out by *The Economist* showed that Lebanon had the highest per capita expenditure on public education in the whole world, and the lowest on military defence. Yet between 1968 and 2005, Lebanon had become a pawn between Syria and Israel because of its military weakness.

La Fontaine, the French author of fables, ended one of his better known stories by writing sarcastically, *"La raison du plus fort est toujours la meilleure!"* "The reason (or excuse) given by the stronger party always seems the better one!"

Apparently, one day the wolf was hungry and had his mind set on eating the little lamb. But he had compunction about taking the life of so helpless a creature. So he accused the lamb of muddying the stream he was drinking from. "How could I be muddying your water, when I am fifty feet below you," said the little lamb. "Well then, you must have insulted me last year," accused the wolf." "How could I have insulted you a year ago? I am only three months old!" "Well then, your father or mother must have done it; and besides, I am not going without my dinner tonight," said the wolf; and with that, he jumped on the defenseless lamb and devoured him without further ado.

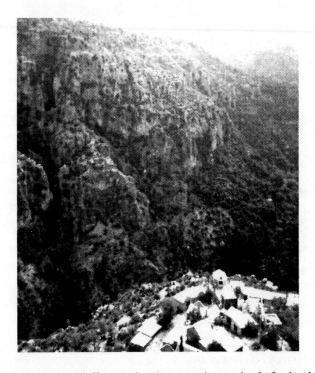

Hanging over a cliff in Lebanon are the makeshift shacks of Palestinians, refugees from the wars of 1948, 1967, 1973, 1982, 1992, and 2002-05.

THE GLORY OF ANCIENT EGYPT

The day following my mother-in-law's remark, we went to visit the great Roman ruins of Baalbeck and then beyond to Egypt. We were driven at night to the shores of the Nile. There we witnessed the most spectacular *Son et Lumière* (Sound and Light) spectacle we had ever seen in our many travels. We were sitting in a beautiful, huge outdoor restaurant when the show started. The pyramids were gloriously illuminated with red lights, and the Sphinx with brilliant green. Trumpets sounded the beginning of the spectacle. Then, through a loud speaker placed in the mouth of the Sphinx, we heard the voice of history speaking:

> *When the pyramids were two thousand years old, I, the Sphinx, the ancient guardian of the Pharaohs, was born. As I grew up in age and wisdom, and reached the ripe old age of two thousand years myself, I saw Mark Antony and Cleopatra make love at my feet. And this evening, as yet another two thousand years have gone by, I am welcoming you to the home of civilization, and asking you to meditate on your short lifespan of three score and ten, and to wonder why it is cursed with so brief an existence on this earth.*

A hush descended on the crowd. All of us (my in-laws, Carol, and I) had goose bumps. The very concept of such long history, all gone with the wind, was as awesome as it was devastating. I could not help but recall the sad and desolate lines from Thomas Gray's famous *Elegy*,

> *The boast of heraldry, the pomp of power,*
> *And all that beauty, all that wealth e'er gave,*
> *Await alike the inevitable hour;*
> *The paths of glory lead but to the grave.*
> —Thomas Gray, from *Elegy Written in a Country Churchyard*

After the Sphinx spoke, I saw Dad writing on the paper napkin. He penned a poem that started with the stanzas,

> *My grandparents are gone,*
> *And so have Dad and Mom,*
> *And next I and my own,*
> *To oblivion assigned.*

Thus has Athens gone by;
Thus has Rome bit the dust;
Thus will we in due time,
Bereft of pomp and glory.

—Yousef Zeiter, *Collected Poems, 1968*

MOSTLY MOZART

In 1971, I had taken John Henry, now eight years old, and Philip, six, to Europe and Lebanon. It was wonderful to establish a permanent cultural and paternal, relationship with the boys. The camaraderie has lasted to this day. We flew out of Oakland, California, straight to Frankfurt, Germany, in one of those overnight flights over the North Pole. We got to Frankfurt in the late morning and took a train to Regensburg, passing through Bavaria's historical and picturesque countryside. We passed through Nüremberg with evocations of Wagner's *Die Meistersinger von Nürnberg*, then through Wurzberg, on the way to our destination. Carol had a cousin on her Polish mother's side, married to a German, and they lived in Regensburg. Alfred and Renata met us at the train station and drove us to their home.

Alfred's family name was Wagner, so I had to tell him how much I loved the master of German opera who had that same name. But seeing signs of exhaustion on our faces, they gave us some warm milk to drink and led us to their bedroom, where we slept for a long time. I slept in the middle with John Henry and Philip on either side of me, under a heavy German comforter. We slept for eighteen hours straight, the longest and deepest sleep we ever experienced. Towards the late afternoon of the next day before we woke up and while still covered with the thick German quilt, I experienced several dreams of my past life.

All three of us woke up at the same time, and when we came out from under our German comforter cocoon, we felt very hungry. We took the Wagners, Carol's cousins, to a nearby restaurant, and the boys were so famished that after eating two full dishes of wienerschnitzel (veal), they each ordered one more. I had never seen them eat so much. The next day, Alfred said he had a surprise for us and he drove us to the center of town.

We saw attendants dressed in Mozart-style hats and breeches hurrying here and there all over the main plaza; across from it, close to the Danube, was the "Thurn-und-Taxis" Palace. It belonged to the ancient Bavarian family who invented postal stamps when the Holy Roman Empire was still going strong. Omedio Taxis had started the enterprise of using curriers for letters with stamps around 1290, in parts of Italy and Germany. One of his descendants, Franz von Taxis, obtained the license to use stamps from the Germanic Holy Roman emperor himself. The business was finally sold to Prussia in 1867, at the time of German unification, when Bavaria was no longer independent.

We entered the Palace and found ourselves slowly moving in a long line, to pay final tribute to the last prince of the Thurn-und-Taxis line. He had just died the day before and was laid in state in an open casket in the large hall. We entered the hall and saw a memorable scene that John Henry and Philip have never forgotten. We could only get to about fifty feet from the casket because surrounding it was a massive sea of wreaths and flower arrangements. That was a truly royal lying-in-state scene. In the center of the huge hall could be seen the deceased old prince. He had a handlebar mustache, full sideburns, but a well-trimmed beard, and was opulently dressed in imperial regalia. It was as if we were at the funeral of Emperor Franz Joseph of Austria-Hungary in 1916.

We left the palace mesmerized. We thanked Alfred and Renata for their kind hospitality and drove away to see the Königschlössen (King's castles) of Ludwig II, the so-called mad king of Bavaria. So we headed towards Neushwanstein, not far from Füssen in southern Bavaria. We had rented a Mercedes in Regensburg that we planned to drive to these Disneyland castles and to Salzburg and Vienna later on. We had planned to get back to Frankfurt in one week to board a plane to Lebanon. The boys were anxious to see the country of their father's origin, after having heard all his stories about it.

On the way to King Ludwig's castles, I parked the car on the side of the road in front of a field of poppies and other wild flowers; the colors were vivid and they extended as far as the eye could see. From the field we could see the Disney-like castles in the distance. The car radio was playing the music of Siegfried's Rhine Journey, from the beginning of the Dawn of the Gods (*Gotterdammerung*), the last of the Ring Cycle. The narrator on the car radio was none other than Karl Haas, the same narrator heard back home on Public Radio. I raised the volume and opened all four car doors so the boys could listen while they ran into the field of flowers. I can still see them running through the poppies with the breeze swaying the flowers back and forth and the castle beyond making a fitting backdrop to this whole impressionist scene. My mind went back to when as a child Dad took me to a prairie full of flowers and I imagined the cars to be toys moving slowly on the far-away horizon. It could have been a Monet, or rather a fuzzy Renoir, with all the air and breath of impressionist art.

When we arrived at the gate of the main castle, people looked tiny in comparison to the high towers and turrets. As we entered the castle, we noticed a group of Americans and other English-speaking tourists surrounding a young guide, probably a German university student. She was explaining to them about Ludwig II of Bavaria and his castles. We were standing in the first hall, next to the group. Ludwig II was Wagner's greatest admirer and had frescos of scenes from the master's operas painted on all the walls. On the wall in front was a fresco of Siegfried slaying Fäfner, the dragon, with fire coming out of the dragon's nostrils. On the wall to the left was another fresco showing Brünhilde being awakened by a kiss from her savior and lover-to-be, Siegfried. The lovers were surrounded by the circle of fire that Wotan had willed. On the right wall was the dead Siegfried, lying on the funeral pyre with Brünhilde on her white horse, Crane, ready to gallop into the fire to die with her husband and be swept away by the swelling waters of the river Rhine.

We were standing next to the group of English-speaking tourists, when all of a sudden, we all heard eight-year-old Philip, all excited, exclaiming at the top of his voice, "Daddy! Daddy! Look at Siegfried slaying Fafner, the dragon. Oh! Look over there at Brünhilde surrounded by the circle of fire. And there's Siegfried, dead on the funeral pyre."

His knowledge of the scenes surprised everybody, particularly the German guide. Carol and I had taken the children to the operas in San Francisco so they were familiar with the stories. The guide asked me where we were from. I told her, from California. She remarked to me, "I've never seen an American tourist recognize any of these frescoes."

From the King's Castle in Bavaria, we drove to Salzburg. It was actually the first time I had ever been there. So, it was a first for all of us. Yes, I had identified with Mozart since childhood, so much so, that I was positive I would not live beyond thirty-six years of age—Mozart's life span! Yes, I had imagined I was a musician when I was ten and went on to compose in my mind symphonies in the Mozart style (a great illusion to be sure), piano concerti (quite shy of Mozart's twenty-seven) and one violin concerto. Yes, I adored Mozart and knew for sure that he was God's second reincarnation through the divine music he wrote—yet I never expected to be affected as deeply as I was in Salzburg. I shed a tear or two every time we visited a Mozart Memorial in Salzburg, whether it was the "Mozarthaus," the Mozart Museum, the Palace of the Archbishop of Salzburg or even the tomb of his wife, Constanze Weber Mozart Niessl at the cemetery (nobody knows where Mozart himself was buried). I felt so close to Mozart's spirit that I was emotionally overcome by his phantom presence all over his native city.

After Mozart's death, his widow, Constanze, went on to marry an architect by the name of Niessl, and lived another fifty years beyond him. She was not alone in this phenomenon. Clara survived Robert Schumann by fifty-odd years, Cosima survived Wagner by fifty-one years, and Alma survived Gustav Mahler by fifty-five years. How much would the world have gained if these life spans of husbands and wives were reversed? With no disrespect for these musicians' wives, I sometimes wonder why God takes away the more talented early in life, and leaves the less fruitful behind. In the movie *Amadeus,* Salieri, gone mad following Mozart's death, kept repeating, "*Mediocrities, mediocrities, mediocrities! All I see left behind are mediocrities! The world is now full of mediocrities.*"

Imagine what Mozart might have composed had he lived his wife's long life? What would he have written following his great Symphonies # 38, 39, 40, and 41, after his mystical late string quintets, and after his divine Requiem? Yet God likes to shower His talents on various people and in various countries. The wonders of the universe are like the wonders of the variety of Renaissance, Baroque, Classical, Romantic, post-Romantic, and contemporary music, spread among many countries of origin and many individual talents. To wit, Bach's mathematical fugues; Mozart's sublimely inspired operas; Beethoven's titanic power; Schubert's melodious spirit; Brahms' majestic nobility; and Tchaikovsky's blend of Orient and Occident in his Russian brooding style. Oh! What diversity! What awesome beauty! A whole universe of color and emotion contained within the realm of serious music. Yet while in Salzburg, I thought that Mozart towered above all these others, if only for the variety of his compositions, encompassing all genres and all depths of feeling, hidden beneath a wealth of melody never heard before or since.

So, my eyes were often wet in Salzburg, and my heart was appreciative of the man who has given me so much happiness over the years, far beyond what friends, books, paintings, career, or money could have ever given me.

MORE WONDERS

Several years later, I took Philip (who was enrolled at California Polytechnic University's architecture school at the time) back to Europe. But he couldn't get out of his mind a teen-age infatuation with a girlfriend back home. So I phoned Carol from Malaga, Spain, and asked her to send Suzie to me and I'd send Philip back home. She did so, and Suzie was delighted with everything she saw. Philip stayed with us until we got to see Italy and Rome, then flew back home. Suzie and I went on to visit the Holy Land, since we couldn't go to Lebanon because the civil war was still raging there. Tel Aviv was an ugly bore—another Pittsburg or Newark. But Jerusalem and Bethlehem were marvels of architecture, history and religion. We were booked to stay at the Sheraton, but we found a little community of Lebanese Maronite Nuns right next to the American Consulate. For a donation of $20 per day, we had lodging, breakfast, dinner, supper, and could attend Mass every morning. At one time the nuns had run a girls' school, but most of the Christians, pressured by both Israelis and Moslems, had emigrated, leaving the nuns very few students to teach. So now, the donations from lodging pilgrims were their only sustenance.

The nuns told us the story of my great Uncle Abuna Boutros' martyrdom, all over again, when they learned who we were. I could picture the old Abbot sitting at my Grandmother Marzuka's humble home, telling me he would play backgammon with me when I got older, but, alas, now that I am older, he's dead. Life's sadness engulfed me at that moment and I shared the experience with Suzie, when she asked me, "What's wrong Dad?" We returned home edified by what we saw of the land where Christ walked.

Another summer I took the family to Vienna and we saw its many sights: St. Stephen's, Karlkirche, the Hofburg, the Scheinborn Palace, the Statsoper, and so on. We even went to Freud's original office and saw his well-preserved couch. It was still covered by his original multi-colored blanket. Then we returned to Frankfurt, took a trip on the Rhine from Meinz to Cologne and visited its huge Dom (Cathedral), my favorite church in the whole world in grandeur and conception. We have made several similar trips since, and that cathedral is still my favorite Gothic structure anywhere. It was started in 1200 as a cooperative work of devout medieval guilds, and wasn't completed till 1850. I thought that is the time span the Church operates in.

While on the Rhine, I saw from the corner of my eye a dark sky looming beyond the famous Lorelei rock. I told the children that Donner (the god of lightning and thunder) will protect the Rhine Maidens from us—Nibelung invaders on the boat—by bringing on a storm of thunder and lightning. And sure enough! Half an hour later, as we approached the curve on the Rhine that marks the Lorelei Rock, heavy lightning and a thunderstorm hailed our arrival. All the kids on the boat thought I was a prophet.

CHAPTER 22

HELP IS ON THE WAY

My nephew Joe joined my practice, the Zeiter Eye Clinic, in July 1981. He had helped me on a few occasions in the office for the three years that he was in residency at UC Davis Medical Center. While in college, Joe used to make jewelry—thus experiencing the kind of hand coordination needed in eye surgery. When he came home to visit, I would take him with me to the operating room when I had emergency surgery at night. He often watched me take out intraocular metallic foreign bodies using a scanner and a giant magnet, and he saw how there were methods of operating without further injuring the eye during the procedure. Other specialists tried to lure him into specializing in their fields (cardiovascular and orthopedic surgeons who were friends of the family), but he opted for eye surgery because of my example and the certainty that he would have a niche in his uncle's practice. A few months after he joined me, the nurses at Dameron Hospital found and attached to the surgical microscope a nicely printed poster that read:

**YOU CAN FORGET MANY THINGS,
BUT YOU CAN'T FORGET YOUR UNCLE HENRY.**

I have no idea where they got that poster from, but it's been stuck on the operating microscope at Dameron Hospital for over twenty years. I am surprised the other ophthalmologists haven't taken it down or complained. I think I know why it was posted in the first place. I once told the surgical nurses, while I was operating, with Joe present, the origin of the word *nepotism*. The Roman Emperors routinely prepared a nephew (the son of a sister) to succeed them, because they knew for certain that he was of their own blood, whereas their own children might not have been their own due to the prevalent licentiousness at court. *Nepos* or *nepotinus* in Latin means grandson or dependent. The term was sometimes used for a son or for a close nephew. Well, Joe was like a son to me and the future inheritor of my practice. Now-a-days, "nepotism" connotes a political favor for a relative, any relative, but the true derivation of the word is to the nephew. It was about two months after Joe had joined me that I explained to the surgical staff what the word nepotism meant, and it was shortly after that that the "YOUR UNCLE" poster was taped to the operating microscope.

A GUARDIAN ANGEL

My brother Tony had five children. In 1973, one of them, Edmond, who was to be valedictorian of the graduating class at St. Mary's High School, succumbed to leukemia before he was able to graduate. The family was devastated; he was only seventeen years old. Nothing would console my brother Tony or my sister-in-law Madelyn. Shortly after, my brother's older son, Joe, applied to UC Davis medical school, the same year that the celebrated Allan Bakke had applied. Bakke was the plaintiff in the famous Supreme Court lawsuit about reverse discrimination at universities. Joe had studied one year at the University of Guadalajara Medical School because he was initially denied admission to UC Davis. Armed with photos of his deceased son Edmond, my brother Tony somehow got an appointment to see Dr. Tupper, Dean of UC Davis Medical School.

Only Tony could have gotten an appointment with a medical school dean. Tony is not afraid of anybody and can be, to put it mildly, both pushy and persuasive—he always takes the offensive and most of the time gets his way. So he was ushered into the dean's office that day by the secretary, and he immediately placed the dead Edmond's photo on Dean Tupper's desk. "This is my son, Edmond, who would have had no trouble getting into your medical school; I am sure of that!" He said to the dean. "He always had A+ in all the subjects he ever took. But he is dead now; so he cannot apply to your school. But his brother Joe has applied for the second time to your school. You have his application somewhere on your desk, I'm sure. Please, lift the darkness that has fallen on our family's eyes and accept Joe into your medical school. He's been a hard worker since he was a child."

Dean Tupper was astounded by Tony's directness, and it didn't take him long to decide. Besides, Tony wouldn't accept any promise of "we'll see". The dean leaned over his desk, looked at Tony straight in the eye and said to him, "When I was a young man, I applied to the University of Michigan Medical School, never expecting I would be accepted; but a guardian angel, a benefactor, came out of nowhere and was instrumental in my getting in. I'm repaying him through your son right now, for that favor of long ago. Your son is in! Go home now, but keep all this to yourself." And that's how Joe got into medical school at UC Davis, a difficult school to get into. I have always suspected he was the one who took applicant Bakke's place that very year. Bakke eventually became a *cause célèbre* and sued all the way to the Supreme Court. In any case, Joe went on to graduate in medicine and four years later completed his ophthalmology residency at the same UC Medical Center.

He came to join me when he finished his training in eye surgery. He passed his ophthalmology boards on the first try and I was so proud of him for that feat. Many flunk the Board the first time around. I could see from the first operation at which I assisted him that he was going to make a first-rate surgeon. He had the golden hands. I knew that with a little more experience and some pointers, he would be able to handle complications when they arose. It is not the routine cases that distinguish a good surgeon from the rest. Rather, it is the successful handling of complications when they arise that makes that distinction.

Several months after Joe joined me, I took him to San Francisco to watch Dr. Max Fine perform corneal transplants. Normally, young eye doctors are not trained to do transplants in their basic residency. Over a three-day period we watched Dr. Fine and his partner, Dr. Picetti, perform nine procedures. I wanted Joe (and myself) to see a master at work. We came back with a set surgical procedure and the newest techniques in mind. Shortly after, we received a call from the eye bank in Houston: "We have six corneas available, if you have the patients to use them on." I always had a prioritized list of patients who needed a transplant, since I would receive a call every few months about a cornea being available. Nobody had ever heard of six donor eyes available at the same time!

A CORNEAL TRANSPLANT MARATHON

In those days, most corneas were offered to major university surgical centers. So what was different this time? All the ophthalmic surgeons who performed corneal transplants around the country happened to be at the annual meeting of the American Academy of Ophthalmology in Miami. Providentially, on Friday, one day before the meeting, we were offered the six corneas. All the other specialists were on airplanes flying to Miami for the meeting. I told the eye bank to send us the eyes (but not before I had called six patients on my list and made sure they were available as standbys for the surgery). I then called Dr. Luis Arismendi, the administrator of Dameron Hospital, and explained the situation to him. I needed to operate right away, because the corneas won't last over 48 hours. He was very pleased that we had chosen his hospital for such an unusual number of corneal transplants and gave us the green light. On Sunday morning at 9:00 a.m. we started operating, using the six corneas. We didn't finish until 6:00 p.m. that evening. Dr Arismendi had promised us enough assistants and circulating nurses to do the job properly, including two anesthesiologists who were to rotate between two operating rooms.

We started our marathon at 8:00 a.m. because we needed one hour of preparation before our 9:00 a.m. scheduled surgical time. I would trephine (cut) the patient's cornea on the operating table, while Joe was preparing the donor cornea on a sterile side table. We would both be ready at the same time to place the donor cornea on the recipient patient's eye, and then place sixteen "10-0" nylon sutures (finer than human hair), to achieve a fluid-tight approximation of the circular wound. We were as efficient as can be that day.

On Monday morning we went to the hospital to change dressings, and all the corneas were clear and beginning to heal. On Tuesday, two more corneas were made available, and on Wednesday, three more. (The National Meeting was still in progress.) We ended up doing eleven corneal transplants in about five days, a feat unheard of in any major university center, let alone in a city the size of Stockton.

One of the patients, Michael, a seventeen-year-old young man with *keratoconus* (thinning of the cornea), turned out to be the nephew of Marian Jacobs, a relative of ours and the owner of a public relations firm in town. Dameron Hospital happened to be one of her accounts, so she wanted to publicize the surgical marathon and Dameron. She called Marge Flaherty, the society editor of the local newspaper, and told her about the series of operations. She further mentioned that her nephew had been successfully operated on by the same doctor about whom Marge "had written an article, eight years before when he conducted the Stockton Symphony Orchestra." Marge did remember and immediately phoned me and interviewed me.

The following Sunday's edition of the *Stockton Record* contained a front page photograph of Dr. Joe and I changing the dressing of the young man who was Miss Jacobs's nephew. The whole front page of the local news section was dedicated to the story of the eleven transplants, the hospital team who performed them, and the unusual circumstances surrounding the marathon.

Both Joe and I were surprised by the article and we expected two consequences from it: first, a great publicity coup; and second, the wrath of the other ophthalmologists. Both premonitions took place. The practice grew by leaps and bounds; and, for a whole year, we were questioned about the indications for the surgery and the appropriateness of the news article. We were put on review until the investigation was complete, but the committee eventually found that everything we did was in proper order and that, besides, we gave new sight to many people who would otherwise have had to travel out of town for surgery.

JOE AND CATHY

Dr. Joe married Cathy Vassar during his internship year. She was the cutest surgical nurse you can imagine and worked in the eye operating room at Dameron hospital. She was young and beautiful, always fit and trim, with long blonde hair and blue almost Eurasian-looking eyes. I didn't know that Joe was dating her at that time, but she soon became my niece-in-law and was happily married to Joe, my partner. She gave birth to two children, Elisa and Joe Jr., now both grown and in their early twenties. Joe Jr. is in second year at Wayne Medical School and intends to specialize in eye surgery and join our practice one day. Elisa wants to become a nurse.

When residency at UC Davis was over, Joe and Cathy moved to a comfortable house in Riviera Cliffs, an upscale residential area in Stockton bordering the San Joaquin and Calaveras Rivers. Joe was doing well in practice. Within a few years, Joe, emboldened by success and a steady income, wanted to move to a larger, more opulent house. Cathy was happy in her home in Riviera Cliffs and actually didn't want to upgrade, but went along with Joe to please him. Joe soon found a home that he wanted to buy, on about three acres of land fronting the Stockton Deep Water Channel. He had plans drawn and proceded to level the house almost completely and at great expense to erect a new two-story mansion in its place.

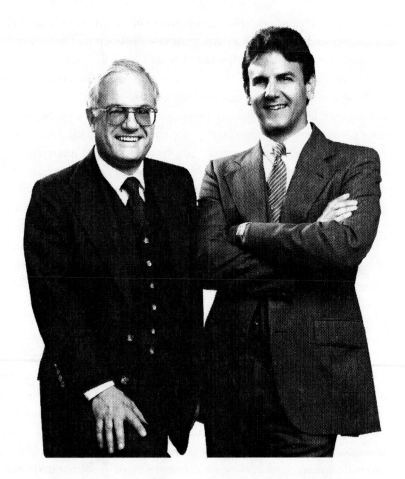

Dr. Joe and Uncle Henry, taking a moment to rest during a
medical convention in 1990, a few years before Dr. John Henry,
and Drs. Wong and Canzano joined us in the practice.

After ten years, Joe's marriage appeared to be on the rocks. Among other
things, Cathy resented Joe being at his parents' place for lunch during weekdays
and became aloof from Joe's immediate family. She also didn't feel good about
his long absences on frequent vacations, with boyfriends she didn't approve of.
Having seen all this happen, I chose a somewhat slow day at the office to take
Joe for a walk around downtown to listen to his side of the story.

When I heard Joe's tale—and having learned from my previous experience—
I advised him to stick with his wife, to understand her position and her innate
fears, and to slightly lessen the parental visits for the sake of his own marriage—

at least for the time being. I explained to him that a girl leaves father and mother and marries into an unknown situation, expecting the husband to protect and comfort her and to put her first in his life. I told him that her apparent resentment of his constant daily relationship with his parents, brothers and friends had some basis in reality.

I spoke with Cathy on several occasions then, and told her that Joe was a good husband who respected his parents, but loved her and the children much more. I also told her that Joe kept her in the style to which she had become accustomed and that was why he worked so hard for her and the children. I emphasized to her that, just because Joe saw his parents often, didn't mean he loved her any less or that he would forsake her. Then, I suggested to Joe that we hire Cathy as our surgical supervisor—after all, she was a nurse and it would keep her occupied now that the children were in school all day. Besides, I thought her presence would brighten up the office.

In the office, Joe was a tiger. He was efficient beyond my dreams and a great surgeon, but he hated to manage the finances. At the same time, his trips and vacations with his male friends increased in frequency. He felt he was entitled to his outings and his pleasures since he worked so hard in the office. So the absences continued and Cathy continued to complain even more than before. Eventually, Cathy started working less and less, and came only sparingly to the office. Joe felt she wasn't doing enough to justify keeping her on the payroll and told her to stay home. One day Cathy came to me in tears. I could see that she was unhappy and angry. Finally, their differences reached a climax.

A few days later, I was in Joe's private office discussing the practice, when an agent-server came in and presented Joe with some papers. I wanted to leave, but Joe asked me to stay. He asked the agent what the papers were for, and was told, "Your wife's petition for divorce." He signed them right there and then. And that was the beginning of an unhappy divorce. I felt sorry for both of them and for their children. I loved the whole family.

When I recall the pain and suffering I went through over several years, and the supreme effort Carol and I had made to keep our marriage together—eventually to see it become successful beyond our dreams—I was sorry to see their marriage ending in a divorce. I believe divorce is a tragic affair, particularly difficult for the children to endure, and rarely a good solution.

Joe is as busy as ever in the office and gets along royally with his partner and cousin, John Henry, my oldest son, and with the new associates, Drs. John Canzano and Richard Wong. They make up a group of well-trained surgeons and caring physicians. The surgical practice has grown by leaps and bounds and Dr. Joe has become the best refractive surgeon in the Central California Valley. He is always his gregarious, generous, open-hearted, and very personable self. Cathy is still pretty, trim, and pleasant; no longer resentful, but I think still unhappy about the experience.

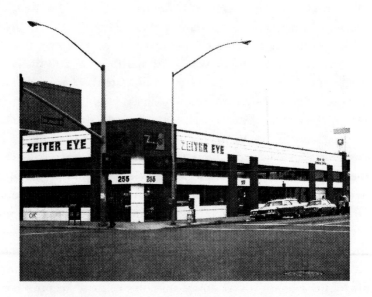

Zeiter Eye offices and surgical center in the center of downtown Stockton, California; it is the headquarters and nerve center for seven other medical offices located around San Joaquin, and two other adjoining counties.

CHAPTER 23

END OF AN ERA

On Sunday, November 30, 1986, we invited Dad over for lunch. Carol prepared for him *kibbe*, stuffed squash with yogurt and a Lebanese salad with lemon and olive oil. She had learned how to cook many varieties of Lebanese food from Dad in the first place, as well as from Irene and Madelyn, my brother's wives. Dad was delighted, but he looked a little tired. After all, in six days he would be entering his ninety-fourth year of life. He was always interested in world geography and history. I couldn't believe that his mind was still alert at his advanced age. I asked him if he still remembered the population of various capitals and large cities around the world. I wanted to test the agility of his nonagenarian mind. "Dad I want to see if your mind is still working," I said to him. He smiled and answered every question, giving me the populations as of around 1970, the last time he must have looked them up. But he was right on, for the populations of big cities as they were around that date.

Then I asked Dad if he remembered what day of the week he was born. He didn't know. So I took him to the computer room and told him, "We're going to find out right now." He was astonished that this could be done on a machine. I ran through a program with him that confirmed December 6, 1893, as a Wednesday. He was dazzled! He fixed his eyes on me and said in his typical biblical style, "Lord, now you can let me go, I've seen it all!"

He was close to the mark when he said that. Two days later, on Tuesday afternoon, Yvonne and Charlie Zeiter, with whom he had lived, quite close to us, called me to say I had better come over right away. Dad had just had a stroke or a heart attack. They lived less than a mile from us. I hurried over there and saw him lying on the floor of the living room, unconscious. The life rescue team arrived at the same time I was checking his pulse. It was rapid but regular. They carried him to the ambulance with the sirens blaring. While I was sitting in the back of the ambulance with him, I meditated on life's twists and turns. Here was a man who had traveled all over the world; sired and educated seven successful children; made and spent money; wrote poetry and prose; and contemplated God and the universe; and now he is lying quiet and barely alive in the back of an ambulance far away from his beloved Lebanon. What is one to think of life?

Shakespeare, in several of his plays (including *Falstaff* and *Julius Caesar*), remarks on how this or that personage lies dead, occupying a tiny space of earth, while when alive the whole world could not contain him. Dad stayed alive but comatose for three days, a holy number. On the third evening, I was in the hospital room with him, keeping vigil with the nurse on duty who was monitoring the EKG. Madelyn had called Tony, Edmond, and Mike (who had come from Canada) to come over to her house and have supper. They asked me to go with them and eat, but I wanted to stay close to Dad a while longer. I was relating to the nurse the story of his extraordinary life, when she suddenly directed the EKG screen towards me. After a few small spikes, the EKG went flat. Dad took his last breath with a deep expiration from an open mouth, and in a flash he was gone to see his Maker.

I knelt beside the bed, held his cold hand, cried and prayed as I meditated, accepting the inevitability of God's will:

> *O Lord, how great are your works!*
> *How deep are your designs!*
> *The foolish man cannot know this*
> *And the fool cannot understand.*
> *The just will flourish like the palm tree*
> *And grow like the Cedars of Lebanon.*
> *Planted in the house of the Lord*
> *They will flourish in the courts of our God,*
> *Still bearing fruits when they are old,*
> *Still full of sap, still green,*
> *To proclaim that the Lord is just;*
> *In him, my rock, there is no wrong.*
> —Psalm 92

Dad lived up to the beginning of his ninety-fourth year, and yet it was over just the same! Mom had died in 1959, twenty-seven years earlier, and it seemed like yesterday. Up to this moment Dad was still alive, like an erect solid wall shielding me from the next world. But now that he was gone, there was no longer a wall separating me from death. I felt very vulnerable. My siblings and I were now next in line to face the inevitable—the one certain thing in this world. Dad was buried in Stockton, far away from the crypt where his father and mother lie.

The old saying, "Two things are for sure in this world, death and taxes," comes to mind. I've always felt it was a dubious saying. Taxes are not unavoidable. A person who is free of greed, a philosopher at heart, pays no taxes because he has no income. St. Francis of Assisi, St. Dominic, and St. Ignatius of Loyola never paid taxes, yet they still died. The rich in this country do a good job avoiding taxes by using shelters, but they do not avoid death. And the crooks, the mafia and the thieves don't pay taxes at all, and if caught, will flee the country without ever paying. But sooner or later, they all will die. The poets often speak of death's inevitability: "So do our minutes hasten to their end," as Shakespeare puts it.

Coming back to Dad, the wise philosopher now dead in front of me, I recalled how when he witnessed me arguing an obvious point with an obtuse person, he would say to me, "Son, remember the old Lebanese proverb, 'I argued with a wise philosopher and won, but when I argued with a donkey, I got nowhere and lost.'" He frequently quoted to me his favorite four verses:

> *He who doesn't know, and knows he doesn't know is ignorant: teach him.*
> *He who knows, but doesn't know that he knows is asleep: wake him.*
> *He who knows, and knows that he knows is wise: follow him.*
> *But he who doesn't know and thinks that he knows is a fool: shun him.*

Actually, it was when I was relating this wise saying to the attendant nurse in the room that Dad expired. He was the man who first taught me to love philosophy (*philo,* love; *sophia,* wisdom) and the man who had influenced my life more than any other. Will I be able to avoid death, or *half* of it? Impossible! As Pascal said in his Wager, "It is the one absolutely inevitable thing in the world."

We buried Dad and I was given the wooden cross on top of the casket before he was placed in the tomb. That was my second wooden cross. The first one was at my mother's funeral years before. I still have both crosses. I also removed the wedding ring from his finger at the same time—the one I began wearing three years later when John Henry at his wedding borrowed (irrevocably!) the one I had kept from Mom.

Following Dad's internment, I went home and played Mozart's Requiem as I often do at such sad moments, and as I had done when I learned of my mother's death twenty-seven years earlier.

FAITH, HOPE AND CHARITY

One month after Dad died I drove to the Camaldolese Monastery at Big Sur, high on the coastal mountains overlooking the Pacific Ocean. It's such an impressionist scene that whenever I am there I flash back in my mind's eye to the Mediterranean Coast where I grew up. I spent a weekend in Big Sur and lapsed into my mystical thoughts. It is at these times that I feel closest to the Source of my being. I had been to the monastery before, but since Dad passed away, I return to that place of peace and holiness more often. The priests and brothers are holy, humble, and they sing beautifully during the daily services. This is especially true of Father Isaiah, the son of my friend Henry Teichert, who gave up his position in a successful development company, voluntarily disinherited himself, and entered the monastic life. How often I have wished I was in his shoes!

Since Carol and I started a Charitable Foundation, we have sponsored several of the student monks at the monastery through their seminary and post-graduate studies. Most of our scholarships, however, go to students at Thomas Aquinas College in Santa Paula, California, and a few go to Christendom College in Front Royal, Virginia, where our daughter Suzie and her husband live. Our favorite charity though is the Stockton Homeless Shelter which takes in families who are poor and destitute. His whole life Jesus was for helping the poor (not institutions). Carol spends most of her time now helping out in this Christ-like cause.

The establishment of the Foundation was a stroke of intuition. I was driving back from Lake Tahoe alone one day when the idea occurred to me like a thunderbolt. I phoned my tax attorney, Richard Calone and my accountant, John De Gregori, about its feasibility, and both said with the same voice: "Let's do it!" We sold our shares in a number of companies and transferred the proceeds to the foundation. It was just at the right time—the shares plummeted shortly thereafter.

Following that experience, we have put into practice what we learned: God rewards those who are charitable tenfold, not only spiritually, but financially as well. Over the next ten years, every time we transferred shares of stock to a charity, their policy is to sell the stock immediately and lock in the profits. And many times after they sold, the price of the stock would drop dramatically. Of course, we make the gift for God's sake, not because we have any knowledge that the stock's price is going to drop. That's precisely why the whole thing is uncanny!

I often sit on a bank facing the ocean, when I am visiting the monastery. In 1992, while overlooking the vast Pacific, I penned a little poem:

> We pray to Thee, all forming Creator,
> We revere Thy image and Thy bounty.
> We exist through Thee, our Benefactor,
> And love Thee in spite of our poverty.
>
> O dear Lord of heaven, and of this earth,
> We do not know Thee, nor understand Thee.
> Only by Thy working on us since birth,
> Do we see Providence, and now thank Thee.
>
> Now that we are old, and often stumble,
> We remain thankful for all your wonders.
> Give us Lord more years, to make us humble
> Save us, Thy poor, in spite of our blunders.
>
> Forgive us Lord. You always have and will,
> You see our confusion and our failures.
> We pile them up; no space is left to fill,
> Help us believe in all Thy saving cures.
>
> Have mercy Lord! Our faults we hope You'll mend,
> And save us from our deserved damnation.
> For Thou art for ever our final end,
> And will not leave us in tribulation.
>
> For all this we thank Thee, and praise Thee Lord!

As I get older peace and tranquility become my quest. One of the better things I came to see with age is that polemics and argumentation are often fruitless. I had always doggedly stood for what I thought was right, but now I find that I have a limited appetite for involvement. For one thing, I no longer get enthusiastic or upset when my favorite sports teams win or lose. Oh, I still watch games every now and then, but I also have no problem turning off a ballgame when the score is tied and the game is in the ninth inning. I am no longer anxious about who is going to win. Indeed, I have tried to shun all anxiety whatsoever and follow the cue of Pope John Paul II who often quoted the wisdom of the late saint, Padre Pio: "Pray, have hope, and do not worry." Besides, ninety percent of what we worry about never comes about. Instead, like St. Paul, I try to keep my worries fixed only on one thing—that "after having preached virtue to others, I myself do not get rejected":

> *While all the runners in the stadium take part in the race, the award goes to one man. In that case run so as to win! Athletes deny themselves all sorts of things. They do this to win a crown of leaves that withers; but we a crown that is imperishable. I do not run like a man who loses sight of the finish line. I do not fight as if I was shadowboxing. What I do is discipline my own body and master it, for fear that after having preached virtue to others I myself should be rejected.*
>
> —Saint Paul, *I Corinthians*, 9:24-27

Few things in life need our constant attention, and even these things are rarely under our control. This applies particularly to one's offspring. One's children want independence after being told what to do for the first eighteen years of their lives. I try now to keep quiet. My sister-in-law Betsy told us a cute anecdote the other day. Apparently when she went to visit her married daughter Mary (a psychiatrist) the last time, she was determined not to give any advice or spout any suggestions. "I kept my vow faithfully by keeping my mouth shut," she told us. When she was ready to leave, she said, her daughter bid her farewell with the words: "Thanks for all your advice Mom!" *Das ist das leben* (C'est la vie!)

Now the children's children are even further removed from our injunctions. The young actually distance themselves from the old and the wise, as if only their peers (who know nothing!) can teach them about life. Of course, that's nothing new—It's been like this for ages. Yet, we love to see them grow and mature under our very old and tired eyes, and win prizes and succeed. Yes, we do enjoy our grandchildren more than anything on earth, because we recognize the beauty of their innocence, after having spent the better part of our own life losing it.

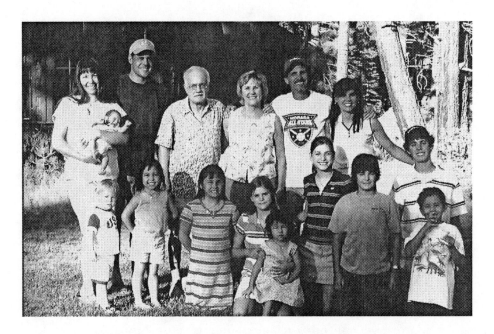

A family portrait, with children and grandchildren—Absent, are Camille, and Suzie and Tony with their two sons. Our progeny is getting older, and the grandchildren plentiful and all beautiful.

A LITTLE MUSIC, A LITTLE OPERA

As music has remained my life-long passion, one of my most enjoyable avocations has been in relation to the Stockton Symphony Orchestra. I joined the board in 1964. In those days the symphony hall was still in the old Stockton High School. But in 1974 a new auditorium, specifically designed for symphonic and operatic performances was inaugurated at the new Delta College. Carol and I worked hard to help raise money to build the new auditorium.

I will never forget the inauguration concert. As Maestro Won's baton came down for Wagner's *Die Meistersinger Overture*, Harold Willis, board member, Peter Ottesen, manager, and I, were standing in the back of the auditorium jumping for joy at every note. We had all worked so hard to help build the new auditorium with its 1600 red velvet seats. The program continued with Beethoven's great Violin Concerto with its fate-filled opening five drum beats, and concluded with a rousing performance of Mussorgsky's *Pictures at an Exhibition* as orchestrated by Maurice Ravel. What a joy it was to be involved in a grand enterprise such as this one, and see it brought to fruition before our very eyes and ears!

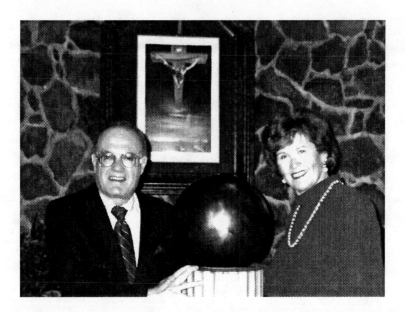

Carol and I in our previous home in Stockton, prior to attending the dedication concert of the new auditorium of the Stockton Symphony Orchestra in 1972. On the wall is Salvador Dali's *The Crucifixion, According to St. John of the Cross.*

In 1972, I became president of the symphony and hired Max Simoncic as manager. Max was a music theory instructor at Delta College and a well-known composer. In gratitude for our friendship he composed and dedicated to Carol and I a string quintet, and the premiere was a local event to which two hundred people were invited. Following the concert Max kindly subtitled the work, the *"Zeiter" String Quintet.* Max would often visit our house and compose variations on the piano on any tune I would whistle. When I marveled about how he did this with such agility, he informed me that most composers keep in their head thousands of combinations and permutations of any succession of musical notes in the various musical keys, and are able to come up with them and rearrange them at any particular moment. I was awe-struck by such creative ability.

Max left the symphony to work full time at Delta College. Then Peter Ottesen was hired. He remained manager of the Symphony for over twenty years. During that time, Peter and our selection committee hired Kyung Soo Won as symphony director who brought the symphony to an astounding level of proficiency and prestige.

One year, Kyung Soo Won was teaching a course in conducting to candidates for a master's degree in music at the University of the Pacific Conservatory. He knew how much I loved symphonic music, so two weeks before the course started, he asked me if I would like to participate. I was delighted. I studied hard with him and practiced all the motions of conducting, and then rehearsed several times, first to piano accompaniment and then in front of the whole orchestra. There were three pieces chosen for study that year: Beethoven's Eighth Symphony and Emperor Concerto, and Elgar's *Enigma Variations*. We had already rehearsed all these scores for several months, when on the morning of the concert Mr. Won called me at home and asked me if I would like to conduct any part of the Beethoven Symphony I wanted. So I did conduct it that very night to an almost full auditorium. The following year, I conducted two sections of Mussorgsky's *Pictures at an Exhibition*. The third year, I conducted the *Introduction* and the *Trepak* (the Cossack Dance) from Tchaikovsky's *Nutcracker Suite*. Two words I found describe one's feelings on conducting a symphony orchestra: a*wesome power*.

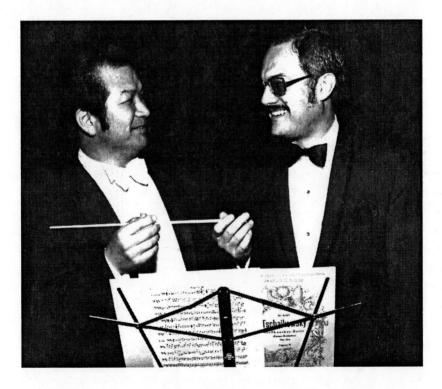

Maestro Kyung Soo Won handing me the baton, prior to conducting the Stockton Symphony Orchestra in Beethoven's Eighth Symphony in 1973.

In addition to conducting, I also found great joy and camaraderie from acting in opera productions in various California Central Valley cities. Eric Townsend, a former professional tenor, now acting director of Valley Opera players asked me several years ago if I would like to play the role of the tavern owner in Puccini's *La Bohème*. Well! Well! I thought. Following several rehearsals with the company, I was ready to become an opera actor. The Stockton Symphony's present director, Peter Jaffe, was the conductor, and he gave me excellent cues. It was fun being back stage with the tenors, baritones, bassos, sopranos and mezzos, and it was even more exciting being on the stage as part of the performance of the opera that Carol and I love the most, *La Bohème*. Acting roles in Bizet's *Carmen*, in Johann Strauss' *Die Fledermaus*, and in Mozart's *Don Giovanni* and later *The Magic Flute* followed each other. I even had a speaking role as Prince Orlovsky's valet in Johann Strauss' *Die Fledermaus*, and a brief singing line in Verdi's *La Traviata* this past year.

But my greatest joy was being on stage in my all time favorite Mozart grand opera, *Don Giovanni*. I had an acting role in all the major scenes, as tavern owner (my specialty now), liquor server, *maitre de chambre*, and finally as Don Giovanni's cook in that fabulous last scene where the Don's brazen and dissolute life leads him straight into the fires of hell and eternal damnation. The scene begins with his cook, and Leporello, his side kick, carving out pheasants and quails, then serving them to him along with various delicate wines, and then watching him savor all the hedonistic pleasures of this world.

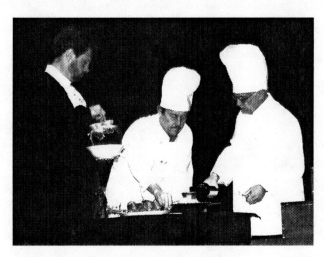

My favorite scene in all opera, the final scene of Mozart's Don Giovanni; just before the entrance of the stone statue, I am seen as the cook preparing the food and the wine for Don Giovanni's insatiable appetite.

I was on stage throughout that scene alongside Leporello (a great basso role) and Don Giovanni (the universal type of the dissolute knave). I was still on stage when, finally, the stone guest (the Comendatore) enters the scene, asking the protagonist to repent of his sins (which he refuses to do), then sending him screaming down to hell amidst the fiery flames, while Satan's miscreants are all over the stage dragging him down to the netherworld of pain and the gnashing of teeth. If I was asked forty years ago what opera scene I would have liked most to perform in, I would have answered unequivocally, "The last scene of *Don Giovanni*, please!" I had known every aria and every note of this opera since medical school. Now, here I was on stage satisfying a long-standing desire.

One year ago, I was a slave in one act, and a priest in another, in Mozart's *The Magic Flute*. I couldn't help but recall when as a child (sixty years ago) I danced to the theme of Papageno's area, in Tripoli, Lebanon. I find myself at a loss to explain such uncanny coincidences. The Greek tragedians call it Fate; and the religious call it Providence.

.

CHAPTER 24

CLINICAL SUCCESS

After Joe became a stable part of our practice, our hope was that my son, John Henry, may be able to join us some day. John Henry had attended Baylor Medical School in Houston. He finished his residency at Kresge Eye Institute and joined us in 1992. In preparation for his arrival, Joe invented the three Z's logo (for the three of us Zeiters) and we enlarged the office and the surgical center to occupy the whole quarter block of what was once the Old San Joaquin Hotel. Six years before, the building had been transformed on a lesser scale to become the Zeiter Eye Clinic, later called simply Zeiter Eye, including our Surgical Center. Credit for the improvements has to go to Dr. Joe, who has a heart full of courage to the point of fearlessness, like his father, my brother Tony. He had originally pushed me to build the Surgical Center in 1986, the year my father (his grandfather) passed away.

Late in 1991, the year before John Henry joined us, we obtained a six-month lease for the building across the street, which we transformed into a makeshift office while we gutted and completely remodeled our permanent quarters. The renovated office building became the pride of downtown Stockton. It had been my purpose for forty five years to stay located in the center of the city to be able to better serve the needs of the poor and disadvantaged, as well as the affluent. Dad had told me upon graduating from medicine, "Son, if you don't help the poor you have no right to claim to be a healing physician." And just the same, the affluent continue to come downtown to see us because Zeiter Eye is a well-established name in the area. When the building phase was over we had enough examining rooms to service all three Zeiter doctors. The whole project took only six months and was designed and supervised by our architect son, Philip, who did a marvelous artistic and structural job transforming an old building to satisfy the new earthquake codes, and still be beautiful and functional to serve our large practice.

I have always been extremely fortunate to have had faithful and devoted help. In 1965, Dr. Barkett suggested that I hire Donna, who turned out to be a heaven-sent office administrator. In her thirty years with us, she rotated through every position in the office until she became office manager. She remained in that position up to her retirement only a few years ago.

Shortly after Donna started, my brother Tony referred his bookkeeper to me. Jane Brause stayed with us for two decades as my personal secretary, bookkeeper, and guardian of secrets. She became a close member of our family. She, too, retired several years ago. I miss her absolute loyalty. She always stood up for me through thick and thin. She's community-minded and, incidentally, healthy as can be, her mother having lived to the ripe old age of 104. Our personnel always felt as though they were part of the family; Erin, the present manager, feels that way after 25 years; Debbie and Apryl, who have been with us for over 22 years, feel the same way. Espy was offered higher-paying jobs with great promises by other ophthalmologists, but she chose to stay with us. At the time, she told me, "I won't leave this office; to me it's like family."

THE COUNTY MEDICAL SOCIETY

Shortly after John Henry joined our practice, I became more involved in the governance of the San Joaquin County Medical Society. It all happened through my impertinence. One day at a meeting for the election of officers, I had the courage to chastise the presiding officers by telling them, "Those who run this medical society are a closed group, who act like members of a 'rotating club', shuffling positions on the same board of governance for years. It has become obvious to the rest of us that the same people have been ruling the roost year after year, and no new blood has been allowed to come in for a long time."

The then president Dr. Peter Salamon replied, "The same people rotate because nobody else wants to do the work, Henry! Would you want to work as hard as we do to run this society?" I said, "You bet your shirt I would!"

Within a year I was asked to be on the Board of the Society. Two years later I was vice-president, and the following year I was elected president. It was an opportune time since I had Joe and John Henry running the practice, which made it possible for me to spend time and effort giving back to medicine part of what I had gained from it. In conjunction with my appointment, the California Legislature wanted to transfer the Medi-Cal program from the state to the counties, if they were willing to take it on. At a well-attended open meeting, I told the Board of Directors that it would be a great advantage if we could control these medical care funds locally, and we would most probably be able to run our own program for indigent care more efficiently. I urged them that we accept the State's offer and become our own bosses.

Fortunately, there was an administrator at the San Joaquin General Hospital, Mike Smith, who was very interested in pursuing this issue with me. He knew that the County Hospital would also benefit since the care of the poor and uninsured has always been the primary function of any County Hospital. Most of these hospitals across the country are located in the poorer area of town. In Stockton, it is the southern fringe of the city. Mike and I became good friends, and we often needled each other about issues that we knew were important to the other person. I was protecting the medical society and the individual doctors' practices; while Mike's interest was in benefiting the county hospital. We engineered the program from the beginning; we hired an experienced manager, Leona Butler, who came up with several great ideas; and the enterprise became a great success story.

GLOBAL CONNECTIONS

For many years between 1975 and 2000, Carol and I flew to Hawaii every January to attend the annual meetings of the Royal Hawaiian Eye Society where often I would speak. These were organized by John Corboy, an active Honolulu ophthalmic surgeon. We would meet the many professionals we had cultivated friendships with over the years. Most of them were in the forefront of ophthalmic progress during an unbelievable era of innovations, inventions, and new surgical procedures in eye surgery (1970-95.) It was a particular pleasure for me to meet with innovative big-time surgeons like Dennis Shepard from Santa Maria, Henry Hirshman, Dick Kratz and Kenny Hoffer from Los Angeles, Charley Kelman from New York, Danny Osher from Cincinnati, Jerry Tenant from Dallas, Al Newman from Florida, and even Federov from Russia, the originator of corneal refractive surgery. The many Barraquers, a great family of eye surgeons from Spain and Colombia, Peter Choyce from England, and of course Federov from Russia, would be there also. It was a fraternity of the most cutting-edge eye surgeons in the world. We all knew each other and would lecture on our latest findings and innovations.

These were the days when the medical insurance companies, and particularly the Medicare administration, could not keep up with the flood of newer and more effective surgical procedures that were introduced on a weekly basis by all of us, i.e. those who frequently attended the Royal Hawaiian Eye Meetings. Eventually the American Cataract and Refractive Surgery Society grew out of this group, and we were all founding members. When my nephew Joe came into practice with me, I would take him to these conventions, and would invite him along to the cocktail parties where he would meet the twenty or so surgeons whose names were on the surgical instruments he used every day.

One year at the Royal Hawaiian meeting, I was asked (impromptu) to lecture on the financial aspect of medical practice. I mentioned everything I could think off to a packed audience of physicians, their wives, and staff. As I was getting down from the podium, I heard a voice telling me, "Henry, you failed to advice them to marry a rich spouse." I turned around and there was Dr. Larry Stocker, an old friend of mine, who taught me pediatric ophthalmology at Kresge Eye and Children's Hospital in Detroit. It turns out that his wife had left him for a golf-pro and moved to Bermuda. Larry was depressed for five years. One day Larry's partner suggested that he join him in Miami Beach to get his *ex* off his mind. In three days he met a woman at a ball at the Fontainebleau; they fell in love, and got married within a month. The woman, as it turns out, was the ex-wife of a well-known Detroit industrialist, one of the richest men in the world. She had gotten half a billion dollars in divorce settlement and was listed at that time in the Forbes four hundred. Larry told me that they were very happy with each other. I told him I would have been happy too under the circumstances! I got a big laugh out of him.

In 1983, I had the privilege of serving as chief surgeon on a medical mission to the Philippines and China. The airplane, a 747 plane known as the *Orbis*, was equipped with the latest operating room facilities, assembled to teach modern surgical techniques to ophthalmologists in third world countries. When we landed in Manila, at two in the morning, I was half asleep but famished, so I called room service in the hotel for a club sandwich. I took one large bite and was fully awakened by the severe pain in my mouth. I had bitten into the toothpick that held the sandwich together, and the top part of the toothpick had gone into my palate and the bottom part into my tongue. They had used a regular toothpick instead of the usually long ones normally used to hold a sandwich together. Well, it wasn't too bad since I finished the sandwich in no time and fell into a deep sleep right away. I was exhausted from the long flight over the Pacific. I woke up early in the morning ready to operate.

The Orbis organization had converted half of the seating section of the airplane into an operating room and the other half into a well cushioned closed-circuit auditorium for local surgeons. We operated on seven patients every morning on the plane; and had about forty local ophthalmologists watching our extra-capsular technique on closed-circuit TV. There were another eighty specialists, assembled in various hospitals in Manila, watching us operate on closed circuit television.

The second night we were invited as VIPs to the Manila Golf and Country Club for a dinner in our honor. Much to our surprise, we were welcomed there by Imelda Marcos, wife of the president of the Philippines at the time. She asked if I we would be kind enough to visit one of the homes for the blind that she sponsored in Manila, to see if any of the residents could be helped. I was driven there after dinner by her chauffeur. There were about fifty blind people in a two-story house, all blind from total corneal opacities due to Vitamin A deficiency. We found we could operate only on two of them (we had two donor corneas), so I chose the two with the least damage, for corneal transplantation the next day. It was fortunate that we had two corneas sent to us that previous day from the Orbis Headquarters in Houston.

There was a knock on my hotel door that night, so I got up from bed and opened the door and standing there was one of the two blind men I had chosen for a transplant. Behind him was Mrs. Marcos's chauffeur, who proceeded to tell me in impeccable English that the blind man was there to give me a massage for as long as I wanted, courtesy of Imelda Marcos. What a surprise! Apparently, in the Philippines, blind people are taught to be masseurs and masseuses. What a great idea this was to help blind people obtain gainful occupation. I said *gracias* to the chauffeur, and *andale* (go to it) to my next day's patient. The man gave me the best massage I ever had, and it went on for about two hours—I don't know for sure how long because the massage put me in a dreamy sleep. He must have left when he saw me go to sleep. What bliss that was! The next day I successfully performed a corneal transplant on this young man.

A few days later, we were flown to Cebu City to continue our surgical mission. On our arrival we were registered at Tambuli, a beautiful resort on Mactan Island. Next day we were taken to the very spot on that island where the Philippine chieftain, Lapu Lapu, killed Magellan and most of his men in 1521. Apparently, Magellan had landed on Mactan Island to gather supplies, not aware that the beach there was a muddy marchland. His soldiers, heavily clad with steel armor and heavy swords, sunk to their knees in the mud and were picked off like fish in a barrel by Lapu Lapu's fighters, using only bows and arrows. Magellan died and is still buried there. He had wisely left enough men on his ship to enable them to continue the voyage to Spain.

Another year I flew to Bogota to do a presentation at the Barraquer Institute on how to place an intraocular lens in the eye following cataract surgery. Surprisingly, at that great center of corneal transplant surgery they weren't using intraocular lenses yet. One night I went into the street to buy Colombian emeralds for Carol and was directed to a second-floor room. I knocked on the door and had to give the secret word, just like in an old Peter Lorre movie. I was let in. The emerald dealer would take envelopes loaded with emeralds out of his pockets and empty them on the glass table, as if they were common pebbles from the beach. I bought some at rock bottom prices as gifts for Carol and staff.

A TROUBLED HEART

Yet all these activities were not to be without a sequel. In May, 2001, we were visiting my old friend from medical school, Dr. Frank Sennewald, who lived during the winter in a little medieval French town in the beautiful Dordogne district of southern France. We were taking hikes daily to visit many of the castles that dot the Dordogne countryside. It seemed that every few kilometers there was a castle perched on a hilltop. I found myself huffing and puffing and stopping every fifty yards to take a breath and relieve a gnawing feeling in my chest. I thought I was just out of shape. I neglected to attend to the warning signs, which, for a doctor, was pretty dumb. Upon our return to Stockton, I was to learn what the problem was.

The first week after our return, I was playing my regular morning tennis doubles game with Dan Canistraci, Bob Unger, and Bill Latham, when in the middle of the first set, I stopped to take a breath and felt pressure in my upper chest. "I was out of shape," I thought again. So we resumed the game and finished the set. Halfway through the second set, the same thing recurred. I stopped, now asking for an antacid, a Tums, or anything to relieve what I thought was heartburn. Dan gave me two Tums, and I felt a little better, enough to resume play. In retrospect, I think it was more the result of my resting a while than my taking the Tums.

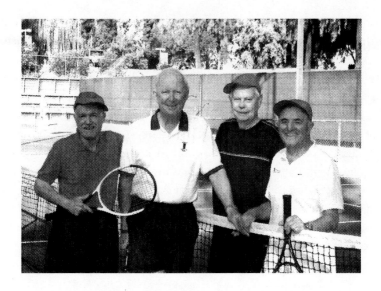

The feared tennis foursome; from the left, Henry, Dr. Bill Latham, Bob Unger, and Dan Canistraci

The same discomfort came back to me early in the third set, and this time I stopped and asked the players on the next court if any of them had nitroglycerine. Don Cerque had some tablets and he gave me two, but the pressure was gone before I was able to put the tablets to use. I told the players let's continue, and I played even more vigorously, wanting to bring the pressure back, to see if the nitroglycerine would relieve the discomfort if it ever came back. That would be diagnostic of angina, I was thinking. How utterly dangerous my thinking process was! What strong denial for a physician! It could have been fatal to voluntarily try to bring the chest discomfort back. I could have died on the court.

I still couldn't bring myself to believe it was my heart. I was rationalizing; after all, my father had lived to be ninety-four. My oldest brother Mike was eighty-one and still fit as a fiddle. Their cholesterol levels had always been below 150 mg. Mine was rarely higher than 200. My mother died of colon cancer, not from a heart attack. Again, what denial!

Well, later that morning, I got to the office, did a few chores and drove to a Salvation Army Board meeting in Lodi where they wanted me to join their board. On the way there, I decided to call John Henry at the office, and tell him about the episodes on the tennis court. I had just left the office and never saw fit to ask Dr. Joe or John for their advice or medical opinion. How foolish it was of me! I, who had spent a good part of my life meditating on life and death and on the passing of time; I, who had undergone years of analysis to understand my motives; I, who philosophized and knew as a physician all the symptoms of angina; that same Henry thought he was immortal; immune from the episodes that kill people—it wouldn't occur to *me*, I rationalized.

When John Henry heard my story, he said to me, "I'm calling Dr. Buhari right now. Keep your cell phone free." Dr. Buhari was my cardiologist. For thirty years I had been joking with him at parties, telling him to take good care of me if my heart ever gave out. He called me immediately and asked me two questions. "Henry, were you exerting when you had the episode?"

"Yes, I was playing tennis."

"How long did the pressure last?"

"About two minutes each time."

"That's angina! When did you have your last stress test?"

"Three months ago, and it was negative."

"That shows you how unreliable these stress tests can be. I am scheduling you for angiography tomorrow afternoon at one o'clock at St. Joseph's Hospital. In the meantime, stay off the tennis court."

I turned my car around towards home. I realized that I needed to be on another Board like I needed a shot in the head! It took this sudden shot between the eyes to convince me of my mortality. Later I recalled that my regular internist, Dr. Navone, had scheduled me for a stress test three months hence, but I had not actually taken the test yet; I had misinformed Dr. Buhari. That was the best mistake I ever made, because it forced him to schedule an angiogram and skip a stress test which might have showed nothing.

The next day, as Dr. Buhari started the coronary arteriogram, my cousin Dr. Barkett showed up, for which I was most grateful. I heard both doctors conversing about the angiogram, and I picked up that the anterior descending coronary was 95 percent occluded; the left posterior and the circumflex about 80 percent. When Dr. Buhari told Carol the news (about thirty minutes later) she thought he was joking. This time it was for real and she was shell-shocked. When Dr. Buhari came to my hospital room to inform me that surgery would be necessary, he said that playing tennis all these years had probably saved my life. Good collateral circulation around my heart from regular exercise had prevented a myocardial infarction (a heart attack). I stayed in the hospital overnight and the next day Dr. Morissey operated on me for six hours. I needed five bypasses and two endarterectomies (roto-rooting the inside of the existing coronaries) so that the bypasses would work. That's how plugged my arteries were. Since I could have died, life could not go on as before. These are the moments when we are chastened and humbled by events not within our control. I could grow or wither from the experience.

After five days, I was discharged from the hospital. The following morning I woke up at 5:00 a.m. and went out to the patio through our back door to the lake-side of our house. I immediately felt the invigorating fresh air. Life never seemed more precious or worthwhile. I could hear the birds singing as I had not heard them sing for years; and I felt the cool breeze pleasantly caressing my face. It all reminded me of my peak experiences. I was still alive! I was breathing, and could still look at my lake! How wonderful it was to be in my own backyard early in the morning, before anybody else had awakened. The early morning silence, interrupted only by the chirping of the birds, was like music to my ears. In the early morning hours, I was transported back to my happy solitary moments of childhood when everything was perceived clearly and crisply. My senses were fully alive again that morning. It was still a little dark, and the sky, the stars, and the lake were all still there, and they seemed more beautiful than ever before.

CHAPTER 25

LIFE

By 2002, I reached a point where I was healthy, happy, and sufficiently satisfied to concentrate on my spiritual welfare. I had overcome marital separation, investment worries, and the children's problems. I was still playing tennis three times a week and almost entirely retired from the practice of medicine and business. I was spending most of every day at home reading, listening to music, and spending time with Carol, the children, and the grandchildren. I found it all quite pleasant. I was making my peace with God and men, with myself, and with my family.

I had undergone a sobering experience, forcing me to realize more fully, the value of health and life. I was brought back full circle to childhood, where I appreciated everything in wonder. I had been too humanly slow in implementing a "change into the new man," as St. Paul phrased it. I've always known where my choice would lead me. Could it really be harder for a rich person to enter the kingdom of heaven? In the last several years, I've been finding out that dispossessing oneself is a difficult task indeed.

> *Have mercy on us Lord, have mercy.*
> *We are filled with contempt.*
> *Indeed all too full is our soul,*
> *With the scorn of the rich,*
> *With the proud man's disdain.*
> —Psalm 123

PROGENY

Now that Philip and Alicia have added six more to the number of grandchildren, we have a total of twelve. We find every one of them a gift from heaven. Playing with them and showering them with affection when they're little, and watching them grow older is a delight—a recompense for the hard work and worries of a lifetime that went into bringing up one's own children. John Henry, Jr., the oldest, is a clone of his father and grandfather. Each grandchild has given rise to charming stories and family lore. The love we give them is returned to us a thousandfold, and we soak it up like a sponge.

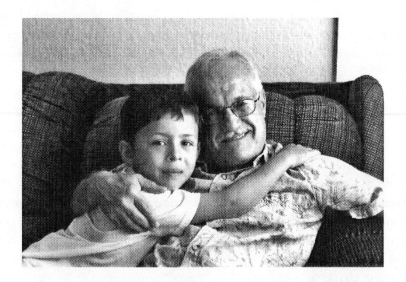

The glory of having plenty of time to spend in love and affection; Zachary tells me that this is also *his* favorite time.

ETERNAL THINGS

Benjamin Franklin named seven virtues for people to live by. Among them, he found humility the most difficult to pursue. He either put it on his face as a mask to impress people, or treated it as a practical measure that would earn him more respect from others. Christ put it best, when asked by his disciples, "Who is of greatest importance in the kingdom of God?" He called a little child over and stood him in their midst and said, "I assure you, unless you change and become like little children, you will not enter the kingdom of heaven. Whosoever makes himself lowly and humble, becoming like this child, is of greatest importance in that heavenly reign."

I decided to be more like I was the days following my First Communion. I am beginning to enjoy the solitude and silence that I experience daily after Mass and Communion. Carol joins me at Mass daily; and reminds me that she cannot live without it. At times I find myself doing nothing more than being immersed in my own quiet thoughts. We spend our summers at Tahoe Donner, surrounded by mountains and the straight, tall evergreens found in the Lake Tahoe area. These trees epitomize to me the seeking and longing for heaven above, beyond our terrestrial daily cares and chores. Oh, yes, I do the chores and take care of things, but lately, I do everything in the spirit of offering it to God above. The pine, fir, and cedar trees I see around me pay the same homage by growing ever taller and taller, seeking the sky above.

I have grown accustomed to looking at everything with the awe of a child, as if discovering whatever I am looking at for the first time in my life. This kind of wonder started with my first philosophy class when Father Dwyer at Assumption College told us, as a lesson in practical metaphysics, to go around all day touching everything we pass by and saying to ourselves, "It is this or that object, it exists! And it is good!" It turned out to be an exercise in wonder and awe at the recognition of everything God has created. "You know, creatures don't necessarily have to be," our professor told us once. "Only God is necessary; all other things are contingent [dependent] on him." It is an exercise in the art of taking nothing created for granted, realizing that it may not be here tomorrow.

The exercise of touching everything and affirming its existence taught me to look at all things, whether new or old, with the wonder of a child—with the intuition that leads to amazement at every new thing one sees. One has to practice this wonderment to make things ever fresh and new in the eyes of a grateful creature, always in awe at the Creator's generosity in making everything, both the good and the not-so-good, the beautiful and the not-so-beautiful, the happy moments, as well as the not-so-happy ones. "O Lord, how manifold are thy works. In wisdom hast thou made them all; the earth is full of thy creatures." (Psalm 103)

The great English Jesuit convert, Gerard Manley Hopkins, often described that *"freshness deep down things,"* as only a child or an intuitive poet could,

> *The world is charged with the grandeur of God.*
> *It will flame out, like shining from shook foil;*
> *It gathers to a greatness, like the ooze of oil*
> *Crushed. Why do men then now not reck his rod?*
> *Generations have trod, have trod, have trod;*
> *And all is seared with trade; bleared, smeared with toil;*
> *And wears man's smudge and shares man's smell; the soil*
> *Is bare now, nor can foot feel, being shod.*
>
> *And for all this, nature is never spent;*
> *There lives the dearest freshness deep down things;*
> *And though the last lights off the black West went,*
> *Oh, morning, at the brown brink eastward, springs:*
> *Because the Holy Ghost over the bent*
> *World broods with warm breast and with ah! Bright wings.*
>   —Gerard Manley Hopkins, S.J., *God's Grandeur* (1918)

He wrote this poem of hope in God's generosity, and as a lament at man's insensitivity, in 1918, when World War I—with horror never seen before— was just ending. Only silence and solitude and long periods of serenity can bring one to perceive and abstract the essence of things—their ever-present newness which fills us with hope and leads us to the perception of the "one thing necessary." It would be good to be able to pass one's life in wonderment at creation, as an exercise in *being* (rather than in *doing*), before we finally face Being Itself. God allows us to experience all this wonder and makes it always available to us. Intuiting being in the universe encourages us to keep our eyes on target, our hopes alive, and our hearts longing for Him, the Being of all beings.

St. Augustine, after a life filled with pleasures of the flesh, intellectual pursuits, and material possessions, exclaimed the truth: "Our hearts were made for thee, O Lord, and they will not rest until they rest in Thee." Pascal and, later, John Henry Newman put it this way: "The heart hath its reasons which reason knows nothing of." It was an intuitive realization of the importance of a perfect blend between reason and emotion, intellect and will, spirit and matter.

FINALLY, ALMOST A MONK—LIKE DAD

For years now, I had been visiting monasteries and attending retreats in an effort to find peace and tranquility. Lately, I have perceived more distinctly the value of learning humility through obedience; gentleness and meekness, through spiritual poverty; and purity through chastity and continence. For me, all of these virtues tend to go against the grain. They surely go against the grain of all of us. Eight years ago I joined the Secular Order of Discalced Carmelites as an aspirant. I was in formation for three years before I was allowed to take temporary promises of obedience, poverty, and chastity (four year ago). All this was in line with my love of St. Teresa of Avila, St. John of the Cross, and Saint Thérèse of Lisieux, all of them Carmelite mystics. I wanted to choose, like Martha's sister, Mary, "the better part"—the part consisting of prayer, contemplation, and with God's grace, union with the Source of my being. On October 15, 2005, I made my permanent (lifelong) promises.

The Carmelites are a contemplative order, inspired by the prophet Elijah, who lived on Mount Carmel in the Holy Land, and Our Blessed Mother Mary. The regular order was founded in the twelfth century. As time went on, the order became lax and had to be reformed by St. Teresa of Avila and St. John of the Cross in 16th-century Spain. It has produced, over the years, great contemplative saints and mystics. Members make binding promises to pursue obedience, poverty, and chastity as a way of surrender to Providence in all things, in imitation of Christ who preached gentleness and meekness to both rich and poor, to the upright and to sinners, to the haughty and to the forlorn. By joining the Order, I have chosen a life of daily verbal prayers leading, I hope, to intense mental prayer and contemplation. However, no true contemplation takes place without God's free gift of grace from above.

I belong to a local lay community whose members have similar objectives. We're in contact with each other and meet formally once a month. We are required to say the Daily Office of prayers three times a day—just as priests, monks, and nuns have done for twenty centuries—and we are required to spend one half hour daily in peace, tranquility, and contemplation. This whole objective formalizes what I have enjoyed doing all my life: reading, praying, and the appreciation of beauty in art and nature. Indeed, all of us, whether religious or not, read and study in order to find *the truth*; practice *goodness* in our lives to develop good habits (towards our families, our neighbors and our nation); and we appreciate and seek *the beautiful* and *the sacred*. After all, what is God, but the essence of Being, Truth, Goodness, and Beauty—the four transcendental values that all ancient cultures had sought since time immemorial and praised in poetry, music, art, and religious rites. These things are not far from the aspirations of all men and women of good will who have come to realize the sacredness of lasting things.

How pleasant, natural, and peaceful to lead this kind of life! Perhaps akin to the stoic life of the noble Greeks and Romans, it has the additional perspective of Christian faith and hope for life beyond this world. As I get older, and I hope wiser, I desire the Eternal more ardently.

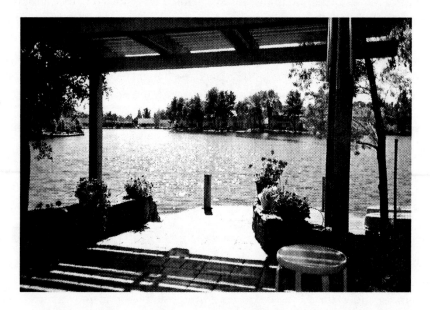

The Lake is my scenic solace in retirement as I read, write, and meditate, while listening to Bach, Beethoven, Berlioz, Brahms, Bruckner, Borodin and Balakiriev, depending on whom I fancy on any particular day.

I still get up early in the morning, say my prayers by the lake, and then get ready to go to seven o'clock Mass. Then I make a short visit to discuss the latest news with my elder brother Tony, who lives next to the church. My tennis doubles game follows, affording me my daily exercise. I shower at the club and snatch a few minutes at the office downtown, where I pick up my mail and share memories with some of the longtime staff members. After completing a few chores in town, I return home to prepare a light lunch, if

Carol is not home from her tennis. I wasn't far off when I said earlier that people in Konigsberg used to set their clocks according to the whereabouts of Immanuel Kant in his daily routine!

The best part of the day are the afternoons when I pick up a favorite book, put a beloved symphony on, and just sit on the deck contemplating the serene beauty of our lake. Sometimes I go back in time to when, as a child, I would enjoy the little pleasures of life. Perhaps I recall going up to the roof in my native Serhel just before sunset to look out over the Kadisha valley and to drink spiritually, so to speak, of the golden alpenglow lighting up the mountain crests. As evening approaches, I turn in for supper and a visit with Carol or the neighbors in our friendly cul-de-sac. Then it is time to go to bed after evening prayers. What a blessing to have the health and peace of mind to enjoy a good night's sleep, in harmony with the life cycle! As Shakespeare puts it for me:

> When to the sessions of sweet silent thought
> I summon up remembrance of things past,
> I sigh the lack of many a thing I sought,
> And with old woes new wail my dear time's waste . . .
> But if the while I think on thee [Carol], dear friend,
> All losses are restor'd, and sorrows end.

And so be it according to Thy will.

Henry J. Zeiter
Lodi, California
September 21, 2005

EPILOGUE

Each person on earth is like a flower in our good Lord's garden. And our masterful Creator, in His goodness and wisdom, makes a continuously rich entourage, teeming with variety and splendor. Some flowers remain simple and blossom into dandelions or daisies, while others grow more extravagant, blooming into carnations or roses. Each is made to complement and support the others in color, size, and style, allowing the fullness of Beauty to manifest Himself within His creation. All the flowers become beautiful, as a thankful homage for their existence.

All people are created to exhibit beauty and goodness in the garden of life. But some are smothered by weeds, and others frozen by darkness. Yet, through God's benevolence and light, most of us grow in harmony with ourselves, each other, and in the love of our wonderful Creator. Some of us become the simple and pure daisy, while others grow to be a splendid rose. And then every once in a great while God, solely for His enjoyment and glory, allows the growth to fullness of the grand sunflower.

—Philip Joseph Zeiter, October, 2005

A LIST OF NAMES

Abdallah, (in Arabic, literally means *slave of God*)
    Sarkis, 1918–78, mayor of Serhel in the 1940s; in Venezuela 1960s
    Tannous, b. 1920, brother of Sarkis; lives in Stockton, CA
Abi-Samra, (Ar., *having a dark hue*), a branch of original Mukari family
    Joseph, 1893–1965, father of Mariam and Jamal; Serhel farmer
    Mariam Thomas, (b. 1928), our maid in the 1940s; lives in Detroit
    Jamal, 1934–2003, Uncle Paul's maid in the1950s; lived in Detroit
Afifeh Prevot, 1893–1975, maid of honor at my parents' wedding
Akrini, Dr., 1890–1950, general practitioner in North Lebanon
Aley, mountain tourist resort near Beirut; population triples in summer
Amato, G., 1875–1948, tailor in Detroit; hired Mom as seamstress, 1923
Ambroise, Frère, 1900–75, Christian Brother and educator, Tripoli, Lebanon
American University of Beirut, founded in 1866; chartered in N.Y. State
Antoinette Bresse Zeiter, 1893–1959; my mother; French for Badwyeh
Antony (Anthony) Abbot, St., 251–356, founder of Eastern monasticism
Antioch, ancient Syrian city; first bishopric of Sts. Peter and Ignatius
    It was annexed by Turkey, the time of the Armenian persecutiom, 1920s
Apryl Gleason, b. 1964, optician for 23 years at Zeiter Eye
Arab, Saba, 1900–80, friend of Youssef Zeiter in Tripoli, 1942-1948
Arak, an anisette liqueur; in fact, the Lebanese national alcoholic drink
Aramaic, also called Syriac, the language of Jesus and the Eastern Rites
Arbeh, village above Serhel in North Lebanon; south of Ehden
Arbor, Al, b. 1933, classmate and professional hockey player
Arismendi, Dr. Luis, 1921–2000, hospital administrator, Stockton
Armstrong, Father, b. 1918, chemistry teacher, Assumption College, 1950s
Assumption College, now Windsor University; school I attended (1950-53)
Assumption College High School, my last year of high school, 1950-51
Austin, Dr. Robert, 1925–90, Stockton psychiatrist and tennis friend
Azar, Jean, b. 1934, elementary school classmate in Tripoli, 1940s
Aziz, (Ar. for *beloved*),

Selma, 1914-65, my landlady at 814 Waterloo Rd, London (1953-58)
Mitch, b. 1932, Selma's younger son and my friend in the1950s
Victor, b. 1928, Selma's older son; a photographer

Baal, ancient Semitic chief deity, symbolizing the forces of nature
Baalbeck, (Heliopolis), city in the Bekaa, Lebanon; site of four huge Roman
          temples
Badwi and Badwyeh are Ar. for *Paduan,* after St. Anthony of Padua
Badwyeh Bresse Zeiter, 1893–1959, my mother; sister of Ramza
Badwi Kafa, 1920-99, a Serhel émigré acquaintance in Caracas
Bakke, Allan, b. 1940, the Supreme Court case against Univ. of California
Baring, Maurice, 1874-1945, British man of letters, and of high culture and
          refined taste
Barkett, (Ar. for *blessings*), the marital family name of Sadi'a, my cousin
          Anthony, 1904–54, husband of Sadi'a, father of Dr Joe and Madelyn
          Henry, b. 1940, the younger son in the Barkett family; a dentist
          Joe, Dr., b. 1928, my friend and mentor; physician and businessman
          Madelyn Barkett Zeiter, b. 1923, my Brother Tony's wife
          Renee, b. 1925, married to Nadim Malcoun, Teresa Malcoun's son
          Sadi'a Rishwain Barkett, 1907–84, my godmother and first cousin
          Sarkis, 1888-1963, grandfather of Dr. Joe Barkett
          Suad (Sue), b. 1935, wife of Dr. Phil Courey, my former classmate
Barr, Murray L., b. 1918, Canadian histologist; discoverer of the *Barr Body*
Barrett, Jim, b. 1926, friend and owner of Chateau Montelena winery
          Judy, b. 1945, an attorney like Jim, her husband
Bashir II, Emir of Lebanon, ruled 1788-1840; fought the Turks' cruelty
Batrun, coastal city in Lebanon; famous for its fruit gardens and mild climate
Bdimane, Kadisha Canyon village; residence of the Maronite Patriarch
Besharre, town overlooking the Kadisha Canyon; birthplace of Khalil Gibran
Beit Minzer, Lebanese village on summit of mountain across from Serhel
Belle River, small town on the St. Clair River, north of Windsor, Canada
Benson, R. H., 1871–1914, Catholic author; was Anglican Archbishop's son
Berdaune, an area of restaurants on the river, in Zahle, Lebanon
Bernardino, Dr. Nicanor, b. 1930, Stockton Philippino physician
Bertoia, Reno, b. 1934, college classmate and Detroit Tigers' baseman
Berytus, old name of Beirut (Fr. Beyrouth) during the Phoenician era
Beuglet, Dr. Ernest, 1900–72, my ophthalmologist in Windsor, Ontario
Bhamdoon, summer resort in the mountains above Beirut
Big Sur, a scenic stretch of the California coast, south of Carmel
Bikfaya, a town in Mount Lebanon over-hanging a series of cliffs
Brais, (aka Breis, Braiz, Ar. for *blondish*), branch of the Mukari family
          Antonio, b. 1920, older brother of my sister Mary's husband Michel

Bacchus, b. 1935, youngest Breis; my childhood playmate in Serhel

Marzuka, b. 1955, daughter of Tannous; named after my grandmother

Michel, b. 1923, married to Mary Zeiter, my sister; lives in Caracas

Tannous, b. 1935, childhood playmate; lives in Stockton; m. to Saida

Brause, Jane, b. 1923, my secretary for many years; married to Robert

Brendmeyer, Dr. Robert, b. 1930, Stockton psychiatrist, 1965–78

Bresse, maiden name of my mother; spelled both as Breiss or Bresse

Badwyeh, 1893–1959, my mother's name: Antoinette in French

François, Père, 1870–1955, Badwyeh's uncle; Franciscan priest

Mariam (Maria), 1865–1916, my maternal grandmother; Italian descent

Nini (Antonio), 1895–1955, great-uncle Philippe's son; Therese's father

Philippe, 1868–1953, mother's paternal uncle; commercial philathelist

Pietro, 1890–1945, Philippe's oldest son; famous wood carver

Yousef (Joseph), 1865–1916, my maternal grandfather; French descent

Brewster, Henry, Dr., 1920–95, Stockton Freudian psychoanalyst

Judy, 1922–98, Dr. Henry's wife

Broummana, one of many red-roofed summer resorts in Lebanon

Brunetta, Dr. Natale, 1912?–1988, surgeon and partner of Dr Barkett

Brünhilde, a Valkyrie demi-goddess heroine in Wagner's *Ring Cycle*

Bruno, Laverne, b. 1944, my first secretary at the Zeiter Eye Clinic

Buckingham, Dr. James, b. 1925, a family practitioner and longtime friend

Buhari, Fram, b, 1944, Stockton cardiologist and personal friend

Butros, Abuna (or 'Buna), 1882–1978, my paternal great uncle and abbot

Byblos (Jbeil), coastal Lebanese city; oldest continuously inhabited city

Caldera, Rafael, b. 1916, my Spanish literature teacher; president of Venezuela

Calone, Richard, b. 1953, knowledgeable tax attorney and friend in Stockton

Camaldolese Order, founded by St. Romuald in Camaldoli, Italy

Camburis, Dr. Angelo, b.1930, surgical resident at Harper Hospital, 1958–62

Canistraci, Dan, b.1929; my tennis doubles partner for the past ten years

Capps, Teresa, b. 1953, my secretary and technician at Zeiter Eye (1968–83)

Caputo, Dr. Nancy, b. 1920, Detroit internist on the staff of Harper Hospital

Caracas, Venezuela; population was 300,000 in 1950; now, five million

Carmel-by-the-Sea, beautiful tourist area on the central California coast

Carmelites, Discalced, re-formed by St Teresa and St John of the Cross, 1500s

Cedars of Lebanon, *Cedrus libani*, huge conifers, 2,500 years old

Cerque, Don, b. 1932, fellow tennis player in Stockton

Chanteur, Fr. Pierre, 1890–1960, rector of Univ. of St. Joseph in Beirut, 1940s

Choyce, Dr. Peter, b. 1920, British ophthalmologist and innivator

Christian Brothers, order founded by St. Jean-Baptiste de la Salle, 1680

Christian Culture Series Award, annual award given to prominent Catholics

Christendom College, a Catholic college in Front Royal, Virginia

Chtaura, a town in Lebanon, near Zahle; a center of wine-making
Church, June, b. 1932, my piano teacher and that of our children
Clark, Dr. Stanley, b. 1920, retired Stockton orthopedic surgeon
Cloud of Unknowing, an anonymous 14th century book on contemplation
Colavito, Rocky, b. 1933, a Cleveland Indians and Detroit Tigers outfielder
Copland, Aaron, 1900–90, American conductor and composer
Courey, (Ar. Khoury, for *priest*) Arabic family name
    Hozen, 1895–1970, uncle of Irene Ziter, my Brother Mike's wife
    Irene, b. 1925, is wife of Brother Mike Ziter; daughter of Shiben Courey
    Mary, 1994-88, Hozen and Shiben's sister; like Hozen, she never married
    Mary Sessine Malik, 1905–2002, Aunt Teresa's daughter; Irene's mother
    Philip, Dr., b. 1934, dentist in Canada and Stockton; classmate and friend
    Sharon, b. 1938, sister of Irene and daughter of Shiben Courey
    Shiben, 1898–1985, head of the Courey family; married Mary Sessine Malik
Craig, Barbara, b. 1936, concert pianist and friend in Windsor, Canada
    Bill, Dr., b. 1934, Barbara's brother; an obstetrician in Ottawa, Canada
Croll, Dr. Maurice, 1915–80, Detroit neuro-ophthalmology professor
Crossen, Dr. Robert, 1922–90, Detroit ophthalmic instructor at Harper hospital

Daniel, Elmoz, 1893–1965, wife of Ragi in Serhel; had no children
    Ragi, 1890–1962, Serhel fresco painter and savant, trained in Rome
Davies, Dr. Windsor, 1910–90, Detroit ophthalmic pathologist at K.E.I.
Dawson, Christopher, 1889–1970, English historian of the Christian West
Debbie Steele, b. 1964, controller and insurance processor at Zeiter Eye Clinic
DeGregori, John, b. 1937, my certified public accountant and friend
DeGroot, Fr. James, 1928–70, parish priest in Stockton in the 1960s
Derrick, Christopher, b. 1921, English author; wrote on liberal education
Donner Lake, California, where the "Donner Party" got stranded in 1847
Dordogne Valley, district in Southwestern France famous for castles and wine
Dorothy Davidson, b. 1932, office nurse to my brother Dr. Mike. 1960s
Dwyer, Father, 1915–75, philosophy professor at Assumption College, 1950s

Ein, Dr, (Ar. for *eye!*), 1895–1960, ophthalmologist in Tripoli, Lebanon
El Mina, port city of Tripoli, Lebanon; site of an old crusader castle
Ellison, Allister, 1920–90, registrar at the University of Western Ontario
Emilia, b. 1917, maid and nanny to Brother Mike's family
Erin McCarthy, b. 1961, present office manager at Zeiter Eye
Espy Arana, b. 1964, insurance processor and typist at Zeiter Eye

Fakhreddine II *Al-Mahni*, ruled Lebanon 1593-1633; encouraged silk trade
Farah, (Ar. for *joy* or *happiness*), like the names *Freud* (Ger.) or *Allegri* (It.)
    Bacchus, 1915–96, son of Mtanios; father of Irene, Brother Johnny's wife

George, 1885–1965, brother of Hanna and Mtanios; lived in New York
Hanna (Ar. for *John*), 1890–1960, Irene's uncle; lived in Serhel
Irene, b. 1935, daughter of Bacchus; married my brother Johnny
Mtanios (Ar. for *Tony*), 1883-1950, married Barbara who was a Mukari
Feisal II, 1934–54, King of Iraq, assassinated; followed by 50-year dictatorship
Felix, Frère, 1914-2003, Christian Brother; teacher in elementary school
Fisher, Dr. John, 1905-80, Canadian pathology professor at medical school
Flaherty, Marge, news reporter (1960-85), for the *Stockton Record* paper
François Bresse, Père, learned encyclopedist and Franciscan Abbot
Frasie Malcoun Zeiter, 1892–1980, wife of my paternal uncle Tannous
Freeman, Joanne, b. 1937, Max's ex-wife and his former secretary
    Max, b. 1936, Stockton attorney, former partner of Bob Rishwain
Fresno, city in California; near Sequoia and King's Canyon National Parks
Freud, (in Arabic that name would be *Farah*)
    Anna, 1895–1982, psychoanalyst daughter of Freud; tutor of Dr. Brewster
    Sigmund, 1856-1939, Viennese neurologist; founder of psychoanalysis
Frey, Dr. James, b. 1920, ophthalmic surgeon at Harper Hospital, Detroit
Friends of Chamber Music, local societies for chamber music performance

Ghios, Donna, b. 1930, secretary at Zeiter Eye Clinic, 1964-70
Gibran, Gibran Kahlil 1883-1931, Lebanese poet, mystic and artist
Graham, John, b. 1925, writer and my English professor in college

Haas, Karl, b. 1920, longtime radio commentator on classical music
Hafiza Sessine, 1900–75, daughter of great-aunt Teresa, Marzuka's sister
Hammer, Laverne Bruno, b. 1944, my first secretary, 1962-64
Harb (Ar. for *War*),
    Joseph, 1896–1964, father of Michel, my friend in Caracas
    Marie, my mother's cousin; married Joseph; doted on only child Michel
    Michel, 1925-1995, suitor to my sister Mary; a close friend in Caracas
Harris, Dr. Robert, b. 1920, psychiatric instructor at my medical school
Hernandez, Sam, b. 1932, internal medicine resident at Harper, 1958-62
Hess, Charles, b. 1925, taught me watercolor painting at Delta College
Hippocratic Oath, code of medical ethics since BC 400 sworn to at graduation
Hirshman, Dr Henry, b. 1934, Long Beach ophthalmologist and innovator
Hopkins, Gerald Manley, 1844–89, English poet; convert to Catholicism
Humboldt Redwood Grove, forest of *Sequoia sempiverens*, in California

Jacobs (Americanized Lebanese family name)
    Marian, b. 1928, in public relations; and matron of culture in Stockton
    Joe, 1938–98, former Stockton interior decorator and sculptor
Jaffe, Peter, b. 1957? Conductor of the Stockton Symphony Orchestra

Jbail, (Byblos), ancient coastal city in Lebanon, site of Crusader castle
    Along with Damascus, probably the oldest city in the world (7000 yrs)
Jiddo, Arabic affectionate term meaning grandfather, like grandpa
John of the Cross, Saint, 1542–91, Spanish poet and mystic of the Reformed
    Carmelites; friend of St. Teresa of Avila; national lyrical poet of Spain; wrote
    the mysticl books, *Ascent to Mount Carmel, Dark Night of the Soul, Spiritual
    Canticle,* and *Living Flame of Love*
John Paul II (Carol Wojtyla), 1921–2005, 265th Pope of the Catholic Church
Johnson, R.A., b. 1935, U.S. Jungian psychologist; writer of popular tracts
Jong, Erica, b. 1942, novelist (*The Fear of Flying*); later denounced her book
Joseph, Blessed Father, 1848–1929, pious parish priest; venerated in Serhel
Jounieh, beautiful city, north of Beirut; on a warm-water Mediterranean bay

Kadisha Valley, deep canyon in Lebanon flanked by scenic red-roofed villages
Karami, Rashid, 1895–1965, former prime minister and statesman of Lebanon
Karm Sadde, village between Serhel and Tripoli; great view of Mediterranean
Kelman, Charles, 1933–2004, famed N.Y. ophthalmologist and inventor
Kibbe, Lebanese dish of ground lean meat with *burghol* (bulgor) and spices
Killyeh al-Islamieh, literally, a Moslem school, with a full curriculum taught
Kimos, family name of Angela, Uncle Paul's wife, in Caracas
    Adele, b. 1918, second wife of Yousef; stepmother to Angela
    Angela Kimos Zeiter, b. 1920, daughter from Yousef's first wife
    Yousef, 1890–1960, married Adele following his first wife's death
Kinsey, Dr. Everett, 1900–92, professor of ocular physiology in Detroit.
Konstantine an-Nahr, 1880-1950, Serhel farmer and my godfather
Kos'haya Monastery, home of about 50 monks in Kadisha Valley, by Serhel
Kresge, Sebastian S., 1867–1966, U.S. retail magnate and philanthropist
Kusba, large city in Lebanon; closer to the Mediterranean than Serhel

La Salle, St. Jean Batiste de, 1651–1719, founder of the Christian Brothers
Latham, Dr. William, b. 1924, Stockton surgeon and traveling companion
Latifa, 1920-90, onetime maid servant of Yousef and Badwyeh Zeiter
Lazarillo de Tormes, Spanish picaresque novel first published in 1554
Liu, Benito, b. 1930, Filipino surgical resident at Harper Hospital, 1958-62
Lorre, Peter, U.S. film actor during mid 20th century; acted in sinister scenes
Luby, Dr, b. 1928, former chief of psychiatry at LaFayette Clinic in Detroit
Ludwig, Dr. Emil, b. 1908, professor of optics at Kresge Eye Institute, 1950s

Madrasat al Hikmeh, (Ar. for *school of wisdom*); college in Beirut
Malach, Beverly, b. 1938, my "Beatrice" in high school in the 1950s
Malcoun, Michel, b. 1919, brother of Nadim and son of Teresa
    Nadim, b. 1923, married to Cousin Renee Barkett; lives in Stockton
    Teresa, mother of above two; was a very close friend of Mom

Malik, Charles, 1906–1987, Lebanese philosopher; former U.N. president
Mansour, George, 1943–88, son of Maria née Zeiter; brother of Yvonne
    Maria, 1900–95, née Zeiter; Yvonne's mother; married George Mansour
    Yvonne, b.1941, married Charles Zaiter, also a cousin
Mariam Abi-Samra, b.1928, house-keeper of Zeiter household, 1940-48
Maronite rite, one of the Eastern rites within the Roman Catholic Church
Marzuka Zeaiter, 1876–1952, scion of our family; my father's mother
McCoy, Fr. Allen, b. 1913, Franciscan priest; leader of the Cursillos, 1960s
McGill University, Montreal; famous for its medical school
Merton, Thomas, 1915–68, U.S. Trappist mystic; *The Seven Story Mountain*
Meza, the inclusive term for the various kinds of Lebanese hors d'oeuvres
Mikhael Yousef, 1876–1941, my paternal grandfather; married Marzuka
Mora, Raul, b. 1940, taught me oil painting at Delta College, Stockton
Morrissey, James, b. 1937, my cardiovascular surgeon; mountain-climber
Mount Lebanon, mountain range, extending the total length of Lebanon
Msahia Zeiter, 1875–1955, spouse of Nehme Zeiter; Yvonne's grandmother
Mujalli, a common Lebanese family name
    Antoine, 1934–78, artistic son of Tamar; was band leader in Germany
    Joseph, 1936–94, son of Tamar and younger brother of Antoine
    Salma, 1893–1978, spouse of Tamar, our next door neighbors in Serhel
    Rose, b. 1925, daughter of Tamar; was friend of my sister Mary
    Tamar, patriarch of the Mujallis, our neighbors in Serhel
Mukari, Yousef Mikhael Zeiter, father of my grandfather Mikhael Yousef
    Mikhael Yousef *Zeaiter*, great-great grandfather; the first *Zeaiter*
    Brais and Abi-Samra, also branches of the original Mukari family

Nahr-al-Kalb, river near Beirut; famous for its etched historic stili (inscriptions)
    by Ramses II (BC 1260), Nebuchadnezzar (BC 585), Antoninus Pius (AD
    150), Napoleon III (1865), others
Navone, Ronald, b. 1950, famed Lodi internist of H. J. Zeiter and A.G. Spanos
Nehme, Ibrahim, 1890–1974, cousin of my mother; lived in Tripoli; died in L.A.
Neushwanstein, (Königschlössen), the famous castles of Ludwig II of Bavaria
Nini, Bresse, 1900–60, cousin to mother; was the son of great-uncle Philippe
Nini, Dr., 1895–1970, Tripoli surgeon; mentor of Brother Mike, 1940s
Nosce, Dr. Louis, b. 1939, Stockton ophthalmologist and good friend

Osius, Dr. Eugene, 1910–98, Chief surgeon at Harper Hospital, Detroit, 1950s
Ottesen, Peter, b. 1944, former manager of Stockton Symphony and a friend

Pascal, Blaise, 1623–62, French philosopher, mathematician; *Les Pensées*
Pascal's Wager: "Only a fool would wager and live as if God did not exist."
Penelope, legendary wife of Ulysses who supposedly remained faithful to him
Penelope Scott, b. 1932, admired lady classmate in College at Western in 1953

Peterson, Camille, b. 1931, Carol's older sister; married to Bob; five children
 Robert, b. 1930, Camille's husband; school principal 1960-90
 Drew, Dr., b. 1960, San Diego orthopedic surgeon; married to Dr. Cyndi
 Rob, Jennifer, Dr. Jeffrey and Dr. Brad, in that order, Camille's children
Philippe Bresse, 1870–1952, my mother's uncle; lived in El-Mina, Lebanon
Philomena Mujalli, 1867–1950, my mother's paternal aunt and sister of Philippe
Phoenicia, ancient kingdom on the Mediterranean, where Lebanon is now
Pearce, Joseph, b. 1958, British author (*Literary Converts*) and biographer
Pieper, Joseph, 1904–2001, German author and philosopher
Pietro Bresse, 1895–1945, son of Philomena, my great aunt; wood carver
Pino, Dr. Ralph, 1870–1965, Detroit ophthalmologist and instructor at K.E.I.
Poisson, Dr. Tom, b.1932, medical school classmate and fellow boarder, 1958
Pope, Alexander, 1688–1744, English poet; master of the *iambic pentameter*
Prevot, Franco-Lebanese family
 Afifeh, 1893–1965, was matron of honor at my parents wedding.
 Francois, b. 1920, oldest son; friend and merchant in Detroit
 Violette, b. 1928, only daughter; still lives in Lebanon
 Maurice, b. 1926, sports medicine physician; lives in Paris
 Robert, b.1923, was chief of U.N. Mission in Mid-East
Punto Fijo, city in Falcon State, Venezuela; the site my brothers' business

Qadisha, another spelling of Kadisha; see Kadisha Valley
Qannubine, a branch of the Kadisha Valley, near Serhel; convent

Ramza Bresse Zeiter, my mother's sister; first wife of Dad; untimely death
Ratto, family we befriended, when we first came to California
 Elsie, b. 1930, Henry's wife; lives in Stockton; four children
 Henry, 1930–75, sold us the cabin on the American River in the 1960s
 Warren, b, 1932, brother of Henry; he had a share early on in the cabin
Retzlaff, my mother-in-law's maiden name
 Harriet, 1906–83, school teacher; Carol's mother, born in Poland
 Murilla, 1915–90, Harriet's sister, thus Carol's aunt; daughter Sandy
 Ted, b. 1920, younger brother of Harriet and Murilla; lives in N.J.
Reinelt, Dr Herbert, b. 1930, retired philosophy professor at U.O.P.
Ridley, Everett, b. 1900, English eye surgeon and innovator
Rishwain, large family in Stockton; related to Zeiters through aunt Ziara
 Ben, 1907–73, a first cousin; son of my Dad's sister, Ziara
 Bob, b. 1938, Ben's oldest son; Stockton attorney, a close friend
 Edmond, b. 1925, son of aunt Ziara and first cousin; five children
 George, 1908–1982, first cousin; married Emily Michaels; four children
 Jimmy, b. 1925, a cousin to the Rishwains; businessman in Stockton
 Joan née Strand, b. 1938, Bob Rishwain's first wife, a close friend

Joe (Shiben) Senior, 1905–98, oldest son of Ziara and first cousin
Joe Junior, b. 1935, son of Joe Senior; attorney married to Connie
Peter, b. 1923, son of aunt Ziara; businessman married Mary Nehme
Raymond, b. 1938, dentist; son of Joe Sr.; married to Georgina.
Rose, b. 1915, Cousin Joe Senior's wife; formerly a Romley
Sadi'a Barkett, 1907–84, married A. Barkett, starting that family branch
Tom, former mayor of Serhel; married my father's sister Ziara
Tony, Dr., b. 1940, younger son of Cousin Ben and brother to Bob
Ziara (Laura), my aunt; had ten children and umpteen grand children
Romano, Dr. Wally, 1930–99, radiology resident at Harper Hospital 1959-62
Ruedemann, Albert D., Sr. 1900-1975, Chief of Ophthalmology at Kresge Eye,
    Harper and Detroit Receiving Hospitals; secretary of the American Academy
    of Ophthalmology (1932–60); president (1960-63)
    Albert D., Jr. 1920-1980, ophthalmologist; son of Ruedemann Sr

Ruiz, Dr. Richard, b1928, senior eye resident, 1960; Chief at Univ. of Texas
Rumi, Jalalud-din, AD 1207-1273, Sufi poet, seer, and mystic
Ryak, town in the Bekaa valley, in the geographic center of Lebanon

Sa'deh, 1900–55, housekeeper in the 1930s in our homes in Serhel and Tripoli
Saida (Sidon), large city in South Lebanon; at one time capital of Phoenicia
Saladin (Salah-ed-Din), AD 1137–93, sultan of Egypt and Syria, 1175-93
Salamon, Dr. Peter, b. 1945, orthopedist, former president of Medical Society
Sanazaro, Dr. Paul, b. 1910, internist at UCSF Medical Center in San Francisco
Sayegh, Dr. Roger, b1933, ophthalmologist friend; Tripoli, Lebanon
Schooff, maiden name of my wife Carol
    Camille Peterson, b. 1932, Carol's older sister; married to Bob Peterson
    Carol Schooff Zeiter, b. 1936; we were married on January 21, 1961.
    Florence, 1903–83, Carol's aunt; sister of George
    George, 1905–78, Carol's father; school teacher of football, baseball, golf
    Harriet (née Retzlaff), 1906–83, Carol's mother; taught high school English
    Judy, b. 1938, Carol's younger sister; married to Dr.Rodney Schroyer
    Ken, b. 1934, Carol's brother; psychiatrist; married to Betsy Currey
    Mary, b. 1960, Carol's niece; a psychiatrist; married to Dr. Ing
    Mildred, 1903–83, Carol's aunt and George's sister, never married
    Henry, b. 1999, Mary's youngest son, named after Uncle Henry Zeiter
Schueurman, Dr Arnold, 1927-1998, former Stockton psychiatrist
Sennewald, Dr. Frank, b. 1931, classmate and friend; married to Nok
    Joyce, Frank's ex-wife; lives in Seattle, a friend of Carol and me
Serhel,my birthplace in Northern Lebanon, 3000 ft in altitude, at the western
    entrance to the Kadisha Canyon; pop. 450
Serra, Dr Joe, b 1931, Stockton orthopedic surgeon and friend

Sessine, my grandmother Marzuka's maiden name

    Bacchus I, 1873–1947, married great-aunt Teresa, Marzuka's sister

    Bacchus II, b. 1935, lives in Serhel and is my close friend and cousin

    Boutros, Abuna, 1882-1978, an abbot; Marzuka and Teresa's brother

    Hafiza, 1893–1960, daughter of great-aunt Teresa; never married

    Marzuka Zeiter, 1876–1952, my grandmother; came to California, 1898

    Philomena, 1905–2002, wife of Simon, son of Bacchus I and Teresa

    Simon, 1905–2002, great-aunt Teresa's son; father of Bacchus II

    Teresa, 1877–1979, my great-aunt; Marzuka's sister; lived 102 years

    Therese, b. 1935, Malcoun family; wife of Bacchus II; five daughters

    Yousef, son of Simon and brother to Bacchus II; lives in Lebanon

Shalita, b. 1933, was a classmate in grade school in Tripoli, Lebanon

Sheina, Fr. Antonios, b. 1917, Lebanese monk, philosopher and hermit

Shepard, Dr. Dennis, b. 1929, California ophthalmologist and innovator

Shroyer, Judy, b. 1938, Carol's younger sister; married to Dr. Rod Schroyer

Sidon (Saida), coastal city in southern Lebanon; one time capital Phoenicia

Siegfried, Nordic legendary hero; main protagonist in Wagner's *Ring Cycle*

Sikich, Georgina, b 1934, college classmate in chemistry class in Windsor

Skinner, Dr. Alan B., 1898–1985, our professor of anatomy in medical school

Smith, Mike, b. 1930, former administrator of San Joaquin County Hospital

Sofar, tourist location in Lebanon, particularly of wealthy Saudis and Kuwaitis

Solis, Anna, 1958–1982, oldest daughter of Dr. Virgilio Solis

    Carlos, Dr., b. 1962, younger son of Virgilio; anesthesiology and psychiatry

    Isabela, 1924–2000, wife of Dr. Solis; mother of the four children

    Patricia, b. 1965, daughter of Virgilio and Isabela; now an architect

    Virgilio, Dr., 1923–2003, fellow physician; was a very close friend

    Virgilio, Jr., b 1960, son of Virgilio; once a medical student at Stanford

Soraya Bresse, 1905–2000, cousin to mother; mother of Therese Harb

Spracher, Joseph, b. 1934, Stockton physician and friend at Dameron Hospital

Starker, Janos, b. 1924, Cellist; best interpreter of Dvorák's *Cello Concerto*

St. Clair, Lake, small lake between Huron and Erie, north of Detroit, Windsor

Stief, Mary, b. 1934, spouse of Dr. Kirwin; Carol's fellow nurse at Harper, 1961

    Kirwin, Dr., 1932–82, my fellow resident and friend in Detroit, 1958-62

Stockton, large city in the San Joaquin Valley; like Lodi, our home for 44 years

Sufis, Islamic "whirling" dervishes known for mysticism; (Ar. *suf,* wool)

Summers, (Americanized name from *Abi-Samra*)

    Joe, Jr., b. 1938, son of Joe Sr., my barber at Harper Hospital

    Joe, Sr., 1920–82, distant cousin from that branch of the Mukari family

Swanson, Evelyn, 1915–85, night nurse at Stockton's old Emergency

Tahoe, a deep blue lake at 6223 feet elev. in the Sierra Nevada of California

Taxis, Omedi, 13th century founder of the *Thurn und Taxis* family line

Franz, 1459–1517, private postmaster to the Holy Roman Emperors
Teresa of Avila, Saint, 1515–82, Spanish Carmelite nun; mystic and reformer
Teresa Sessine, 1877–1979, long-lived great-aunt; sister my grandmother
Therese of Lisieux, Saint, 1873–97, French Carmelite saint of "The Little Way"
Thomas Aquinas, Saint, 1225-1274, Dominican theologian and philosopher;
    encyclopedist of his time: *Summa Theologiae, Summa Contra gentiles*;
    commentaries on the works of previous philosophers; Admirer of Aristotle;
    his philosophy became known as Thomism
Thomas Aquinas College, a Great Books institution, Santa Paula, California
Thomas, Louis, b. 1925, married to Mariam Abi-Samra; lives in Detroit
    Mariam, b. 1928, house-keeper to the Zeiters in Serhel 1940-48
Thurn-und-Taxis, noble German family; couriers and mailmen
Till Eulenspiegel, prankster in R. Strauss' *Till Eulenspiegel's Merry Pranks*
Townsend, Eric, b.1948, operatic tenor, director of Townsend Opera Players
Trappist Order, Benedictine monks vowed to manual work and contemplation
Traverso, Greg, b. 1960, Dean at St Mary's high school, Stockton
    Jack, b. 1934, father of Greg and Douglas; was married to Peggy
    Peggy, b. 1932, Stanford graduate, mother of Greg and Douglas
Tripoli, Lebanon's second largest city on the coast; our winter home, 1930-48
Tschirky, Donna, b. 1948, worked for Zeiter Eye Clinic for thirty years
Tupper, Dr. John, b. 1912, former dean of U.C. Davis Medical School
Tyson, Dr., b. 1920, chief of ophthalmology at Medical School, 1950s
Tyre (Sur), coastal city in South Lebanon; a one time capital of Phoenicia

Ulysses, legendary hero; fought in the Trojan War; wandered his way home
Ulysses, novel by James Joyce about a single day in the life of Leon Bloom
Unger, Bob, b. 1930, engineer, fellow tennis player in our foursome
Ursula, 1870–1955, very devout widow; lived in our apartment in Tripoli

Vatican Council II, gathering of bishops and church leaders 1962-65
Volcker, Paul, b. 1927, U.S. Federal Reserve Chairman in the 1980s

Wagenberg, Dr. Harold, b. 1932, classmate in medical school
Wagner, Alfred, 1930–85, Renata's husband; no relation to the composer
    Cosima, 1837–1930, Liszt's daughter; married von Bulow; then Wagner
    Renata, 1932–85, Carol's Polish cousin; wife of Alfred Wagner
    Richard, 1813-83, German composer of thirteen musical dramas (operas)
Wawona Big Trees, several groves of *Sequoia gigantica* at Yosemite Park
Western Ontario, University of, large school located in London, Canada
Windsor, city at the Southern tip of Essex County, Ontario, Canada
Wolfe, Dr. Leon, 1926–2003, classmate in medical school; Rhodes Scholar
Won, Kyung Soo, b. 1924, former conductor of Stockton Symphony Orchestra

Wooledge, Dr. Barry, b. 1938, Stockton optometrist at Zeiter Eye in the 1970s

Yamouni, Antoine, b. 1933, classmate in Tripoli grade school; now in Stockton
    Josephine, 1893–1975, mother of Antoine and Michel; married to Yousef
    Michel, b. 1936, brother of Antoine and son of Yousef and Josephine
    Youssef, 1895–1972, Antoine's father, immigrated to Venezuela in 1947
Yosemite Park, national park in central east California; majestic mountains

Zablith, Salem, b. 1934, classmate in grade school in Tripoli
Zahle, central tourist city in Lebanon; site of the *Berdauni* Restaurants
Zahtar, the thyme plant, supposedly the origin of the name Zeaiter
Zaiter, one of the variations in the spelling of Zeiter; e.g. Charles Zaiter
Zeaiter, another variation of the Zeiter name; the original true spelling
Zehrie, an upscale area in Tripoli; now it is crowded like the rest of the world
Zeiter, a branch of the original Mukari family – (Consult the Genealogical Chart).
    Ass'ad, 1897–1964, Dad's brother; five children; son Joe married to Martha
    Camille, b. 1968, our youngest daughter; M.Sc. in social work
    Christine, b. 1960, Dr Mike youngest daughter; a master pharmacist
    Dale, Dr., b. 1956, physician, youngest son of Dr. Mike; married to Sheryl
    Edmond Jr., Dr., b. 1963, Edmond and Yvonne's son; chiropractor in Stockton
    Edmond, 1923-1997, older brother; was a Stockton pharmacist; married Yvonne
        Ragi; four children, Michael, Andre, Dr. Edmond, and Laurie Anne
    Henry, b. 1934, son of Yousef and Badwyeh; retired Stockton eye surgeon
    Irene (née Farah), b. 1935 in Lebanon; married to my brother Johnny
    Irene (née Courey), b. 1927, married to Brother Dr. Mike in Windsor
    Joe, Dr., b. 1950, son of my brother Tony and Madelyn; for 25 years my
        partner in practice at Zeiter Eye
    John Henry, Dr., b. 1961, our oldest son; ophthalmologist at Zeiter eye
        married to Lynette, 4 children, John Henry, Danielle, Paul, Sierra
    John Henry Jr, b. 1989, son of John Henry and Lynette; a great pitcher
    Johnny, b. 1927, retired businessman; lives in Windsor; plays mandolin
        and piano; married to Irene Farah, one daughter, Antoinette
    Mary, b. 1925 in Detroit, married to Michel Braiz; One daughter, Ramza
    Mary Lee, b.1954, daughter of Dr. Mike; a physical therapist
    Michael, Dr., b. 1950, oldest son of Dr Mike; M.D.; married to Ruth
    Mike, Dr., b. 1921, my oldest brother; M.D., practices in Windsor
    Mikhael Yousef, 1876–1941, my grandfather, married Marzuka Sessine
    Mikhael Yousef, and Yousef Mikhael, grandfather and father of my
        grandfather
    Msahieh, 1875–1952, married Nehme, my great-uncle; mother of Maria
    Nehme 1874–1930, my grandfather Mikhael's brother; married Msahieh

Paul, Dr., b. 1952, physician, son of Dr. Mike, married to Yvette

Pablo, 1905–98, my uncle and Dad's youngest brother; married Angela Kimos

Pablo Jr, b. 1948, son of Uncle Pablo; married to Michelle; lives in Stockton

Paulette Saade, b. 1940, daughter of Uncle Pablo; married to Edmond Saade

Philip, 1926-2005, violinist and painter; married Lidia in Caracas; three
    daughters, Mary, Paula and Carolina

Philip, b.1963, our youngest son; AIA, architect; married to Alicia; six
    children, Tyler, Zachary, Christia, Alesandra, J. Henry, and Michael

Renee Gaspar, b. 1938, oldest daughter of Uncle Pablo; lives in Venezuela

Suzie, b. 1965, our older daughter; M.A; married to Tony Andres, Ph.D.,
    they live in front Royal, Virginia; two children, Joseph and Dominic

Tannous, 1895–1970, younger brother of Dad; married Frasia; six children

Tony, b. 1922, my brother; a merchant; Dr. Joe's Dad; married to Madelyn;
    five children, Tony Jr, Dr. Joe, my partner, Edmond, deceased, Peter,
    and Madeline.

Yousef, 1893–1986, my long-lived Dad, son of Marzuka and Mikhael

Zetter, another variation of the family name; e.g. Joe and Martha Zetter

Ziara Zeiter, 1891–1944, Dad's older sister; married Tom Rishwain; ten children

Ziter, another variation of Zeiter; e.g. my own brother! Dr. Mike and Irene Ziter

SHORT PRECIS

Dr. Henry Zeiter, renowned eye surgeon and founder of the Zeiter Eye Clinic in Stockton, California, traces the remarkable journey of his life from the small mountain village of Serhel in North Lebanon to California's Central Valley. His story is more than a biography; it is a tour through art, philosophy, music, and culture, as he retells his family history from a land where time stands still, through his family's migration to Caracas, to his education in Canada, and to his family and professional life in Stockton, where, with his wife Carol, he raised four children, pioneered techniques in cataract surgery, led the Stockton Symphony Orchestra, and devoted time, treasure, and talent to a host of charitable, educational, and philanthropic endeavors. Sit with him by the lake and enjoy a moment of leisure, a moment to share the beauty of life, with its triumphs and its tragedies, and a moment to stand in awe of things eternal.

ABOUT THE AUTHOR

D r. Henry Zeiter was born in 1934 in the small mountain village of Serhel, in North Lebanon, a stone's throw from the famous Cedars. He, along with his parents and six siblings spent the summer months in the mountain region, and the winter months in Tripoli, where he attended a Christian Brothers school. There, the students had to speak French, and learn both French Literature and Classical Arabic.

In 1948, the family moved to Venezuela, where Henry attended high school in Spanish. While in Caracas, he fell in love with Spanish Literature and developed a lasting love of classical music and the visual arts. Two years later, his parents decided to move to Windsor, Canada, where Henry's oldest brother had established a medical practice. This meant learning another language— English. He learned it so well, that his professors urged him to major in English Literature, even while taking a premed curriculum. He graduated from college *summa cum laude* while still a teenager.

Henry went on to medical school and graduated *cum laude* at age 23. He did his Internship in Detroit, and his Residency at the Kresge Eye Institute. There, he met Carol, a young nurse, and asked her to marry him on their first date. Shocked at the time, she eventually consented and they raised four children together.

After completing his surgical training in 1962, he and Carol moved to Stockton, California, where his grandmother had immigrated more than sixty years before. Henry established an ophthalmology practice, and, over the next 40 years, would pioneer many new surgical techniques, and perform more than 25,000 operations for cataracts, glaucoma, and corneal transplantation.

Henry's eclectic education and his many-sided interests led to a variety of activities–publishing findings in refereed medical journals; teaching advanced surgical techniques in Third World countries; serving as board member and later as president of the San Joaquin County Medical Society; as president of the Stockton Symphony Association; and for twenty years, as member of the Board of Governors of Thomas Aquinas College, a Great Books institution in Southern California, where Dr. Zeiter is Chairman of the Curriculum Committee.

Now in retirement, Dr. Zeiter remains active in the community, assisting in the musical arts (symphony, opera, chorale and chamber music), helping the Stockton homeless shelter, counseling Youth Authority prisoners, lecturing in local high schools, and sponsoring many Church activities. Yet he still finds time to enjoy his leisure, sitting by the beautiful lake he lives on and watching time go by, as he listens to music, reads a book, or meditates on God's gratuitous gifts to mankind and the amplitude of His magnificent Creation.

Printed in the United States
62873LVS00005B/1-48

9 781599 263069